ARTERIAL MESENCHYME AND ARTERIOSCLEROSIS

ADVANCES IN EXPERIMENTAL MEDICINE AND BIOLOGY

Recent Volumes in this Series

ARTERIAL MESENCHYME AND ARTERIOSCLEROSIS

Edited by

William D. Wagner and
Thomas B. Clarkson

Department of Comparative Medicine
Arteriosclerosis Research Center
The Bowman Gray School of Medicine
Wake Forest University
Winston-Salem, North Carolina

PLENUM PRESS • NEW YORK AND LONDON

Library of Congress Cataloging in Publication Data

International Workshop on Arterial Mesenchyme and Arteriosclerosis,
New Orleans, 1973.
    Arterial mesenchyme and arteriosclerosis.

    (Advances in experimental medicine and biology, v. 43)
    Includes bibliographies.
1. Arteriosclerosis—Congresses. 2. Mesenchyme—Congresses. I. Wagner, William
D., 1943-   ed. II. Clarkson, Thomas B., 1931-   ed. III. Title. IV. Series.
[DNLM: 1. Arteries—Congresses. 2. Arteriosclerosis—Physiopathology—Con-
gresses. 3. Mesoderm—Congresses. W1AD559 v. 43 1973/WG550 I625a 1973]
RC692.I57   1973   616.1'36   74-5207
ISBN-13: 978-1-4684-3245-9   e-ISBN-13: 978-1-4684-3243-5
DOI: 10.1007/978-1-4684-3243-5

Proceedings of an International Workshop on Arterial Mesenchyme and
Arteriosclerosis held in New Orleans, April 2-3, 1973

© 1974 Plenum Press, New York
 Softcover reprint of the hardcover 1st edition 1974
A Division of Plenum Publishing Corporation
227 West 17th Street, New York, N.Y. 10011

United Kingdom edition published by Plenum Press, London
A Division of Plenum Publishing Company, Ltd.
4a Lower John Street, London, W1R 3PD, England

PREFACE

Presently, and in the past, the predominant investigative emphasis among research workers in arteriosclerosis has been on plasma and arterial lipids. Recent data from a number of laboratories suggest that arterial mesenchyme is of considerable importance in the pathogenesis and fate of arteriosclerotic lesions. The significance of some of these observations made it clear that there was need for intensified research on the connective tissue components of the arteriosclerotic lesion and that arteriosclerosis research workers could benefit from a more comprehensive view of the subject.

Because of their experience in the field of arteriosclerosis and their interest in stimulating new directions for research on the lesion, the Committee on Coronary Artery Lesions and Myocardial Infarctions of the Council on Arteriosclerosis, American Heart Association, planned an International Workshop on Arterial Mesenchyme and Arteriosclerosis.

The Workshop brought together scientists expert in connective tissue research and research on arteriosclerosis who presented the current status of knowledge in their areas of expertise.

The Workshop was held April 2-3, 1973 at the Royal Orleans Hotel, New Orleans, Louisiana and was attended by more than 170 people. The twenty papers and discussions presented in this volume summarize the proceedings of the Workshop and represent a comprehensive review of the role of arterial mesenchyme in arteriosclerosis.

The first section of the volume sets the problem in perspective and includes papers by several expert participants who define the mesenchymal components with respect to the arterial wall and the arteriosclerotic lesion. The Workshop then addressed itself to the interaction of lipids with the various connective tissue components such as collagen, elastin, glycosaminoglycans, and glycoproteins. The third section of papers is intended to stimulate interest in tissue culture technology and deals with culture techniques applicable in the study of arteriosclerosis. The final series of papers addresses the pathologic processes resulting from the interactions of connective tissue components and the arterial wall.

We are hopeful that the Workshop and the published proceedings will stimulate investigators to undertake specific new directions in investigating the pathogenesis of arteriosclerosis, including progression and regression of lesions, based on new knowledge of mesenchymal tissues.

One of our aims was to publish and disseminate to other investigators in arteriosclerosis and connective tissue research the information presented at the workshop as soon as possible. In this regard we apologize for any unavoidable form and stylistic imperfections. During the printing process for the book all illustrations were reduced 10% in addition to any reductions listed for figures. Certain remarks of some of the participants were not recorded clearly at the meeting; therefore, to those discussants omitted we apologize.

We should like to acknowledge the following support provided for the workshop and the preparation of the proceedings.

National Heart and Lung Institute (HL 15707), National Institutes of Health

Committee on International Program, American Heart Association

Committee on Coronary Artery Lesions and Myocardial Infarction, American Heart Association

The local arrangements for the meeting were gratefully provided by the staff of the L.S.U. SCOR in Arteriosclerosis under the direction of Dr. Gerald Berenson.

The editors thank the efficient assistance of Mrs. Shirley Pegram, Ms. Suzanne Pickett, and Ms. Martha Van Noppen in the technical preparation of the manuscripts for publication.

William D. Wagner

Thomas B. Clarkson

ORGANIZING COMMITTEE

CLARKSON, THOMAS B.
Chairman

Department of Comparative Medicine
Bowman Gray School of Medicine
Wake Forest University
Winston-Salem, North Carolina

WAGNER, WILLIAM D.
(ad hoc as Assistant
to Chairman)

Department of Comparative Medicine
Bowman Gray School of Medicine
Wake Forest University
Winston-Salem, North Carolina

BERENSON, GERALD S.
(ad hoc for Local
Arrangements)

Departments of Medicine and
Biochemistry
Louisiana State University
Medical Center
New Orleans, Louisiana

ARMSTRONG, MARK L.

Department of Internal Medicine
The University of Iowa
Iowa City, Iowa

CHOBANIAN, ARAM VAN

Department of Medicine
Boston University Medical School
Boston, Massachusetts

DAOUD, ASSAAD S.

Department of Pathology
Veterans Administration Hospital and
Albany Medical College
Albany, New York

FRANTZ, IVAN D., JR.

Department of Medicine
University of Minnesota
Medical School
Minneapolis, Minnesota

GORE, IRA   Department of Pathology
                             University of Alabama
                             Medical School
                             Birmingham, Alabama

MCGILL, HENRY C.   Department of Pathology
                             University of Texas
                             Medical School
                             San Antonio, Texas

STRONG, JACK P.   Department of Pathology
                             Louisiana State University
                             Medical Center
                             New Orleans, Louisiana

WISSLER, ROBERT W.   Department of Pathology
                             University of Chicago
                             Chicago, Illinois

WORKSHOP PARTICIPANTS

BERENSON, GERALD S.

Department of Medicine
and Biochemistry
Louisiana State University
Medical Center
New Orleans, Louisiana

DAOUD, ASSAAD S.

Department of Pathology
Veterans Administration
Hospital and Albany Medical College
Albany, New York

DORFMAN, ALBERT

Department of Pediatrics
The University of Chicago
Chicago, Illinois

FEDOROFF, SERGEY

Department of Anatomy
University of Saskatchewan
Saskatoon
Saskatchewan, Canada

FISHER-DZOGA, KATTI

Department of Pathology
The University of Chicago
Chicago, Illinois

GEER, JACK C.

Department of Pathology
College of Medicine
The Ohio State University
Columbus, Ohio

GROSS, JEROME

Developmental Biology Laboratory
Harvard Medical School
Massachusetts General Hospital
Boston, Massachusetts

HAUST, M. DARIA

Department of Pathology
The University of Western Ontario
London, Ontario, Canada

KRAMSCH, DIETER M.

Department of Medicine
University Hospital
Boston University Medical Center
Boston, Massachusetts

LABELLA, FRANK S.

Department of Pharmacology and
Therapeutics
University of Manitoba
Faculty of Medicine
Winnipeg 3, Canada

MCMILLAN, GARDNER C.

National Heart and Lung Institute
National Institutes of Health
Bethesda, Maryland

MINICK, C. RICHARD
MURPHY, GEORGE E.

Department of Pathology
The New York Hospital-
Cornell Medical Center
New York, New York

MUIR, HELEN

Kennedy Institute of Rheumatology
Bute Gardens, Hammersmith
London, England

PARTRIDGE, S. M.

Agricultural Research Council
Meat Research Institute
Langford, Bristol

RENAIS, J.

Centre de Recherches Cardiologiques
Hospital Boucicaut
Paris, France

ROBERT, LADISLAS

Laboratoire de Biochimie du Tissu
Conjonctif
Faculte de Medecine
Universite Paris-Val de Marne
Creteil, France

ROSS, RUSSELL

Department of Pathology and
Medicine
University of Washington
School of Medicine
Seattle, Washington

STARY, HERBERT C.

Department of Pathology
Louisiana State University
Medical Center
New Orleans, Louisiana

STEMERMAN, MICHAEL B.   Division of Hematology
                              Montefiore Hospital and
                              Medical Center
                              Albert Einstein College of Medicine
                              Bronx, New York

SMITH, ELSPETH B.   Department of Chemical Pathology
                              University of Aberdeen
                              Foresterhill
                              Aberdeen, Scotland

URRY, DAN W.   Laboratory of Molecular Biophysics
                              University of Alabama Medical Center
                              Birmingham, Alabama

YU, SHIU YEH   Veterans Administration Hospital and
                              Department of Internal Medicine
                              Washington University
                              School of Medicine
                              St. Louis, Missouri

CONTENTS

SECTION III

TISSUE CULTURE APPLICATION IN

CONNECTIVE TISSUE RESEARCH

SECTION IV

PATHOLOGIC PROCESSES AND CONNECTIVE

TISSUE INTERACTIONS

SECTION I

THE PROBLEM IN PERSPECTIVE

MESENCHYMAL INVOLVEMENT IN ARTERIOSCLEROSIS

Gardner C. McMillan

National Heart and Lung Institute

National Institutes of Health, Bethesda, Maryland

In this presentation I should like to speak of some of the qualities of vascular mesenchyme and some of the range of its structural responses - including reference on occasion to some of the responses it may not make.

In doing so, I shall use the term differentiation in a broad and unspecialized sense that indicates a local state of structure or function different from its previous condition. It includes, therefore, histogenesis and cytodifferentiation in which potentially reversible differences are evoked from the genome as a consequence of local environment. It is also, however, intended to include the idea of strain differentiation in which the difference has the nature of breeding true in the offspring of the altered cells.

It is probable that most of the changes observed in arteriosclerosis represent modulation or environmental effects on cytodifferentiation, rather than new genetic differences self-reproducing in daughter cells because of changes in the genome or in an epigenetic system. Very little attention has been given to these issues in considering the pathogenesis, localization or regression of arteriosclerosis. They merit study.

A brief and helpful review of the language and nature of differentiation together with instructive comment is given by C.H. Waddington and P. Weiss and others (Abercrombie, 1967).

It is a tautology to note mesenchymal involvement in arteriosclerosis. Angiogenesis occurs from embryonic mesenchyme derived from a mesoderm that gives rise to smooth, cardiac and skeletal

muscle; connective tissue; blood; lymphatics; mesothelium of
pericardium, pleura and peritoneum; joint cavities, bursae and
tendon sheaths as well as other structures. In an ultimate sense,
it is not surprising that common and multipotential capacities
for differentiation can be found among these various tissues of
common origin. Yet, in fact, the varieties of mesenchymal reaction
with differentiation that we recognize as arteriosclerosis are
relatively restricted among those that are possible for mesenchyme
in general or vascular mesenchyme in particular.

Angiogenesis, proceeding beyond the blood island stage, occurs
in a budding network of small endothelial channels. Dominant
channels develop and acquire a condensation or investment first of
tunica intima, then of tunica media and finally a differentiated
adventitia. Such vessels are capable of a great deal of growth,
development, and remodeling; but they have already lost much of
their primitive mesenchymal capacity for differentiation.

In general, we have only the sketchiest of ideas as to what
causes vascular cells to "turn on," or differentiate in particular
ways, and to manifest particular changes in structure and function.
At times we believe that it may be a mechanical force, a biochemical gradient, a neurotropism or some abnormal substance. We may
have reason to speak of genetic factors, species differences for
example, or injury, repair, growth, or remodeling as being involved
in the mesenchymal reactions with differentiation we call arteriosclerosis; but again we have only the most simplistic views about
how these may operate to stimulate individual cells or mixed populations of cells to produce plaques. I hope, indeed, that this workshop may start us on the road to understanding some of these phenomena.

What are some of the variations in reaction and differentiation
that one may see in vessels? To place the problem in proper perspective, I would like to go somewhat beyond arteriosclerosis
proper and include observations about veins, such vessels as the
ductus arteriosus and about several arterial diseases other than
arteriosclerosis. The intent is to discuss a variety of phenomena
and to note that arteriosclerosis has a somewhat restricted range
of morphological expression within these various possibilities.

In the infant, proliferative lesions with some production of
collagen and elastin and a rich formation of mucopolysaccharides
are found in vessels undergoing rapid obsolescence such as the
ductus arteriosus or the hypogastric arteries. Somewhat similar
proliferative lesions in plaque-like form can be found in vessels
such as the coronary arteries. Both may show gaps in elastica
and continuity between media and intima. They share many morphological similarities with the changes that can be observed in the
uterine arteries of childbearing women. I prefer to regard all

three as manifestations of vascular remodeling and development
rather than as arteriosclerosis, although the latter process
involves some of the same cellular activities.

Necrosis is a feature of atherosclerosis, yet it should be
noted that there is a striking form of necrosis of the media of
large arteries that has no apparent connection with it. In
Erdheim's medial necrosis extensive groups of medial cells die and
they do so without eliciting any inflammatory response or any
intimal proliferation. The mesenchyme seems inert. Its response
in this lesion stands in marked contrast to its reactions in luetic
aortitis with its foci of gummatous necrosis of muscle and destruction of elastica, chronic inflammation, and fibrous tissue proliferation in both intima and adventitia.

In the reaction of pulseless disease it is possible to destroy
all media cells, and yet leave a distorted but relatively complete
elastica as a residuum of a vasculitis. In such lesions one may
find arteries encased in a very dense cicatrical adventitia, an
acellular media of compressed elastic fibers and a lumen greatly
narrowed by a thick sclerotic intima. There is no residual
inflammation.

Digital vessels seen in advanced Raynaud's disease represent
a rather similar stenosing intimal mesenchymal response which is
noteworthy for the normality of all layers of the artery except the
intimal one. It may represent the effect of restricted flow in
contrast to hemodynamic wear and tear. Such changes appear to be
late phenomena in Raynaud's disease.

Many investigators regard arteriosclerosis as a process of
injury and repair that shows all the features of low grade chronic
inflammation. The arterial mesenchyme, however, is capable of a
wider range of responses to subacute and chronic inflammation than
is seen in plaques. We have already mentioned syphilitic aortitis
with hyaline intimal thickening. In temporal arteritis there is
granulomatous destruction of the media and giant cells formed around
bits of elastica. The change is associated with great intimal
proliferation. Yet another example is Buerger's disease where one
may see a focally inflamed thrombus in the lumen and a media with
focal destruction and inflammation while the adventitia is excessive
in amount; or the lesions seen in rheumatoid aortitis with fairly
large areas of chronic inflammation that may be diffuse through
the intima and inner media of the aorta.

In atheromas the inflammatory component includes the usual
cells of granulomatous inflammation and as is typical of granulomatous or chronic inflammation, these are or become part of the
local tissue or mesenchyme. On occasion an appreciable number of
polymorphonuclear leukocytes may be found too. It is not uncommon

to find many multinucleated giant cells of foreign body type
around the crystal spaces in the core of an atheroma. The mesenchyme does not always, however, react to crystalline material with
an overt granulomatous response. For example, one can see what
appears to be a crystalline cholesterol sequestrum lying in a
quiescent fibrotic intima of a coronary artery with only a minimal
giant cell reaction.

There appears to be a difference in the reaction of the intima
and the media to the presence of lipid. Although lipid accumulations in the intima are commonly associated with a marked mesenchymal response, apparently similar accumulations in the media may
only elicit necrosis with but little cellular proliferation or
elaboration of interstitial material. Such a contrast can be seen
in cerebral artery atherosclerosis where lipid is often present in
both intima and media out to the adventitia. In such lesions one
sees intimal fibrosis and a focus of medial destruction but little
other medial reaction.

The arterial wall is capable of the features of organogenesis
under the correct conditions. While the ability to form new blood
vessels is not perfect, nevertheless channels with a new intima,
elastica and recognizable media will develop. Examples may be seen
in recanalized thrombi or emboli of large arteries with well defined
media in the recanalized vessels. Sometimes mesenchymal differentiation is incomplete in recanalized thrombi and one can see an
almost amorphous jelly that has failed to form muscle or mature
connective tissue.

Another noteworthy organoid differentiation that may be seen is
osseous metaplasia. It is common in venous thrombi but rare in the
walls of arteries. Much more commonly, mineralization occurs in
relation to elastic or collagen fibers in a non-organoid manner as
simple calcification without the differentiation of special tissues.

(21 illustrations shown but not reproduced).

SUMMARY

My purpose in this review of the reactions of human vessels
has been to point out not only that the vascular mesenchyme is
involved in arteriosclerosis - that seems obvious, but to note
that it can have marked variations in reaction or differentiation
in different vascular diseases. To emphasize the variety of
mesenchymal responses that may occur in vascular development and
disease is also to make plain how little we know about what controls
mesenchymal cells with respect to adopting given structures and
functions. That the circumstances of such differentiation are
likely to be both complex and subtle seems to me to be implicit
in the material I have discussed.

Arteriosclerosis does not comprise this full range of mesenchymal variations, but it does partake of many of them. It is of
interest to note both the ones it does manifest and those that it
could express but does not. I would anticipate that the stimuli
and mechanisms that determine mesenchymal development into different kinds of arteriosclerotic plaques are also likely to be
subtle and complex.

REFERENCE

Abercrombie, M. (1967). In "Cell Differentiation." A Ciba
    Foundation Symposium. (A.V.S. DeReuck and Julie Knight,
    eds.), pp. 3-17. Little, Brown and Company, Boston,
    Massachusetts.

DISCUSSION FOLLOWING THE PRESENTATION BY GARDNER C. MCMILLAN

Dr. Strong: Dr. McMillan, I have never seen a neoplastic
process of a large elastic artery or a medium-sized muscular
artery. I wonder if you have. If your experience is similar to
mine, could you give your ideas on why tumors do not develop in
these vessels?

Dr. McMillan: No, I never have and, indeed, I have many
reservations about the neoplastic quality of many so-called
tumors of blood vessels. I tend to share Willis' view that much
of what passes for neoplasm in vessels is, in fact, hamartomatous
or malformation rather than a neoplasm in the sense of new growth.
I think I will stop there and not try to comment on why neoplasms
of large arteries are not identified.

Dr. Fleischmajer: There is some evidence that smooth
muscle cells can synthesize collagen and glycosaminoglycans, but
is there any evidence that endothelial cells may do the same?

Dr. McMillan: I think I should leave that question for
other speakers on the program because I believe there will be
specific reference by other speakers to their views about the
capacity of endothelial cells to differentiate in the direction of
smooth muscle cells or to differentiate metabolically to form
particular substances. It has been argued for many years, for
example, that they do form polysaccharides. If you will let me
pass that question, I am sure there will be much more cogent
answers from other speakers.

MORPHOLOGY OF MESENCHYMAL ELEMENTS OF NORMAL ARTERY, FATTY STREAKS, AND PLAQUES

Jack C. Geer and William S. Webster

Departments of Pathology and Veterinary Clinical

Sciences, The Ohio State University, Columbus, Ohio

The objective of this paper is to review briefly normal arterial structure and the cells found in the various types of human atherosclerotic lesions, and to contrast the cellular reaction of human lesions with that in certain experimental models. There is a striking similarity between the mesenchymal cell reaction in human lesions and that in the experimental models, indicating that the models are valid for studying certain aspects of the pathogenesis of atherosclerosis. Our studies support the conclusion of many other investigators (Altschul, 1950; Björkerud, 1969; Hassler, 1970; Jores, 1924; Lee et al., 1970; McMillan and Stary, 1968; Poole et al., 1971) that the source of the mesenchymal or smooth muscle cells in the intima is medial cells that have proliferated and migrated into the intima.

NORMAL ARTERIAL STRUCTURE

Arteries of all sizes have three tunics or coats: intima, media, and adventitia. The intima includes the lining endothelium and extends to and includes the internal elastic membrane or lamina. The media extends from the medial aspect of the internal elastic membrane or lamina and includes the external elastic lamina. The adventitia begins at the external elastic membrane and gradually blends into the surrounding interstitial tissue with no defined external limit. Arteries vary in structure with size and anatomical location. The variations are in medial structure and in the presence or appearance of the elastic membranes.

Structures comprising normal arterial intima are difficult to define because with aging there is progressive thickening

9

of the intima, which varies in magnitude between species and
within a given species from one arterial bed to another.
Whether intimal thickening is normal or pathological is a subject
of debate. The intima of most arteries at the time of birth
consists of a single layer of endothelial cells resting on a
basement membrane which is either contiguous to or separated from
the internal elastic membrane by a narrow connective tissue space.
The connective tissue space contains occasional fibrils of collagen
and connective tissue microfibrils. Whether smooth muscle cells
are present in "normal" intima cannot be determined with certainty,
since their presence may represent the beginning of intimal thickening.

Endothelium is a simple squamous type cell with a centrally
placed nucleus. Between endothelial cells there are specialized
cell-to-cell tight junctions or desmosomes (Parker, 1958). Between
the areas of tight junctions the plasma membranes of contiguous
endothelial cells course parallel to one another separated by an
electron lucid regular space. Normal endothelial cells have sparse
cytoplasmic organelles (Parker, 1958) consisting of scattered small
mitochondria (Rhodin, 1962), profiles of granular endoplasmic
reticulum, free ribonucleoprotein particles, and Golgi membranes
(Moss and Benditt, 1970a). There are a variable number of fine
filaments in the cytoplasm which generally are located at the base
of the cell (Moss and Benditt, 1970a). The endothelial plasma
membrane has numerous micropinocytotic vesicles along the lumen
and intimal surfaces and none along the area where two endothelial
cells are in apposition. Adjacent to the basal plasma membrane of
endothelium there is a basement membrane of variable thickness
composed of electron-dense flocculent appearing material. Specialized tight attachment areas have been described between the basal
plasma membrane and the basement membrane (Ts'ao and Glagov, 1970).
Similar areas of attachment have been described also between the
basement membrane and the internal elastic membrane (Ts'ao and
Glagov, 1970).

Structures comprising the arterial media vary with arterial
size. Arteries are classified as elastic, muscular or arterioles,
based upon size and medial structure. The media of elastic arteries is composed of alternating laminae of smooth muscle cells
sandwiched between elastic plates, with intervening connective
tissue spaces containing collagen fibers. Mammalian arterial
media is composed solely of smooth muscle cells (Paule, 1963;
Pease and Paule, 1960; Pease and Molinari, 1960). Elastic arteries
of avian species have, in addition to smooth muscle cells, a cell
in the connective tissue spaces referred to as the interlamellar
connective tissue cell (Cooke and Smith, 1968; Moss and Benditt,
1970a). The media of muscular arteries is composed primarily
of smooth muscle cells in all species with very little connective tissue space between the cells. Large muscular arteries

have scattered small elastic fibers and collagen fibers between
the cells, and small muscular arteries generally show only collagen fibers between the cells.

Smooth muscle cells in arterial media are fusiform with a
centrally placed elongated nucleus and abundant cytoplasm containing primarily myofilaments. Between adjacent smooth muscle
cells the plasma membranes course parallel one to the other with
a regular intervening electron lucid space. There are circum-
scribed points of cell attachments of the nexus type where the
outer leaflets of the plasma membranes fuse, forming a five-layered
junction (Cliff, 1967, 1970). The smooth muscle plasma membrane
is surrounded by a thin basement membrane except at the points
where one cell abuts another (Parker, 1958). Numerous micropinocytotic vesicles are found in the plasma membrane. Myofilaments
in the cytoplasm are arrayed in the long axis of the cell (Rhodin,
1962). Numerous fusiform-shaped densities among the myofilaments
appear to be areas of convergence of the filaments (Pease and
Molinari, 1960). Triangular-shaped densities are found at irregular intervals along the plasma membrane (Pease and Molinari,
1960). Remaining cytoplasmic organelles are rather few and
localized to the region of the nucleus, especially the poles of
the nucleus. These organelles consist of profiles of endoplasmic
reticulum, small mitochondria, and Golgi membranes. The morphologic
features commonly used for identifying smooth muscle cells are
cytoplasmic myofilaments, micropinocytotic vesicles in the plasma
membrane, and a limiting basement membrane.

The amount and composition of adventitial tissue is variable
from one artery to another but generally consists of nerve fibers,
blood vessels, lymphatic vessels, collagen fibers, and fibro-
blastic type cells. Nerve fibers have not been shown to penetrate
the arterial media (Parker, 1958; Pease and Paule, 1960; Pease and
Molinari, 1960; Rhodin, 1962). The spread of nerve impulses in
the media must be from one cell to another, possibly via nexus
junctions (Dewey and Barr, 1962).

INTIMAL THICKENING

Intimal thickening, commonly referred to as diffuse intimal
thickening, is observed in varying degrees in man and all other
species. The thickened intima is composed of smooth muscle cells
and connective tissue. The phenomenon of intimal thickening has
been reviewed in detail recently (Geer and Haust, 1972) and we
will present only some basic considerations. Many investigators
believe that intimal thickening is a function of aging and thus
is a normal developmental phenomenon (Jores, 1922; Geer and Haust,
1972; Karrer, 1960; Keech, 1960; Pease and Paule, 1960). To the
contrary, others (Dock, 1931; Fangman and Hellwig, 1947; Prior and

Jones, 1952; Sappington and Horneff, 1941; Vlodaver et al., 1969; Wilens, 1951) believe this is a pathological process which is interpreted to mean that it predisposes to degenerative changes, especially atherosclerosis. In man the most striking intimal thickening is found in proximal portions of the extramural coronary arteries where the thickness of the intima may be three or more times that of the adjacent media by age 20 years (Geer et al., 1968b). Coronary artery intimal thickening has been studied in populations with high and low prevalence of coronary heart disease and has been found to be similar in magnitude (Geer et al., 1968b). This observation supports the thesis that the thickening is a normal developmental phenomenon, but does not negate the possibility of the thickening predisposing to atheroma formation when factors that cause such also are present.

Intimal thickening has not been studied extensively by electron microscopists. Smooth muscle cells are readily found in the thickening intima and may be the only cell type present. The smooth muscle cells near the region of the internal elastic membrane in the intima closely resemble in shape and size those in the media, but are aligned at a right angle to those in the media (Gross et al., 1934). Toward the endothelium the smooth muscle cells become smaller and more variable in shape, becoming stellate. The stellate cells were described originally by Langhans (1866) and in the past have been referred to as Langhans' cells. It appears at present that these cells are derived from smooth muscle, but this has not been proved. There are variable numbers of elastic fibers and collagen fibers in the thickened intima. These connective tissue fibers are found in greatest number and size in the region of the internal elastic membrane (Gross et al., 1934). The number and size of elastic and collagen fibers diminishes toward the endothelial surface.

THE FATTY STREAK LESION

Fatty streak type lesions are the most exhaustively studied of all the forms of atherosclerotic lesions. Observations of human fatty streaks and experimental models allow us to describe with some degree of accuracy the histogenesis of the fatty streak type lesion. Fatty streaks are focal rather discrete lesions. Because of the focal occurrence of the lesions, many investigators have proposed an "initial lesion" that predisposes to lipid accumulation. The cause or causes of the initial lesion are unknown and the morphological expression has been described variously as intimal thickening, focal intimal edema, accumulation or alteration of intimal connective tissues, mural thrombosis, and endothelial alteration caused by or associated with platelet aggregation (Geer and Haust, 1972). These morphological expressions are not mutually exclusive; indeed, many combinations or sequences of changes are possible. There is rather general agreement on the sequence of changes that occurs with lipid deposition in the intima. Initially the lipid is observed as stainable granules in the interstitial space (Anitschkow, 1933; Ashoff, 1925; Duff, 1935b; Duff and McMillan, 1951; Geer, 1966). This is followed by the appearance of lipid vacuoles in stellate and fusiform-shaped cells in the intima and later the appearance of foam cells.

The principal cell found in human fatty streak lesions is smooth muscle (Geer et al., 1960, 1961; Haust et al., 1962). This cell, in addition to accumulating lipid in the lesion, also has been proved to be the one responsible for elaboration of the elastin and collagen found in the intima (Ross, 1972). Nearly all investigators agree on these roles for smooth muscle in fatty lesions. There is controversy with regard to the origin of the intimal smooth muscle cells. Most investigators believe the intimal smooth muscle cells are derived from medial smooth muscle cells that have proliferated and migrated into the intima (Björkerud, 1968; Buck, 1963; Hassler, 1970; Lee et al., 1970; Murray et al., 1966; Poole et al., 1971; Spaet and Lanjnieks, 1967). Morphologic evidence to support this view in the main is the demonstration of smooth muscle cells that appear to be passing through fenestrations of the internal elastic membrane into the intima (Buck, 1963). Tritiated thymidine uptake studies support a medial source of intimal smooth muscle cells (Björkerud, 1969; Hassler, 1970; Lee et al., 1970; Spaet and Lanjnieks, 1967). Others hold that endothelium is the source of intimal smooth muscle, offering histochemical and immunochemical evidence of myofilaments and actomyosin in endothelium (Becker and Murphy, 1969; Puchtler et al., 1968). For a time there were a number of investigators who held that the source of the smooth muscle cells in the intima was a circulating cell that entered the intima and subsequently differentiated (Ghani and Tibbs, 1962; O'Neal et al., 1964; Still, 1966; Still et al., 1967). Recent studies have shown rather well that a circulating cell is not the source of intimal smooth muscle (Hassler, 1970; McMillan and Stary, 1968; Poole et al., 1971; Ross et al., 1970; Sparagen et al., 1962). Another postulated source of intimal cells is a special population of native subendo-thelial cells which is geared to respond to injury (Moss and Benditt, 1970c).

There are numerous readily recognizable smooth muscle cells in human fatty streak lesions. These cells are identified by the presence of myofilaments primarily. Intimal smooth muscle cells differ morphologically from those in the media by being smaller and irregular in shape. Typically, the cell has a rather large cell body with an ovoid nucleus and a variable number of short, blunt cytoplasmic processes that extend into the surrounding connective tissue space. Relative to cytoplasmic area, the intimal smooth muscle cells contain more numerous mitochondria, profiles of endoplasmic reticulum, and fewer myofilaments than do medial

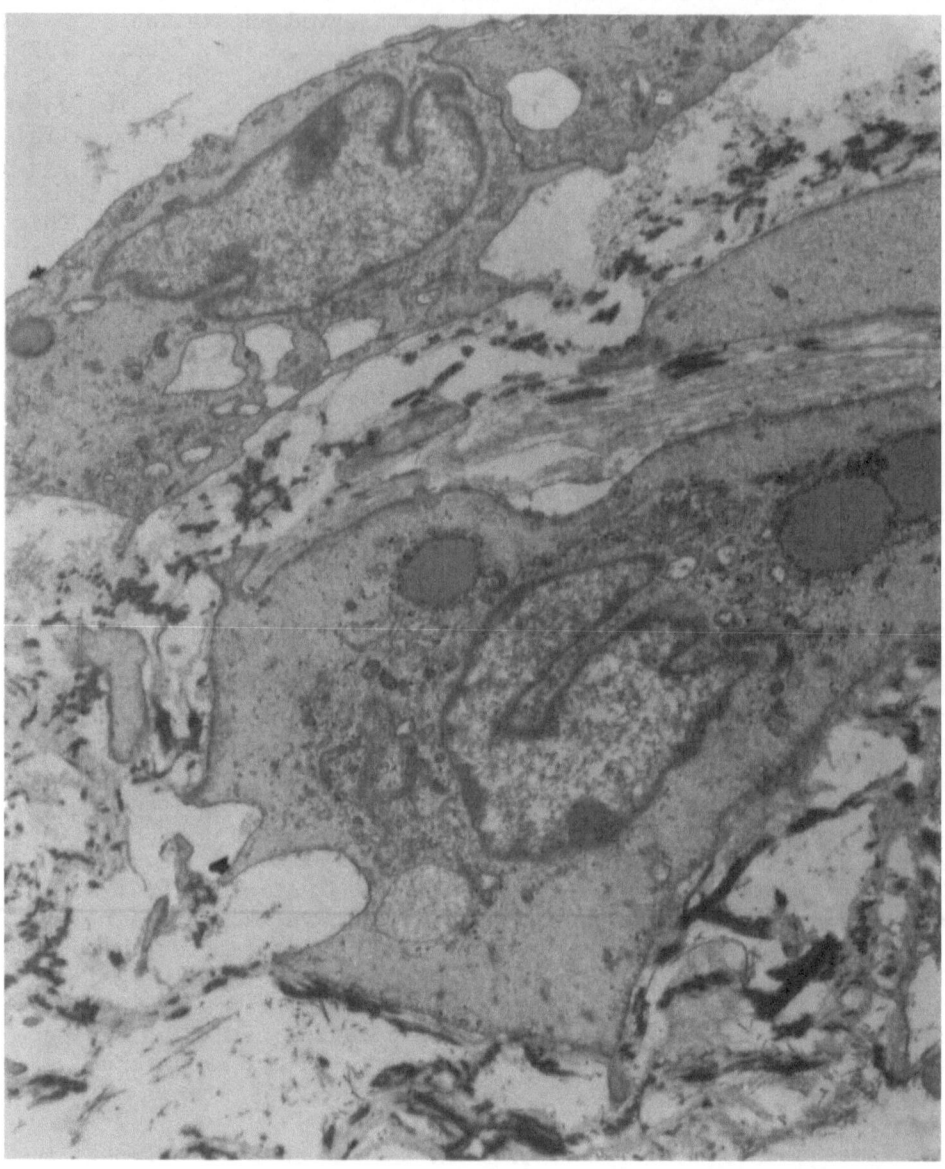

Fig. 1. Human aortic fatty streak. Endothelial cell at upper
border has lipid inclusion in cytoplasm. Smooth muscle cell
in center of micrograph contains three lipid inclusions and is
well differentiated. In the interstitial tissue there are
electron dense newly forming elastic fibers surrounded by microfilaments. (x 10,000).

cells. Myofilaments are found near the plasma membrane. The
intimal cells frequently have rather large cisterns of granular
endoplasmic reticulum and prominent Golgi apparatus. The number
of lipid inclusions in smooth muscle cells is variable. Some
cells have numerous lipid inclusions and have been termed
"myogenic foam cells" (Balis et al., 1964). The lipid inclusions
are homogeneous, electron dense and have no demonstrable limiting
membrane. Usually, but not invariably, the lipid containing
smooth muscle cell has abundant mitochondria and profiles of
endoplasmic reticulum (Figures 1 and 2).

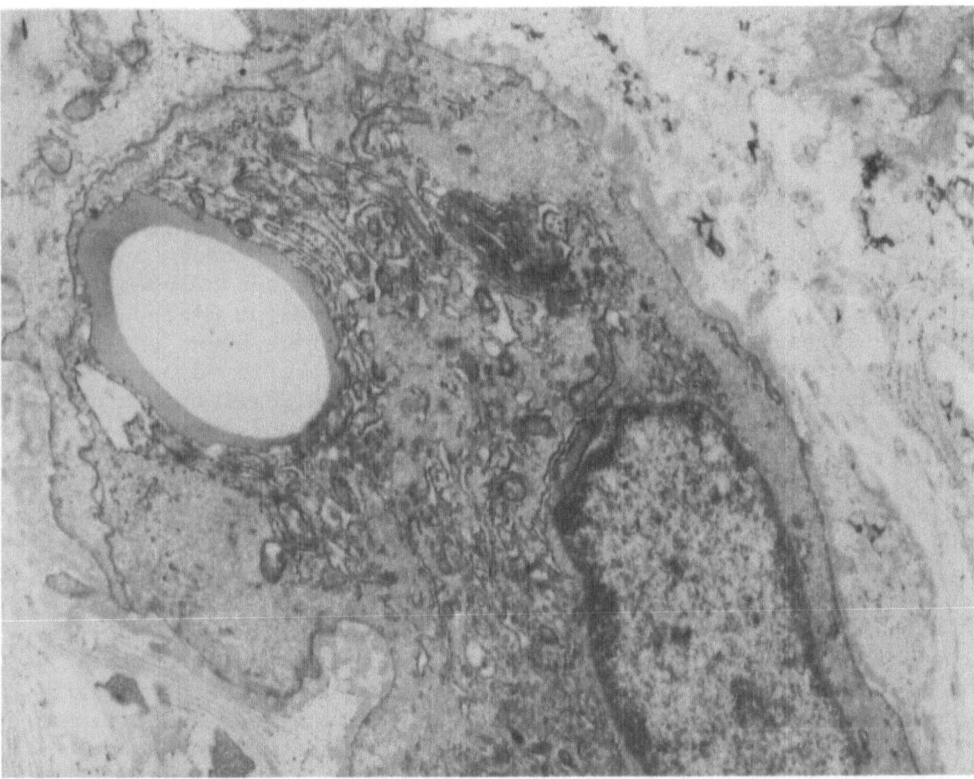

Fig. 2. Human aortic fatty streak. Smooth muscle cell with
single lipid inclusion and numerous cytoplasmic organelles. There
is electron dense extracellular lipid in the upper right corner
of the field. (x 14,900). (Reproduced with permission from Geer,
J.C., and Haust, M.D. Monographs on Atherosclerosis: Smooth
Muscle Cells in Atherosclerosis, ed. by Pollak, O.J., Simms, H.S.,
and Kirk, J.E., S. Karger, Basel, vol. 2, 1972).

A variable number of cells are found in fatty streak lesions
that have some features of smooth muscle but their identity
is in question either because they lack myofilaments or because
cytoplasmic filaments present cannot be positively identified as
myofilaments. The cells typically have a stellate configuration
with a cell body that varies from one with very little cytoplasm
to abundant cytoplasm. Cytoplasmic organelles usually are numerous
and primarily are elongated mitochondria and profiles of granular
endoplasmic reticulum, many of which are cisterns containing a
flocculent appearing material. These cells are widely referred
to as "modified smooth muscle cells" because of their resemblance
to smooth muscle and the presence of what appear to be transitional
forms of recognizable smooth muscle. Modified smooth muscle cells
usually have a partial limiting basement membrane and show a
variable number of micropinocytotic vesicles in the plasma membrane
(Figure 3). They may have lipid inclusions in their cytoplasm,
but the number of such inclusions is usually less than that seen
in recognizable smooth muscle.

The classical foam cell is a very large ovoid cell with a
central oval or kidney-shaped nucleus and cytoplasm that is a
honeycomb of lipid vacuoles of rather uniform size (Figure 4).
In the electron microscope the cell has no limiting basement
membrane. There are numerous thin villous processes of cytoplasm
extending from the cell. The plasma membrane has no micropinocytotic vesicles. The lipid inclusions are membrane bound and
typically are less electron dense than those seen in adjacent
smooth muscle cells. The foam cell has a large Golgi apparatus.
The origin of the foam cell is in debate. Many workers believe
the cell is derived from smooth muscle (Geer, 1960, 1961; Haust
et al., 1962; Parker, 1960); and others contend it is derived from
a blood monocyte that has migrated into the intima (Balis et al.,
1964; Balis et al., 1968; Geer, 1965a,b, 1966; Geer and McGill,
1967; Geer et al., 1968a; Still and Marriott, 1964). Another
school of thought is that the cell is derived from endothelium
(Altschul, 1944, 1954; Kuntz and Sulkin, 1949; Pallaske, 1930;
Schonheimer, 1924; Wacker and Hueck, 1913). Discussion of this
difference of opinion is not within the province of this presentation; however, we offer the following as facts with regard to foam
cells. The cell has none of the identifying features of smooth
muscle. Myogenic foam cells that still retain identifying features
for smooth muscle are present despite the accumulation of a large
amount of fat.

Human fatty streaks contain rather numerous ovoid cells with
a centrally placed oval or kidney-shaped nucleus, and cytoplasm
containing a small number of ovoid mitochondria and profiles of
smooth endoplasmic reticulum (Figure 5). The cells have no
basement membrane. There are numerous thin microvillous cytoplasmic
processes extending a short distance into the connective tissue

space. Because of the resemblance between this cell and a blood
monocyte, some investigators have thought these cells to be monocytes (Geer et al., 1961; Haust et al., 1962; Parker, 1960). In
view of the function of monocytes, it was logical to hypothesize
these cells as the precursors of foam cells. Present evidence
allows for no firm conclusions with regard to the origin of this
monocyte-like cell or any role in the formation of foam cell. It
is equally as plausible that the cell is an immature muscle cell,
and later we will present evidence for this possibility.

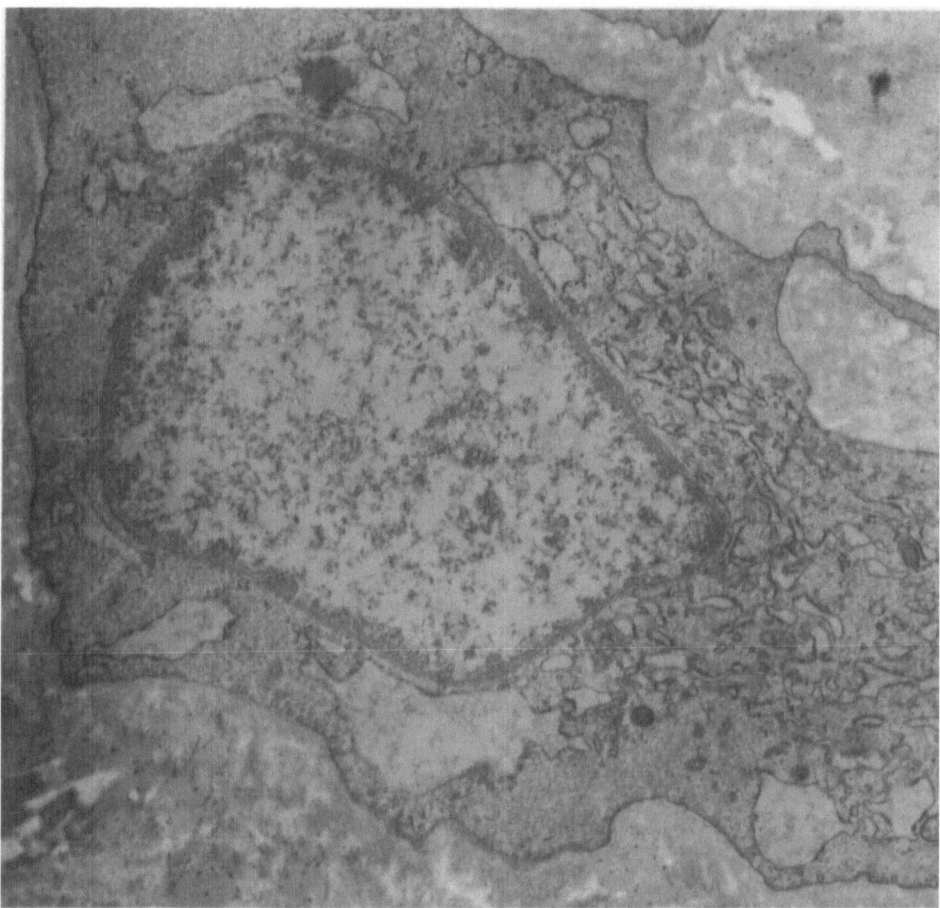

Fig. 3. Modified smooth muscle. There is rather extensive
granular endoplasmic reticulum present with cisternae containing
moderately electron dense flocculent material. Note micropinocytotic vesicles, lack of basement membrane, and filamentous
cytoplasm near plasma membrane. (x 18,750).

Endothelial cells are a constituent of the fatty streak
lesions and are identified by their anatomical position lining
the vessel surface. Most investigators have described endothelium
overlying fatty streaks to be more complex in structure than that
overlying normal intima (Balis et al., 1968; Cooke and Smith, 1968;
Daoud et al., 1968; Geer, 1965a, 1966; Geer and McGill, 1967;
Geer et al., 1968; Parker and Odland, 1966; Still and Marriott,
1964). The endothelial cell is larger in size and contains an
increased number of cytoplasmic organelles (Figure 1). Whether
a down-growth of endothelium is a source for cells within the

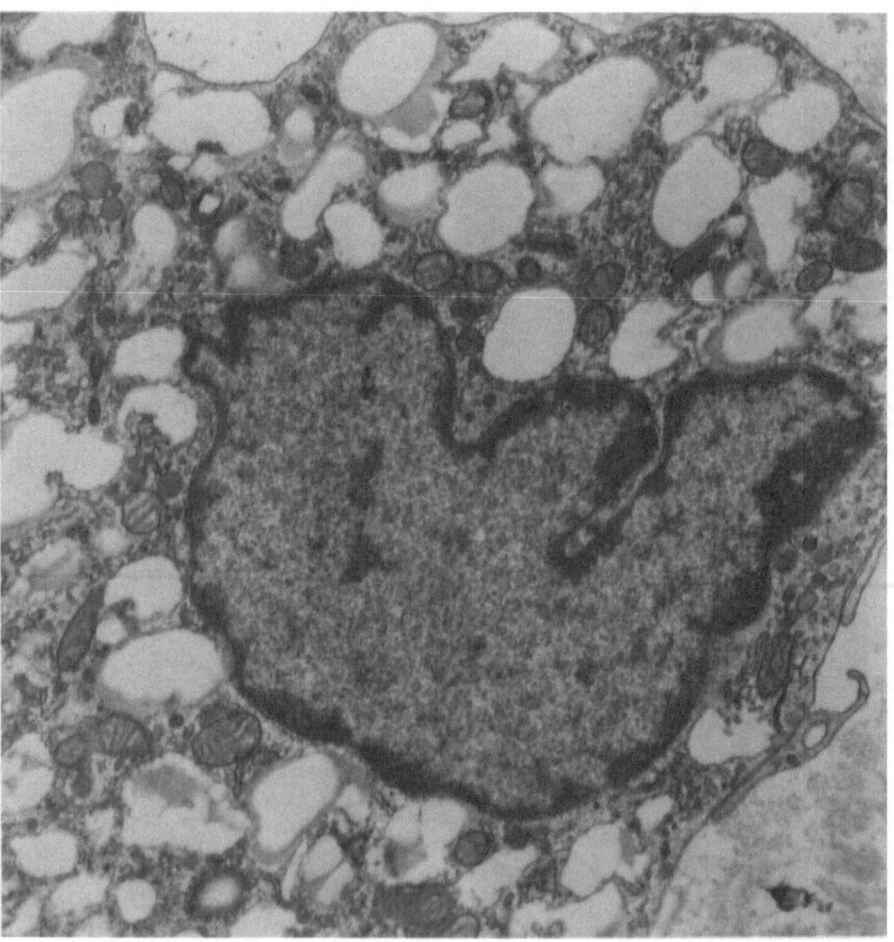

Fig. 4. Foam cell in human aortic fatty streak. Lipid inclusions
are rather uniform in size and typically are less electron dense
than those in smooth muscle cells. (x 18,750). (Reduced 15% for
reproduction).

intima is an unresolved question. We have not found evidence to
support such a source.

Human fatty streaks contain, in addition to the aforedescribed
cells, cells that can be identified positively as mast cells
(Geer, 1965b; Geer and McGill, 1967) by the cytoplasmic granules
which contain cylinders of whorled membranes. Mast cells are
present in small number.

The relative numbers of the various cells found in human
fatty streaks cannot be stated with any degree of certainty.
Quantitative studies have not been done and probably will not be
done for a long time to come, since it is reasonable to expect the
cellularity of lesions to change as the lesion ages, and we have
no way at present of accurately assessing the age of any given
fatty streak. Smooth muscle is the predominant cell in most human

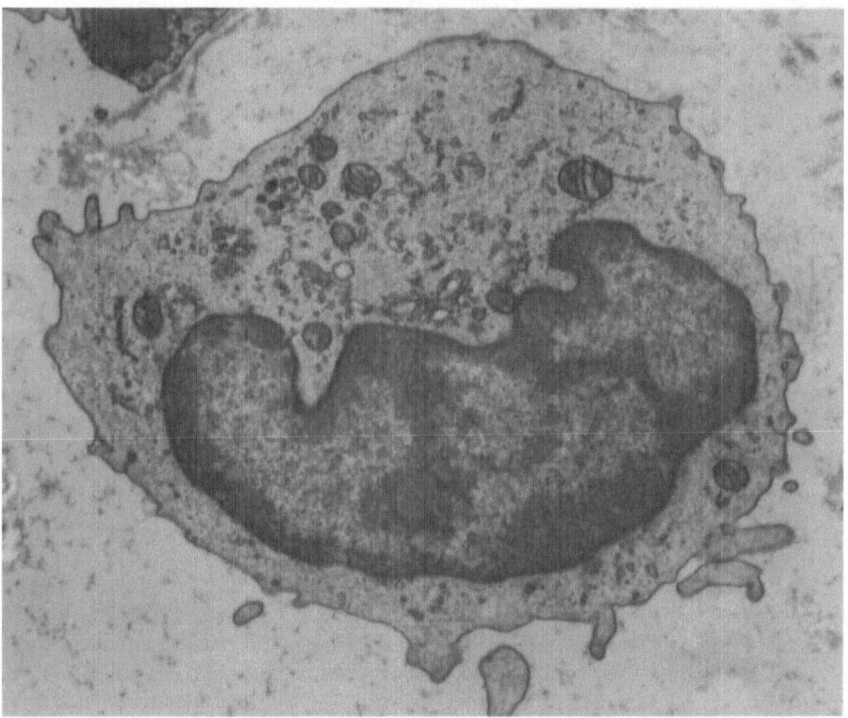

Fig. 5. Undifferentiated cell in human aortic fatty streak.
(x 13,600). (Reproduced with permission from Geer, J.C., 1965,
Lab. Invest. 14, 1764-1783).

fatty streak lesions. Foam cells are very abundant in some
lesions and quite sparse in others. Modified smooth muscle cells
vary in number depending on the depth of intima being observed.
Modified smooth muscle cells are most prevalent near the lumen.

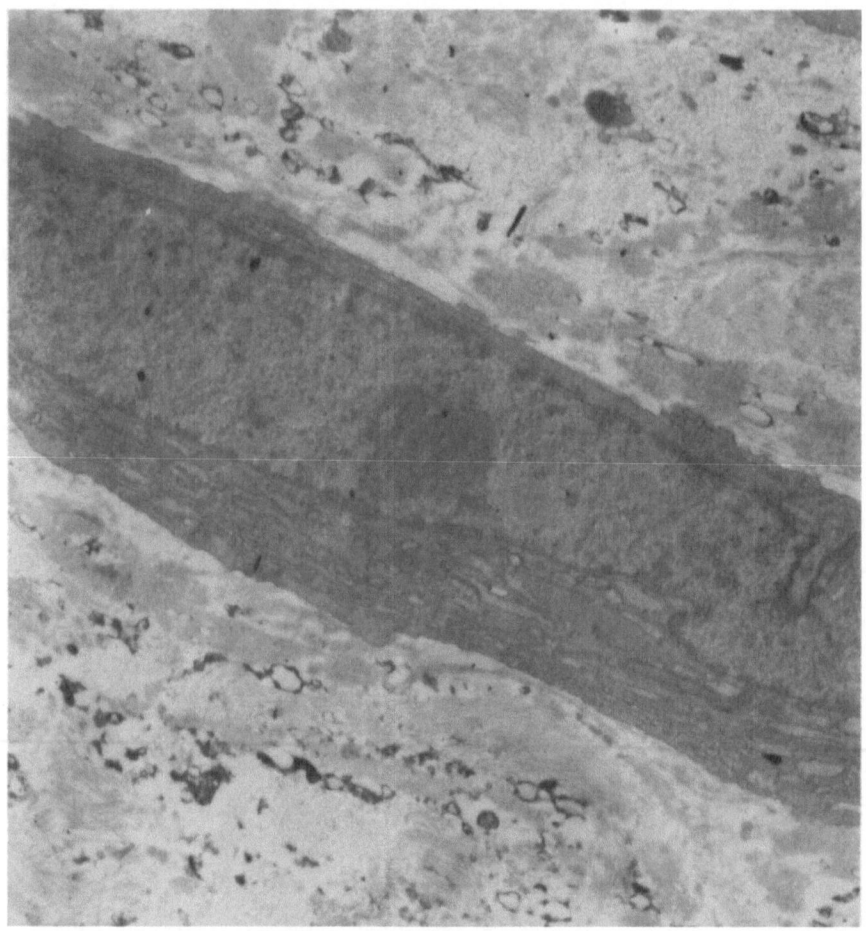

Fig. 6. Human aortic plaque lesion. Portion of long and slender
smooth muscle cell contains extensive profiles of granular endo-
plasmic reticulum and myofilaments adjacent to the plasma membrane.
There is abundant electron dense extracellular lipid. (x 14,400).
(Reproduced with permission from Geer, J.C., and Haust, M.D.
Monographs on Atherosclerosis: Smooth Muscle Cells in Athero-
sclerosis, ed. by Pollak, O.J., Simms, H.S., and Kirk, J.E., S.
Karger, Basel, vol. 2, 1972).

The monocyte-like cells are variable in number and no regional localization within the intima has been described.

FIBROUS PLAQUE LESIONS

The mechanism by which fibrous plaques form is unknown. The plaque lesion is an elevated, mound-like, white thickening in the intima. The most characteristic histological structure in the lesion is the band of fibromusculoelastic tissue forming the cap of the lesion beneath the endothelium. The lesions usually, but not always, have a core of extracellular lipid. Whether fatty streaks sometimes or ever develop into plaques has been and remains a point of controversy. It has been proposed that necrosis of lipid-containing cells occurs in fatty streaks and that the lipid released into the extracellular space somehow stimulates connective tissue deposition resulting in the fibrous plaque (Abdulla et al., 1967; Geer and McGill, 1967; Geer et al., 1968b; Haust, 1971a; O'Neal et al., 1961; Still and O'Neal, 1962). By electron microscopy, cells are seen in some fatty streak lesions with coarsely granular, electron dense cytoplasmic inclusions, swollen mitochondria, and disrupted plasma membranes (Geer et al., 1968a). These degenerative changes are an indication of cellular necrosis. In human lesions the cells undergoing necrosis are almost exclusively smooth muscle.

There have been few electron microscopic studies of fibrous plaques but the findings are generally in accord. The cells in the fibromusculoelastic cap are smooth muscle (Cooke and Smith, 1968; Ghidoni and O'Neal, 1967; Haust and More, 1966; Haust, 1970, 1971b; Marshall et al., 1966; Moss and Benditt, 1970a,b; Simpson and Harms, 1969). The smooth muscle cells are extremely long and slender with few cytoplasmic processes extending into the surrounding tissue. There are numerous mitochondria and profiles of granular endoplasmic reticulum in the central portion of the cytoplasm, and myofilaments within a narrow rim of cytoplasm near the plasma membrane (Figure 6). Fewer micropinocytotic vesicles are observed in the plasma membrane than in medial smooth muscle. The number of cytoplasmic lipid inclusions is variable. Near the endothelium there have been described unidentified cells similar to the ovoid (monocyte-like) and modified smooth muscle cells seen in fatty streaks and intimal thickening (Moss and Benditt, 1970b,c). Foam cells may or may not be found. The core of the lesion or atheroma is composed of electron dense debris and occasional clefts presumed to have been cholesterol crystals (Marshall et al., 1966). The cells in fibrous plaques are the same as those found in fatty streaks, except for mast cells which, to our knowledge, have not been described in human plaques.

EXPERIMENTAL LESIONS

Intimal lesions having features similar to human plaques can
be produced experimentally by a variety of methods (Florey et al.,
1961; Ghani and Tibbs, 1962; Hassler, 1970; Hoff and Gottlob, 1968;
Jorgensen et al., 1967). The experimental lesions appear as focal
intimal thickenings characterized by a band or zone of fibromusculoelastic tissue beneath the endothelium. The intimal thickening
basically is a scar and is the common reaction of arteries to
nearly all forms of injury (Geer and Haust, 1972). We have
compared the cellular reaction in two forms of arterial injury
produced experimentally with the cellular reaction that is
observed in human atherosclerotic lesions.

One form of arterial injury was a dietary induced one resulting
in the so-called regressing fatty streak observed in rabbits
(Anitschkow, 1933). Fatty streak lesions were induced in rabbit
aortas by feeding 1% cholesterol added to pelleted rabbit chow
for a period of four weeks, after which the rabbits were fed the
same chow without added cholesterol. Lesions were obtained by the
sequential killing of rabbits after cessation of cholesterol
feeding for a period of 120 days. The changes that occur in the
foam cellular intimal lesions following cessation of cholesterol
feeding have been described in detail by light microscopy
(Anitschkow, 1933; Duff, 1935a). During the period in which no
cholesterol is fed, the lesions rich in foam cells at the end of the
period of cholesterol feeding,undergo a metamorphosis which, in
brief, is a marked reduction in the number of foam cells associated
with the appearance of a fibromusculoelastic cap beneath the endothelium and a core of extracellular lipid including cholesterol
crystals. By electron microscopy the rabbit foam cells are quite
similar to those found in human lesions. The only striking
difference between the cells of the two species is that the rabbit
foam cell typically contains numerous and large, coarse, electron
dense cytoplasmic inclusions similar to those in human intimal
smooth muscle cells undergoing necrosis. Similar inclusions are
found in human foam cells but are much less numerous, and smaller.
The loss of foam cells from the rabbit lesion is due in part to
necrosis of the foam cells and probably to migration of foam cells
from the intima (Geer, 1966; Geer and Haust, 1972). Foam cells
penetrating the endothelium have been observed in rabbit lesions
(Parker, 1960; Geer and Haust, 1972) and in lesions from a number
of other experimental models (Marshall and O'Neal, 1966; Still and
O'Neal, 1962). As the number of foam cells diminishes, stellate-
shaped cells and smooth muscle cells appear in the intima in large
numbers. The stellate cells are morphologically quite similar to
modified smooth muscle cells in human lesions. These cells in
rabbit lesions contain variable numbers of lipid inclusions. The
stellate cells have numerous profiles of endoplasmic reticulum with

large cisterns containing flocculent appearing material. In the
adjacent interstitial tissue there are numerous collagen fibers
and newly formed elastic fibers. The elastic fibers are identified
by the parallel arrays of microfilaments, among which the amorphous
elastin matrix is seen. There can be little question that these
cells are elaborating fibrillar connective tissue precursors.
Near the endothelium there are very elongated smooth muscle cells
morphologically identical to those seen in the cap of the human
fibrous plaque. The rabbit lesion is strikingly similar to the
human plaque both by light and electron microscopy. The source
and identification of the stellate cells in the rabbit lesion
cannot be proved with the regression model. No morphological
evidence supporting an endothelial origin was found. Though the
identity of the cells could not be proved, their close resemblance
to smooth muscle cells is highly suggestive of an origin from
smooth muscle.

The problem of cell identification and source has been studied
using models of traumatic arterial injury wherein the exact time
of injury is known and the repair reaction can be observed sequentially. We have utilized the suture placement model reported
recently by Poole et al., (1971) and electrocauterization
(Schlicter, 1946; Ssolowjew, 1929). Both injuries resulted in
focal intimal thickening with the formation of a fibromusculoelastic zone beneath the endothelium (Webster et al., 1973). The
cellular changes found in both forms of injury were identical,
indicating that the form of injury has little or no effect on the
subsequent reaction. In both models tritiated thymidine administration was employed to observe the location of cells synthesizing
desoxyribonucleic acid and thus presumably dividing. Labeling was
evident earliest in the endothelial cells and medial smooth muscle
cells immediately surrounding the zone of intima injury (suture or
electrocoagulated arterial wall). The increased labeling in these
injured areas, in comparison to non-injured areas of media and endothelium, was readily evident 48 hours after injury. Labeling in
these areas rapidly declined to near normal levels by five days
following injury. Between three and four days after injury labeled
cells appeared in the intima and significant levels of labeling
remained in the intima until 10 days after injury. The finding of
early labeling in medial cells adjacent to the intimal injury, and
later the presence of labeled cells in the intima, supports the
medial origin of intimal smooth muscle cells. On the basis of
labeling studies alone, the same tentative conclusion could be drawn
for endothelium as a source of intimal cells, but concomitant light,
electron, and scanning microscopic studies (paper to be published)
did not support the hypothesis that endothelium is a source for the
cells found in the intima.

The intimal cells observed by electron microscopy changed in
morphology as the lesions evolved. At the early time period most

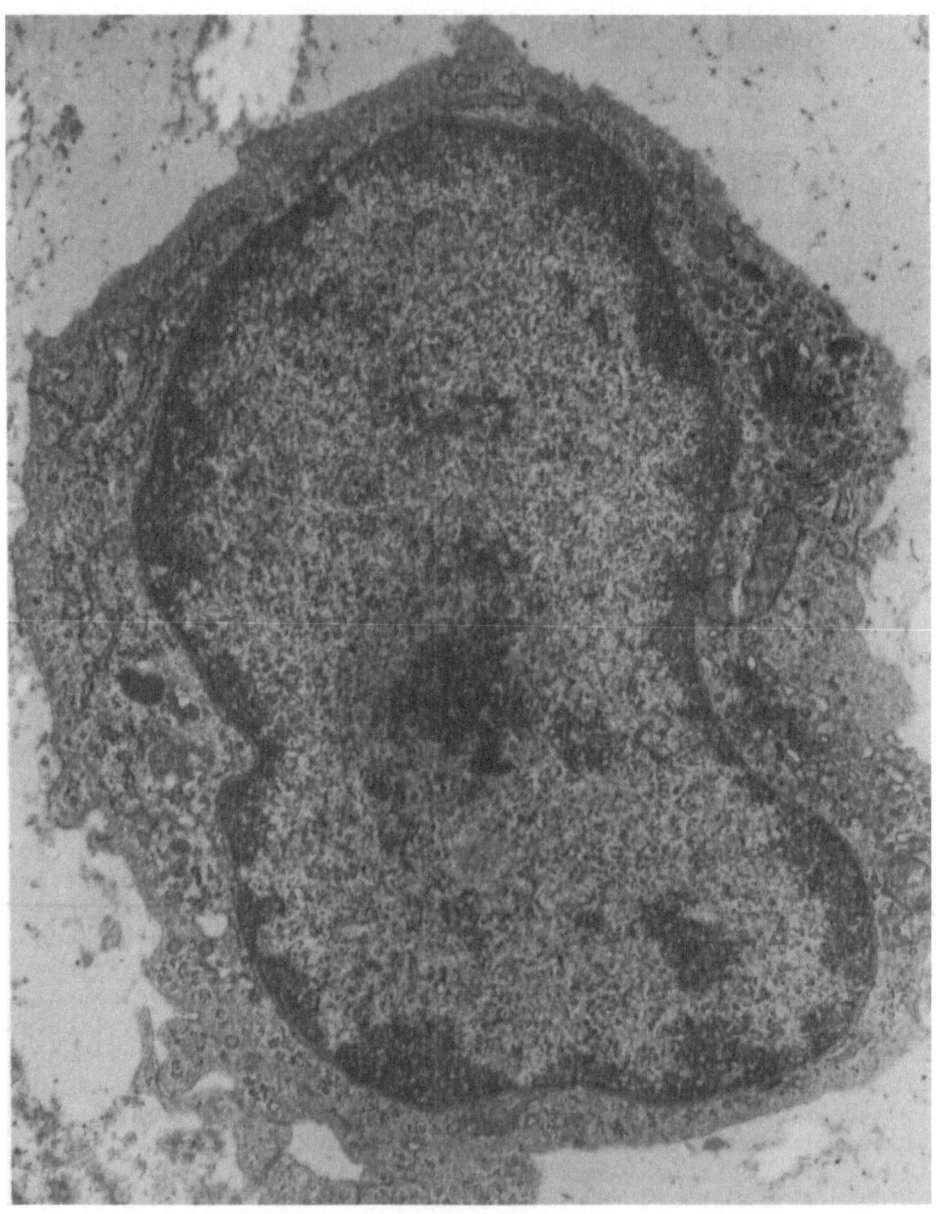

Fig. 7. Rabbit aorta. An undifferentiated cell beneath suture
at the intima-media junction. The lesion is 3 days old. The cell
has no basement membrane. Prominent Golgi apparatus and occasional
mitochondria are present in the cytoplasm. Some free ribosomes
are organized into granular endoplasmic reticulum. (x 15,500).

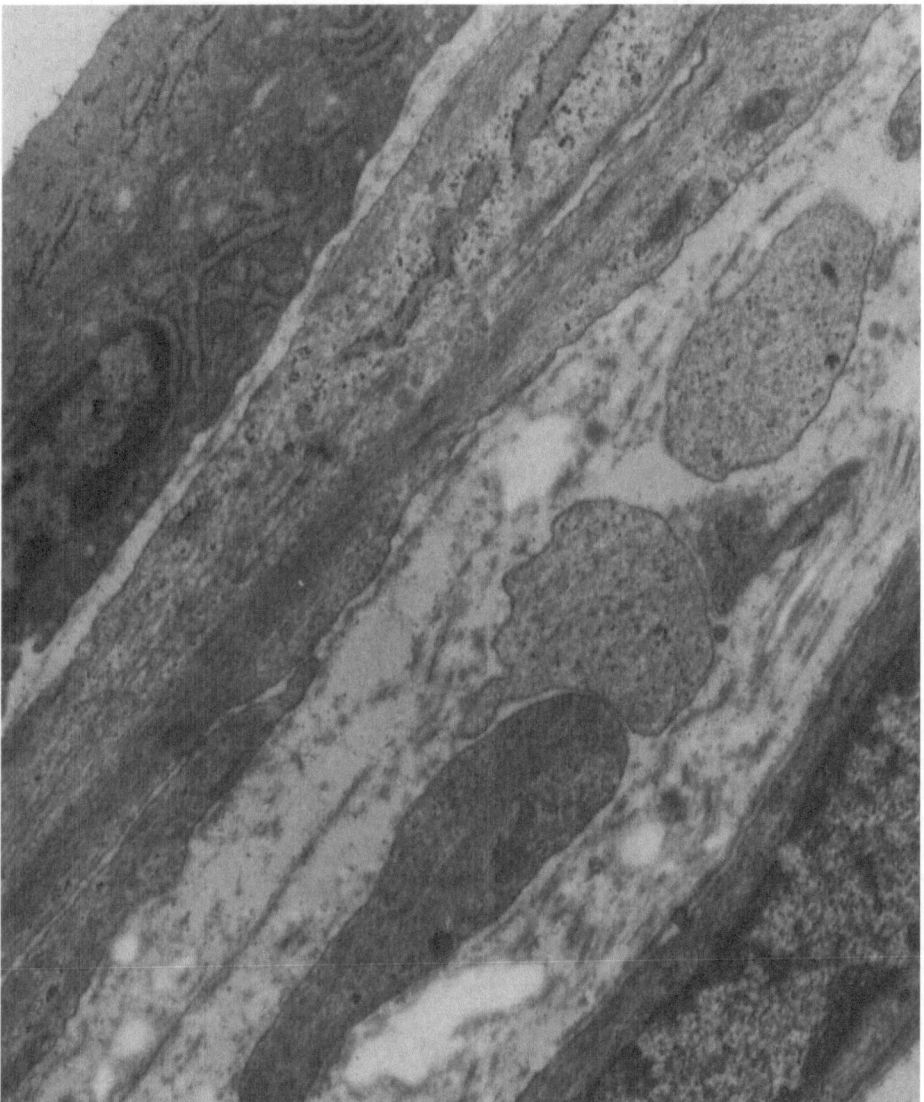

Fig. 8. Rabbit aorta. Superficial portion of 21 day old intimal
lesion induced by electrocautery. The endothelial cell (E) contains
abundant granular endoplasmic reticulum and numerous mitochondria.
Several elongated intimal cells have characteristic features of
smooth muscle, i.e., prominent basement membrane and myofilaments.
Newly formed bands of collagen fibers and electron lucent islands
of elastic fibers are present between cells. (x 21,200).

of the intimal cells were undifferentiated, appearing as ovoid or
stellate-shaped cells with a rather large nucleus and sparse
cytoplasm (Figure 7). The cytoplasm contained scattered ovoid
mitochondria and profiles of granular endoplasmic reticulum and
numerous, free ribonucleoprotein granules. Later the cells had
more abundant cytoplasm containing numerous profiles of granular
endoplasmic reticulum and were associated with the appearance of
collagen and newly forming elastic fibers in the interstitium.
Still later, numerous readily recognizable smooth muscle cells
were present. In the fibromusculoelastic zone beneath the endothelium, the smooth muscle cells were very elongated and morphologically identical to those seen in the regressing rabbit fatty
streak and the human fibrous plaques (Figure 8). The sequence of
cellular changes during the repair reaction in the rabbit aorta
leaves little room for doubt concerning the identification of the
modified smooth muscle cell as smooth muscle. Further, the cells
found in the very early stages of repair were indistinguishable
from the monocyte-like cells found in human fatty streaks, suggesting that at least some of these cells in human lesions are
smooth muscle in the undifferentiated state.

SUMMARY

Smooth muscle cells are the principal, and perhaps the only,
reacting intimal cells in the evolution of atherosclerotic lesions.
The cells accumulate lipid and thus play a role in reacting to
lipid deposition. Smooth muscle cells elaborate the precursors
of both collagen and elastic fibers. The source of intimal smooth
muscle cells probably is medial smooth muscle cells that have
proliferated and migrated into the intima. The origin of foam
cells in fatty streak lesions remains to be proved. The role of
mast cells in the human fatty streak lesion is unknown.

ACKNOWLEDGEMENTS

Studies of the authors were supported by research grant
HL 11897 from the National Heart and Lung Institute, National
Institutes of Health, U.S. Public Health Service; National
Institutes of Health General Research Support 5409, Project 7139;
and the Harkers Fund.

REFERENCES

Abdulla, Y.H., Adams, C.W.M., and Morgan, R.S. (1967).
J. Pathol. Bacteriol. 94, 63.

Altschul, R. (1944). Arch. Pathol. 38, 305.

Altschul, R. (1950). "Selected Studies on Arteriosclerosis,"
Charles C Thomas, Springfield, Illinois.

Altschul, R. (1954). "Endothelium," Macmillan, New York.

Anitschkow, N. (1933). In "Arteriosclerosis, A Survey of the
Problem" (E.V. Cowdry, ed.), pp. 271-322. Macmillan, New
York.

Aschoff, L. (1924). In "Lectures on Pathology," pp. 131-153.
Paul B. Hoeber, New York.

Balis, J.U., Haust, M.D., and More, R.H. (1964). Exp. Mol.
Pathol. 3, 511.

Balis, J.U., Chan, A.S., and Conen, P.E. (1968). Exp. Mol.
Pathol. 8, 90.

Becker, C.G., and Murphy, G.E. (1969). Amer. J. Pathol. 55, 1.

Björkerud, S. (1969). Virchows Arch. Abt. A. Pathol. Anat. 347,
197.

Buck, R.C. (1963). In "Atherosclerosis and Its Origin"
(M. Sandler and G.H. Bourne, eds.), pp. 1-38. Academic
Press, New York.

Cliff, W.J. (1967). Lab. Invest. 17, 599.

Cliff, W.J. (1970). Exp. Mol. Pathol. 13, 1972.

Cooke, P.H., and Smith, S.C. (1968). Exp. Mol. Pathol. 8, 171.

Daoud, A.S., Jones, R., and Scott, R.F. (1968). Exp. Mol. Pathol.
8, 263.

Dewey, M.M., and Barr, L. (1962). Science 137, 670.

Dock, W. (1931). J. Amer. Med. Ass. 131, 875.

Duff, G.L. (1935a). Arch. Pathol. 20, 81.

Duff, G.L. (1935b). Arch. Pathol. 20, 259.

Duff, G.L., and McMillan, G.C. (1951). Amer. J. Med. 11, 92.

Fangman, R.J., and Hellwig, C.A. (1947). Amer. J. Pathol. 23,
    901.

Florey, H.W., Greer, S.J., Poole, J.C.F., and Werthessen, N.T.
    (1961). Brit. J. Exp. Pathol. 42, 236.

Geer, J.C., McGill, H.C., Jr., Strong, J.P., and Holman, R.L.
    (1960). Proc. Soc. Exp. Biol. Med. 19, 15.

Geer, J.C., McGill, H.C., and Strong, J.P. (1961). Amer. J.
    Pathol. 38, 263.

Geer, J.C. (1965a). Amer. J. Pathol. 47, 241.

Geer, J.C. (1965b). Lab. Invest. 14, 1764.

Geer, J.C. (1966). In "Cerebral Vascular Diseases" (C.H.
    Millikan, R.G. Siekert and J.P. Whisnant, eds.), Vol. 5,
    pp. 37-52. Grune and Stratton, New York.

Geer, J.C., and McGill, H.C., Jr. (1967). In "Atherosclerotic
    Vascular Disease" (A.N. Brest and J.H. Moyer, eds.),
    pp. 8-22. Appleton-Century-Crofts, New York.

Geer, J.C., Catsulis, C., McGill, H.C., Jr., and Strong, J.P.
    (1968a). Amer. J. Pathol. 52, 265.

Geer, J.C., McGill, H.C., Jr., Robertson, W.B., and Strong, J.P.
    (1968b). Lab. Invest. 18, 565.

Geer, J.C., and Haust, M.D. (1972). "Smooth Muscle Cells in
    Atherosclerosis". Monographs on Atherosclerosis (O.J.
    Pollak, H.S. Simms and J.E. Kirk, eds.), Vol. II, Phiebig -
    S. Karger, Basel.

Ghani, A.R., and Tibbs, D.J. (1962). Brit. Med. J. 1, 1244.

Ghidoni, J.J., and O'Neal, R.M. (1967). Exp. Mol. Pathol. 7, 378.

Gross, L., Epstein, E.Z., and Kugel, M.A. (1934). Amer. J.
    Pathol. 10, 253.

Hassler, O. (1970). Lab. Invest. 22, 286.

Haust, M.D., Balis, J.U., and More, R.H. (1962). Circulation 26,
    656.

Haust, M.D., and More, R.H. (1966). Circulation 34, 14.

Haust, M.D. (1970). In "Atherosclerosis: Proceedings of the Second International Symposium, 1969" (R.J. Jones, ed.), pp. 12-20. Springer-Verlag, New York.

Haust, M.D. (1971a). Hum. Pathol. 2, 1.

Haust, M.D. (1971b). In "Concepts of Disease" (J.G. Brunson and E.A. Gall, eds.), pp. 451-487. Macmillan, New York.

Hoff, H.F., and Gottlob, R. (1968). Virchows Arch. Pathol. Anat. Physiol. 345, 93.

Jores, L. (1922). Deut. Med. Wochenschr. 48, 649.

Jores, L. (1924). In "Handbuch der Speziellen Pathologischen Anatomie und Histologie". Band II, Herz und Gefässe (F. Henke and O. Lubarsch, eds.), pp. 608-786. Julius Springer, Berlin.

Jorgensen, L., Rowsell, H.C., Hovig, T., and Mustard, J.F. (1967). Amer. J. Pathol. 51, 681.

Kadar, A., Veress, B., and Jellinek, H. (1969). Exp. Mol. Pathol. 11, 212.

Karrer, H.E. (1961). J. Ultrastruct. Res. 5,1.

Keech, M.K. (1960). J. Biophys. Biochem. Cytol. 7, 533.

Kuntz, A., and Sulkin, N.M. (1949). Arch. Pathol. 47, 248.

Langhans, T. (1866). Virchows Arch., Pathol. Anat. Physiol. 36, 187.

Lee, K.T., Lee, K.J., Lee, S.K., Imai, H., and O'Neal, R.M. (1970). Exp. Mol. Pathol. 13, 118.

Marshall, J.R., Adams, J.G., O'Neal, R.M., and DeBakey, M.E. (1966). J. Atheroscler. Res. 6, 120.

Marshall, J.R., and O'Neal, R.M. (1966). Exp. Mol. Pathol. 5,1.

McMillan, G.C., and Stary, H.C. (1968). Ann. N.Y. Acad. Sci. 149, 699.

Moss, N.S., and Benditt, E.P. (1970a). Lab. Invest. 22, 166.

Moss, N.S., and Benditt, E.P. (1970b). Lab. Invest. 23, 521.

Moss, N.S., and Benditt, E.P. (1970c). Lab. Invest. 23, 231.

Murray, M., Schrodt. G.R., and Berg, H.F. (1966). Arch. Pathol.
    82, 138.

O'Neal, R.M., Still, W.J.S., and Hartroft, W.S. (1961).
    J. Pathol. Bacteriol. 82, 183.

O'Neal, R.M., Jordan, G.L., Jr., Rabin, E.R., DeBakey, M.E.,
    and Halpert, B. (1964). Exp. Mol. Pathol. 3, 403.

Pallaske, G. (1930). Frankfurt. Z. Pathol. 40, 64.

Parker, F. (1958). Amer. J. Anat. 103, 247.

Parker, F. (1960). Amer. J. Pathol. 36, 19.

Parker, F., and Odland, G.F. (1966). Amer. J. Pathol. 48, 197.

Paule, W.J. (1963). J. Ultrastruct. Res. 8, 219.

Pease, D.C., and Molinari, S. (1960). J. Ultrastruct. Res. 3,
    447.

Pease, D.C., and Paule, W.J. (1960). J. Ultrastruct. Res. 3,
    469.

Poole, J.C.F., Cromwell, S.B., and Benditt, E.P. (1971).
    Amer. J. Pathol. 62, 391.

Prior, J.T., and Jones, D.B. (1952). Amer. J. Pathol. 28, 937.

Puchtler, H., Sweat, F., Terry, M.S., and Conner, H.M. (1968).
    J. Microsc. 89, 95.

Rhodin, J.A.G. (1962). Physiol. Rev. 42, Suppl. 5, 48.

Ross, R., Everett, N.B., and Tyler, R. (1970). J. Cell Biol.
    44, 645.

Ross, R. (1972). In "The Pathogenesis of Atherosclerosis"
    (R.W. Wissler and J.C. Geer, eds.), pp. 147-163. Williams
    and Wilkins, Baltimore.

Sappington, S.W., and Horneff, J.A. (1941). Amer. J. Med. Sci.
    201, 862.

Schlicter, J.G. (1946). Arch. Pathol. 42, 182.

Schönheimer, R. (1924). Virchows Arch., Pathol. Anat. Physiol. 251, 732.

Simpson, C.F., and Harms, R.H. (1969). J. Atheroscler. Res. 10, 63.

Spaet, T.H., and Lenjnieks, I. (1967). Proc. Soc. Exp. Biol. Med. 125, 1197.

Sparagen, S.C., Bond, V.P., and Dahl, L.K. (1962). Circ. Res. 11, 329.

Ssolowjew, A. (1929). Z. Gesamte Exp. Med. 69, 94.

Still, W.J.S., and O'Neal, R.M. (1962). Amer. J. Pathol. 40, 21.

Still, W.J.S., and Marriott, P.R. (1964). J. Atheroscler. Res. 4, 373.

Still, W.J.S. (1966). Lab. Invest. 15, 1492.

Still, W.J.S., Ghani, A.R., and Dennison, S.M. (1967). Amer. J. Pathol. 51, 1013.

Taylor, C.B., Baldwin, D.R., and Hass, G.M. (1950. Arch. Pathol. 49, 623.

Ts'ao, C., and Glagov, S. (1970). Lab. Invest. 23, 510.

Vlodaver, Z., Kahn, H.A., and Neufeld, H.N. (1969). Circulation 39, 541.

Wacker, L., and Hueck, W. (1913). Muenchen. Med. Wochenschr. 60, 2097.

Webster, W.S., Bishop, S.P., and Geer, J.C. (1973). (In Preparation).

Wilens, S.L. (1951). Amer. J. Pathol. 27, 825.

DISCUSSION FOLLOWING THE PRESENTATION BY JACK C. GEER

Dr. Kramsch: Jack, I have two questions. You talked about lipids being incorporated into the cells. At any stage in the atherosclerotic lesions did you find lipid associated with connective tissue, collagen, or elastin, and if so, is this also true in the fatty streaks? Also, in those cells that have filled extensively with lipids, did you find any evidence of connective

tissue synthesis? I question whether the cells filled to the brim
with lipids still can fulfill the function of synthesizing lipids
and proteins?

Dr. Geer: The answer to the first question is yes. We do
see lipids associated with connective tissue and with elastin.
The lipid is the amorphous extracellular type of lipid tending,
at least in some cases, to be concentrated in the internal elastic
membrane or lamina. Regarding the second question as to whether a
lipid-filled cell can synthesize connective tissue, I do not know.

Dr. Fleischmajer: Do you think that the modified smooth
muscle cells are responsible for the collagen deposition rather
than the smooth muscle cells? Fritz et al.[1] suggested a cycle
whereby fibroblast-like cells differentiate into modified smooth
muscle cells which eventually may differentiate into smooth muscle
cells. Is there some evidence that this mechanism may be operative
in atherosclerosis?

Dr. Geer: The question, as I understand it, is whether the
modified smooth muscle cells have a greater connective tissue
synthesizing capacity than that of well differentiated smooth
muscle. My impression is yes, but I have never really specifically
studied this point.

Dr. McGill: I have one question, Dr. Geer, regarding this
modified smooth muscle cell. Would you venture a guess as to
which way it is going? Is it differentiating into smooth muscle,
or is it dedifferentiating from smooth muscle?

Dr. Geer: I can't prove it one way or the other, but I
think it is clearly evident that it is differentiating toward the
muscle cell.

Dr. Kramsch: Dr. Geer, several times you have mentioned the
increase in rough endoplasmic reticulum, particularly in the
modified cells. Did you also notice an increase in smooth endoplasmic reticulum, particularly in the foam cells?

Dr. Geer: In the fully developed foam cell, practically
everything you see is lipid. However, the foam cell has a large
Golgi, that is of course composed of smooth membranes.

Dr. Ross: The term modified smooth muscle disturbs me. I
gather that the basis for the term modified means that it has a

---

[1]Fritz et al. (1970). Exp. Molec. Pathol. 12, 354.

large amount of rough endoplasmic reticulum (RER). Is that the
principal change that one sees? If that is the case, then I think
that one has to point out that the amount of RER in these cells
does not serve to identify the cells at least as best we understand it -- now, all cells, not just smooth muscle cells, can
develop a RER. For example, in going from the so-called fibroblast to fibrocyte, or from the active pancreatic acinar cell to
the inactive one, or from the active salivary gland cell to the
inactive one, all show in one state a large amount of RER, and in
the other state relatively little; in one state a well developed
Golgi complex, and in another relatively little.

All this tells us, I think, based on other studies of amino
acid incorporation during protein synthesis, is that the cell has
now developed a certain aspect of its machinery to make secretory
proteins. The secretory proteins differ from one cell type to
another, but the machinery has the same general morphology. I
don't think this is necessarily a cellular modification so much as
an expression of the fact that the particular ability of the cell,
which is already genetically built in, had been turned off and
becomes turned on again under special circumstances. I think it
is a normal component of cell stimulation to make a specific
secretory protein that has already been genetically built into
the cell. The term modified bothers me because it implies the
cell is doing something it shouldn't normally do, whereas, I
think the smooth muscle cell normally during development makes
all these connective tissue proteins and when it does, it has
more RER. When the cell stops making protein, the RER disappears
and if the cell becomes stimulated again, the RER reappears.

Dr. Geer: I certainly agree with you. I feel the term
modified smooth muscle has been used only in the morphological
sense as a description and not to infer that anything in the
cell is really modified biochemically.

REACTION PATTERNS OF INTIMAL MESENCHYME TO INJURY, AND REPAIR IN

ATHEROSCLEROSIS

M. Daria Haust

Department of Pathology, University of Western Ontario
London, Ontario, Canada, and Sir William Dunn
School of Pathology, University of Oxford, Oxford,
Great Britain

The role of the arterial wall itself in the inception and progression of atherosclerotic lesions had been disregarded for many decades. It became apparent, however, that one had to take into consideration factors pertaining to the organ in which atherosclerotic tissue changes took place, if one hoped to account ultimately for all features of the disease process. For example, the striking variations in the degree and extent of involvement and type of atherosclerotic lesions in different arteries or in various segments of the same artery, and the range in severity in different individuals of the same age group or in the many populations of the world, cannot be accounted for by any one theory on the etiology and pathogenesis of atherosclerosis (Haust and More, 1972), or by the more modern approach of "grouping" of factors, such as those referring to several blood constituents or to hemodynamics (Haust, 1971a). The key issue is then, if by taking into consideration the factors of arterial wall at least some of the remaining problems can be solved.

Mural arterial factors have been studied by many means: by analyzing in great detail the normal structure of different arteries and various levels of the same artery; the mode of nutrition, metabolic requirements, and permeability in general and local terms; enzymatic activity under normal and atherogenic conditions; fibrinolytic properties of normal and atherosclerotic arteries; the "behaviour" of given arterial segments transplanted into a different position; and application of innumerable forms of injury known or expected to produce changes of the endothelium or the intima as a whole. Thus, a large body of knowledge has accumu-

lated on the nature and reactivity of the arterial wall, but it is
difficult to extrapolate from this knowledge to the conditions under
which atherosclerotic lesions begin and progress in man.

A way to study human mural arterial factors that may be operational in atherosclerosis is by "dissection" and subsequent
detailed analysis of all forms of atherosclerotic lesions with
regard to the reaction of the individual components of the intima
to injury, and the repair features. Such analysis may be carried out
most profitably in terms of general (pathology) tissue reactions,
and these compared with responses to injury of similar cells and
tissues elsewhere in the body in order to ascertain whether there
may be some peculiarity of the intimal reactivity. It is such
peculiarity that should be concentrated upon in future efforts to
study atherosclerosis.

The present communication is concerned with the above aims.
A short section defining some terms of reference used in this
account precedes the actual presentation.

DELINEATIONS AND TERMINOLOGY

Mesenchyme and the Origin of Arteries

The term mesenchyme was coined by Hertwig (1881) for the non-
epithelial cells with amoeboid characteristics, which lie between
the epithelial (both ectodermal and endodermal) and mesothelial
(mesodermal) layers of the embryo. Mesenchyme is largely, but not
exclusively, derived from embryonic mesoderm, i.e., the last layer
to appear in the embryonic disc between the two other layers (the
ectoderm and the endoderm). However, mesenchyme begins to develop
from the mesoderm only when the latter reaches the stage of division into the paired somites, intermediate mesoderm on each side,
and mesodermal epithelia lining the intra-embryonic coelom. At
that time the ventro-medial portion of each somite loses its
epithelial appearance and forms a loosely arranged tissue called
the mesenchyme. The remaining portion of the somites forms dermo-
myotomes, later giving origin to skeletal muscle and mesenchymal
components of the skin.

In addition to the somites, the intra-embryonic coelomic
(somato and splanchno-pleuric) mesoderm also contributes to the
mesenchyme. Cranial to the somites, the embryo possesses a diffuse mesenchyme derived from an extension forward of the paraxial
mesoderm, but possibly also derived from the ectoderm (mesectodermal mesenchyme) and from prochordal plate (endodermal origin).

The above data (Hamilton et al., 1962) are of importance as they indicate that the specificity of the contributions by each of the three embryonic disc layers in general is not as rigid as was formerly believed and, specifically, that the mesenchyme is not derived exclusively from the mesoderm but from the ectoderm and perhaps even endoderm. Actually, this is not as extraordinary as it may appear when one recalls that the main precursor of the mesenchyme, i.e., the mesoderm, develops from a regional differentiation of the embryonic ectoderm in the caudal region of the embryonic disc (= primitive streak) (Hamilton et al., 1962).

The embryonic mesenchyme may be considered as the "filling tissue" between the germ layers of the embryo and later that of various organs; it gives origin to all connective tissues proper, lymph glands, spleen, myocardium and visceral musculature (including that of blood vessels), the endocardium and endothelium of blood vessels, lymphatics, the various blood cells, synovial membranes, connective tissue sheaths of muscle, tendons and nerve endings, and others (Hamilton et al., 1962).

The primitive mesenchymal cells are stellate with numerous processes of different sizes which contact intimately those of adjacent cells to form a network. Some investigators regard the mesenchyme as being largely syncytium in which the processes of adjacent mesenchymal cells are fused to form a protoplasmic continuity; most maintain that, while there is contiguity of the processes, there is no protoplasmic continuity. A structureless, semi-solid, jelly-like substance fills the meshes of this network. The mesenchymal cells possess characteristics of amoeboid cells and in early stages of the development they may be concerned with the transport of foods to, and metabolic waste products from, the developing organs and tissues. They also exhibit phagocytic properties. Although the mesenchymal cell is capable of differentiation into many types of cells, an apparent complete differentiation into a given cell line does not preclude a subsequent transformation into another cell line (Hamilton et al., 1962).

The aortae and their muscular coats, as well as the embryonic heart and the vitelline and allantoic vessels, develop from the mesenchyme derived from the visceral (splanchno-pleuric) mesoderm. Other vessels which form later from the mesenchyme of the parietal (somatopleuric) mesoderm of the body wall, limb-buds, and head, acquire their muscle coat from the surrounding differentiating mesenchyme, although their endothelial component may be formed by sprouting from the original vessels (the endothelium thus also being derived from visceral mesoderm) (Hamilton et al., 1962). It may be said, therefore, that the smooth muscle components of the walls of the (primitive) aortae (and their principle derivatives) have a different origin than those of other arteries of the

body. It is tempting to postulate that the difference in derivation may have some implication in the reactivity of the smooth
muscle components in the postnatal life.

The intima of the large elastic and medium size (muscular)
arteries, i.e., arteries affected by atherosclerosis, consists of
an endothelium resting upon a basement membrane and of a variable
amount of extracellular components of connective tissues (microfibrils, collagen fibrils, elastic tissue elements and the ground
substance) embedded in which are smooth muscle cells (Movat et al.,
1958; More and Haust, 1968; Haust, 1971a; 1971b). It follows,
therefore, that the entire intima is of mesenchymal nature.

                    Injury, Reaction and Repair

Injury should be defined strictly as the (actual) act upon
living tissues by a stimulus which exceeds the physiological
limits of either intensity or duration. Factually, however,
injury has been equated with the stimulus itself as defined above.

Except for some direct physical forms, e.g., the cutting of
tissues, or a blow, crash, and so on, most other "acts" of injury
cannot be witnessed or appreciated and may be recognized only by
their consequences upon, or manifestations in tissues. These
consequences or "traces" consist of several components: (1) the
immediately visible effect of injury (discontinuity in tissue,
hemorrhage, or burning, etc.); (2) the latent effect upon tissues
(fatty metamorphosis, atrophy, formation of intracellular "inclusions," etc.); (3) active tissue response (inflammation) to
dilute and/or eliminate the injurious agent; and (4) the repair
(an attempt at returning to homeostatic conditions, if necessary
by replacement of damaged tissues).

The above sequence of events seldom, if ever, proceeds step
by step. Rather, some tissue reactions, as well as certain forces
of repair, may set in immediately following injury or even before
the injury ceases (Table I). Indeed, many forms of injury, such
as some biological agents and foreign particulate matter may not
be successfully eliminated, and thus the repair process could not
"wait" for elimination prior to beginning its operation. Consequently, the phase of tissue reactions may overlap with the period
of injury, and the phase of repair may overlap with both the phases
of injury and tissue reactions (Table I).

The term "reaction" (to injury) embraces the second and third
steps listed above if a separate nomenclature is employed for step
four (repair) and in recognition that the first step is an imposed,
i.e., passive effect upon tissues and thus not a reaction. In the

TABLE I

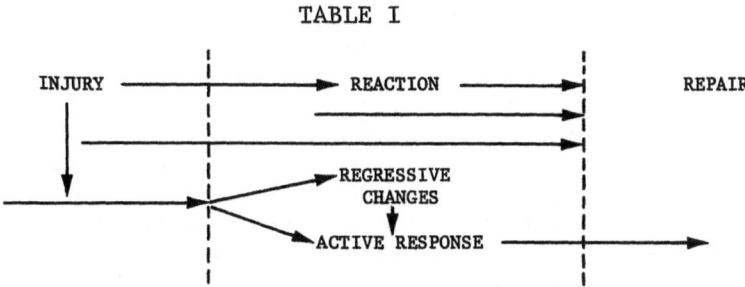

following presentation the term "reaction" as defined above will
be employed.

THE CONCEPT OF INJURY IN ATHEROSCLEROSIS

When one assesses the "profile" of research activities,
particularly that of scientific writings in the field of atherosclerosis, it becomes apparent that there is a successive replacement of one popular era by another. Regretfully, some of these
popular eras reflect a rather superficial and hollow "hang-up" on
a catching phrase or a new but single aspect of the broad spectrum
of atherosclerosis; often, no attempt is made to relate data being
offered on the "fashionable" subject to the overall problem of
atherosclerosis. One may recall that the "age of theories" in
atherosclerosis which lasted over several decades was followed in
rapid succession by the eras of low-density and then very low-
density lipoproteins, mural metabolism, the smooth muscle cells,
permeability, platelets, and many others. Astonishingly enough,
some techniques became at one time or another an end in themselves,
rather than tools of investigation. One may remember the various
eras of gas liquid chromatography, fluorescent antibody techniques,
electron microscopy, and recently the tissue culture technique -
to name only a few.

Of late, we have entered the era of "injury and repair" in
atherosclerosis with all its stimulating aspects, but also many
of the pitfalls of a fashionable phrase, as mentioned above. To
avoid some of such pitfalls, it will be of utmost importance
to test first the applicability of the terms injury, reaction,
and repair, as defined in the preceding section, to all stages of
tissue changes known in atherosclerosis; and second, to assess
what the concept of injury means with regard to the entire atherosclerotic disease process and possibly its prevention.

Any form of atherosclerotic lesion may be viewed at any stage of development as a morphological expression of an outcome, or a sum of offensive (injury) and defensive (mural, particularly intimal reactions and repair) forces operating at a given time in a given focal point of a specific arterial segment. It has been accepted, however, that forms believed to be the early lesions of atherosclerosis, i.e., fatty dots and streaks, gelatinous elevations, and microthrombi (Movat et al., 1959; Haust, 1971c), largely represent the phase of mural reactions, whereas the advanced forms, i.e., fibrous and atherosclerotic plaques (Haust et al., 1959; Haust and More, 1972), are in large measure the outcome of repair. In the latter forms certain tissue reactions may take place secondarily. "Pure" forms of lesions are not the commonest however; the lesions of "mixed" type are more numerous.

For a better understanding of certain unusual features of the various atherosclerotic lesions (for terminology see: Haust and More, 1972, Table 1.2) in terms of reactions and repair, it is desirable to recall briefly some peculiarities of structure and function of the artery as an organ. The following account pertains to the elastic and muscular arteries. This subject was considered in an extended version elsewhere (Haust, 1970; 1971a).

Arteries perform as active organs and not merely tubes through which blood is propelled passively. They distribute blood from the heart to the tissues thus functioning without interruption, and they are at all times exposed to a high blood pressure. This constant exposure and the physiological necessity of maintaining a sizable lumen in the diastole are perhaps the two most important factors determining the structure and the mode of nutrition of the elastic and muscular arteries. The intima and the media (with the exception of the outer third of the media in elastic arteries) are avascular, being nourished largely by perfusion from the lumen. The perfusion of necessary nutrients from the lumen, as well as the transmural clearing of metabolites allowing them to reach the lymphatics in the external coat of the arterial wall, is greatly facilitated by the action of the alternating systolic stretch and diastolic recoil. There is an explanation for the avascularity of the inner wall. Were the thin-walled capillaries from vasa vasorum to extend through the media into the intima, they would collapse under the high pressure to which the arterial wall is submitted since their intraluminal capillary blood pressure is very low. On the other hand, if the inner wall were supplied by the "high pressure" capillaries (connecting with the arterial lumen) as is occasionally observed in disease, it would be subject to hemorrhages from rupture of the thin-walled capillaries exposed directly to the intraarterial (luminal) high blood pressure.

It is believed that under normal conditions, in addition to the necessary nutrients, small amounts of albumin and some lipo-proteins enter the intima from the lumen (Duncan, 1963) and are drained effectively along with mural metabolites. In the process of propelling all substances across the arterial wall the acid mucopolysaccharide-rich ground substance most certainly does play an important role. The homeostasis of the arterial wall depends in large measure not only upon the status of the ground substance but also upon other connective tissue elements of the area.

The many factors involved in the transmural transport, the effective clearing of the wall and thus maintenance of homeostasis, relate to the arterial wall itself, the circulation and properties of the blood. Under normal conditions these factors are in balance. But even normally this balance is very fine, indeed, since in the absence of lymphatic capillaries in the inner coats the arterial wall may not be able to rid itself of substances as readily as other tissues do. Focal intimal accumulations of local metabolites and substances derived from blood may result. These difficulties are compounded with age because the arterial (particularly intimal) connective tissues degenerate much earlier than do those at other sites of the body, and because of the progressive increase in diffuse intimal thickness (Jores, 1924; Wolkoff, 1924; Gross et al., 1934; Movat et al., 1958; More and Haust, 1968). Both factors add further to local difficulties in adequate nourishment of the inner arterial wall and clearing of undesirable substances.

The above problems become aggravated under adverse conditions (following injury) for several reasons. Owing to the peculiari-ties of structure and function, the arterial wall has a very limited scope and range (versatility) of defense mechanisms and the defense forces are hampered not only by the lack of mural capillar-ies but also by the fact that the artery is never at rest and thus an important healing-promoting factor is absent.

If we apply the concept of injury to atherosclerosis, what does this really mean in terms of lesions as they present them-selves, in terms of experimental data, and some clinical facts as we know them (e.g., that hypertension and hyperlipidemic condi-tions aggravate them)?

On the basis of the nature of tissue reactions observed as lesions it may be postulated that the injury operating in athero-sclerosis is not severe but rather subtle. This is indicated by the fact that the lesions are limited (in a focal fashion) only to the intima rather than extending throughout the mural thickness and they are not characterized by a prominent necrosis or intense cellular infiltrations, both features usually associated with severe injury. Because of the arterial peculiarities it is possible

that the endothelium and other intimal components may be susceptible to injurious factors of very low grade which elsewhere in
the body are considered as being stimuli within physiological
range.

Which are the injurious factors that may be operating in
human atherosclerosis? These injurious factors probably include
many forms of physical, chemical, metabolic and biological agents,
and these may be as diverse for the arterial wall, as they are elsewhere in the body. Some factors may have predilection for certain
arteries or even arterial segments. Certain injurious factors
may be operational in the inception of atherosclerotic lesions,
whereas others may be promoting the progression of lesions, and
still others may act at both levels, or even be instrumental in
the precipitation of clinical manifestations (see Table 1.3,
Haust and More, 1972).

Experimentally, many forms of injury have been employed to
produce tissue reactions resembling human atherosclerotic lesions
in a great variety of animal species, and the interested reader
is referred to several reviews on the subject available in the
older and more recent literature (Duff, 1935; Hueper, 1944;
Taylor et al., 1950; Bruce and Bing, 1965; Gutstein, 1965; Roberts
and Straus, 1965). The sophistication in experimentation with
various methods and in different animal species that has been
achieved of late permits one to study selectively almost any
aspect of atherosclerosis. Thus, in more recent years experimentation has been extended to test many factors implicated in
some way in human atherosclerosis, e.g., the properties of platelets, the state of thromboplastic-fibrinolytic systems, the role
of saturated versus unsaturated fatty acids on cholesterol levels
and on the morphology of lesions, the role of certain phospholipids
on thrombosis, the organization of thrombi, altered hemodynamic
forces and their influence on lesions, the alleged regression of
lesions, the influence of sucrose administration on plasma lipid
profiles and on lesions, and many others.

Much has been learned from experimental data; however, it is
important to stress that the experimentations with various forms
of injury and with various species has failed to produce lesions
identical to those of human atherosclerosis in all aspects. This
should be perhaps anticipated, as human arteries are peculiar to
man, and each species has its characteristic arterial tree. In
keeping with the belief that among other factors the arterial wall
determines the nature and extent of the reaction (and its outcome)
to injury, it should be expected that the consequences of even
"identical" injury in different arteries would be different. If
in addition, one takes into account a wide range of factors implicated in atherosclerosis, the levels and profiles of plasma

lipoproteins, blood pressure and profiles of flow, plasma proteins, properties of platelets and many other) that differ considerably from species to species, how is one to expect identical intimal lesions in any two species? Beyond this problem many other important and basic answers have not been obtained from animal experimentations, e.g., why some animals of the same species on identical experimental regime develop lesions, and others do not.

The many factors that have been considered injurious to either endothelium or the other intimal components always may be related either to those of hemodynamics, the arterial wall itself, or to the components of blood (normal constituents and elements in transit) (see Figure 1, Haust, 1969). Regardless of the nature and derivation of the injurious agent, it may act upon the intima largely in the following ways: injurious elements derived from the luminal site (either blood or hemodynamic factors) may act upon the endothelium in such a way that its selective and differential permeability is abolished with the resulting indiscriminate (in amount and/or composition) influx of blood components into the intima. The degree of the endothelial damage may be reflected in the amount and nature of the substances entering the intima. Substances with large molecular size (the beta lipoproteins, fibrinogen) will enter the intima in addition to those of small molecular size following severe injury, whereas the latter substances alone may be allowed through the endothelium when the injury is only minor. Considerable quantities of accumulated blood constituents in either case present problems in draining and clearing in the avascular intima; in addition, the large molecular substances precipitate in the intima (e.g., fibrinogen is converted to insoluble fibrin by arterial thromboplastins) further impairing the clearing process, and damaging the local cells and the extracellular connective tissues by either exerting pressure upon them or impairing their metabolism. Alternatively, the injurious agent may be not damaging to the endothelium, leaving it unaltered and instead acting upon the underlying intima. The so-damaged intima, however, will have a secondary effect upon the endothelium with resulting changes of permeability as outlined above. Finally, the injurious factors may be derived directly or indirectly from the arterial wall itself (in inborn errors of connective tissues, other metabolic disorders, or altered neurovascular function) affecting via intimal changes the endothelial permeability.

Altered endothelium with or without underlying intimal changes will promote the deposition of mural thrombi that may vary in size from submicroscopic, microthrombi, to larger forms. But mural thrombi also may form when the normal equilibrium of factors promoting thrombosis on one hand and those of fibrinolysis is shifted to the former.

The inception of the three forms of early lesions may follow
any form of injury to either the endothelium, the underlying
intima, or both. We have, however, very little factual information regarding particularly the initiating factors in man.
Mechanical trauma (hypertension), toxemia, collision of formed
blood elements with subsequent release of permeability factors,
and hypoxia resulting from the turbulence and eddies in the
blood stream are a few of the currently favoured forms of injury
presumably operating in atherosclerosis.

How does the concept of injury in atherosclerosis relate to
some well documented clinical observations, for example that
hypertension and hyperlipidemic states aggravate the disease?

Hypertension (Gutstein, 1965; Bruce and Bing, 1965) may
operate at the very inception of lesions as a mechanical injury
to the endothelium, intima, or both with consequent mural thrombosis. Overstretching the intima may "drive", in the phase of insudation, an increased amount of blood proteins into the intima.
Hypertension may cause focal turbulence and eddies which in turn
alter (it is thought by local hypoxia) the endothelium and/or the
intima, or by causing increased collisions of formed blood elements
with the release of factors promoting increased permeability.
Hypertension may also contribute to the growth of lesions, as it
is believed that it may cause minute ruptures in the internal
elastic lamina with subsequent proliferation of intimal connective
tissues (Hass, 1955; 1963). It may promote the growth of lesions
by increasing the incidence of hemorrhages (Paterson et al., 1960)
from capillaries that may develop at the base of larger lesions
and by causing fissuring of lesions and intraatheromatous hemorrhages it may be a force in complicated lesions. Hypertension is
also an acknowledged factor in precipitating the clinical manifestations in atherosclerosis.

Plasma lipids of particular composition and/or increased
levels were thought to be injurious to the endothelium by exerting
a "toxic" effect; however, if the lipids were "toxic" to the endothelium or subjacent intima the argument that the fatty change
would be diffuse rather than focal is not entirely valid in view
of the present day knowledge on local differences of the arterial
wall. Lipids may be acting through a variety of routes. Certain
plasma lipids promote thrombosis and thus atherosclerosis either
by altering the fibrinolytic systems or by influencing the platelets.
The coagulation of blood may be promoted by high content of dairy
fat in the diet and hyperlipemia (Duncan and Waldron, 1949; Mandel
et al., 1958), by saturated long-chain fatty acids (Connor and
Poole, 1961), and by phospholipids rich in phosphatidyl ethanol-
amine (Poole and Robinson, 1956). The turnover and adhesiveness
of platelets was said to be increased, whereas the survival of

platelets shortened by diets rich in eggs and dairy fats (Mustard, 1967). Alimentary lipemia and butter intake have an inhibiting influence upon fibrinolytic activity (Billimoria et al., 1959; Greig, 1956). Furthermore, when in the process of insudation significant amounts of the large size lipoproteins enter the intima, their presence creates serious local problems and most certainly prevents a complete restitution to normal conditions; in this sense they are directly injurious to the intima.

PATTERNS OF INTIMAL REACTION IN ATHEROSCLEROSIS

There appear to be three distinct morphological patterns of reaction to injury in atherosclerosis and these are observed at times in "pure" form. These are: the fatty dots and streaks, gelatinous gray elevations, and microthrombi. The first two of these focal lesions are visible by an unaided eye on the intimal surface, whereas the third is usually detectable on microscopic examination only.

If the individual lesion, in its purest form, be the point of departure in considering the nature of reactions then it may be stated that the fatty dots and streaks are a gross reflection of a focal fatty metamorphosis of a variable number of intimal smooth muscle cells, and the gelatinous elevation represents either a serous or sero-fibrinous insudation. The microthrombi either are composed largely of fibrin, platelets, or both components.

Detailed examination of these lesions, especially by special methods (antibody techniques, electron microscopy, etc.), discloses that the reaction patterns are more complex than mentioned above, either because the injury in operation was capable of eliciting more than one form of reaction, or because one reaction induced another in due time. For example, a fatty streak may contain in addition to its hallmark (fat-containing smooth muscle cells), an insudate that may be serous or sero-fibrinous; necrotic cell remnants which presumably released fat into the extracellular space; extracellular fat in a granular form suggesting luminal derivation and subsequent precipitation in tissues (some of which may be identifiable biochemically or immunologically as beta- or prebetalipoproteins); and native connective tissue fibers in various stages of degeneration. Either the "pure" lesion or one with some or all of the above additional changes may also show the presence of a superimposed microthrombus. Similarly, the lesion that appears on gross examination as a gelatinous elevation may in addition to its hallmark (serous or sero-fibrinous insudate) show the presence of a variable number of fat-containing smooth muscle cells, damaged native connective tissue elements, and small amounts of extracellular fat. It in turn may also be covered by a

microthrombus. When all of the above changes are present it
becomes a difficult task to decide whether the lesion commenced
as a small fatty dot or streak, or a gelatinous elevation. Conceivably, when a lesion begins as a "pure" microthrombus, secondary
changes in the underlying intima may be those of fatty metamorphosis of smooth muscle cells (as a consequence of local hypoxia,
lack of nourishment, or both, because of the overlying thrombus),
or those of local edema (possibly a consequence of the release
of permeability factors from platelets of the thrombus), or both.

Thus, local injury may be followed by either increased focal
permeability with consequent insudation of blood components into
the intima, deposition of microthrombi, or both. Fatty dots and
streaks may be the result of local hypoxia for whatever primary
reason that causes fatty metamorphosis of intimal smooth muscle
cells, or the latter change may be a secondary consequence of
either insudation or thrombus deposition. A detailed account on
the possible fate of each early "pure" and mixed lesion is given
in detail elsewhere (Haust, 1971c). And finally, one may often
observe features of reaction as well as those of repair in the
same lesion (Table I); for example, in large fatty streaks, mononuclear cells are present in the lesions in addition to native
smooth muscle cells. Many of the mononuclear cells contain fat
and this is interpreted by some investigators as indicating phagocytosis, and thus represents a feature of repair. The various
tissue reactions manifested in the three different lesions are
indicated in Table II.

TABLE II. INTIMAL REACTION PATTERNS TO INJURY IN ATHEROSCLEROSIS

Early Lesions	Tissue Changes (Applicable Only)	Advanced Lesions
1. Fatty dots and streaks	1. Degenerations - fatty metamorphosis	
2. Gelatinous elevations	2. Inflammations (insudation) - serous - sero-fibrinous	1. White fibrous plaque
	3. Atrophy	
3. Microthrombi	4. Necrosis	2. Atherosclerotic plaque - fibrous cap - atheroma
	5. Circulatory Disturbances (transmural) - thrombosis - oedema	

THE PROCESS OF REPAIR IN ATHEROSCLEROSIS

The nature of repair and the ultimate outcome of the entire
process depends, among other factors, upon the characteristics of
the injurious agent, duration of exposure to it, the type of
initial local manifestations and mural reactions, and the status
of the host. In addition, the mobilization of the mural defense
mechanisms depends in large measure upon the structural, functional,
and metabolic status of the arterial wall.

The aim of the repair process is to restore the affected area
to normal structure and function. In terms of the early atherosclerotic lesions this _restitutio ad integrum_ would presuppose that
in each of the three early forms the tissue reactions are relatively
simple and, ideally, reversible, or that very minimal loss of
tissue components occurred. It is reasonable to postulate that
upon return to homeostasis the fat-containing smooth muscle cells
of fatty dots and streaks are capable of metabolizing the accumulated fat in analogy to other sites of the body, such as the kidney
and liver. Having "freed" itself of the intracellular fat, the
area returns to normal. Similarly, when the gray gelatinous elevation represents accumulation of serous fluid containing only
albumin (but not fibrin) and no significant changes of the native
connective tissue fibers are present, the fluid may be absorbed
into the circulation completely and promptly and again, _restitutio
ad integrum_ is achieved. Finally, deposited microthrombi may
undergo lysis, but if the microthrombus was deposited on altered
or necrotic endothelium, its lysis would probably follow only the
regeneration of the endothelial lining, and the area will also be
restored to normal.

Failing the restitution to normal structure, the forces of
repair concern themselves with the formation of repair tissue and
clearing the area of debris (Table III). The tissue of repair in
atherosclerosis is rather unique as it is avascular and consists
largely of smooth muscle cells, collagen fibrils, and elastic
tissue elements arranged in parallel fashion to the lumen - all
features identical to those of normal intima. The elaboration of
this kind of repair tissue may be interpreted as an attempt at
physiological adjustment of a pathological process simulating the
normal intima. The repair tissue blends imperceptibly with the
components of adjoining normal intima and is often molded in its
shape to conform, at least to some extent, to the contour of the
luminal aspect of the intima.

The connective tissue formation in the process of repair is
the result of several operating factors: a component of it is no
doubt intended as a replacement of native connective tissues,
damaged and lost as a consequence of injury; a large portion of it

represents the outcome of organization of exogenous proteins
deposited either upon (thrombi) or into (sero-fibrinous insudate)
the intima; finally, some investigators still maintain that
certain lipids deposited into the intima in the process of atherosclerosis have a proliferative effect upon the local connective
tissues.

When forces involved in the organization of the exogenous
proteins as well as those of the clearing of tissue debris (and
fats) in the affected area are adequate, the outcome of the repair
process is one of the so-called advanced lesions, the white fibrous
plaque. The other, more common advanced lesion is the atherosclerotic plaque consisting of a centro-basal atheroma and the
superficial fibrous cap. It is believed that this lesion emerges
when the forces of either organization or the clearing of tissues
are not adequate (More and Haust, 1961). There is no reason to
assume that one or the other of the three forms of early atherosclerotic lesions culminates exclusively in either one of the two
advanced lesions. A summary of potential factors that may contribute either to the fibrous or the atheromatous components of the
atherosclerotic plaque is provided in Table IV.

Beyond the distinct peculiarities of functional adaptation
mentioned above, the tissues of repair in atherosclerosis manifest
an interesting biological phenomenon. The cells responsible for
the organization of exogenous proteins and for the elaboration of
all connective tissue elements are smooth muscle cells rather
than fibroblasts. It is probable that the need for a contractile
cellular element in an area which will ultimately become the seat

TABLE III

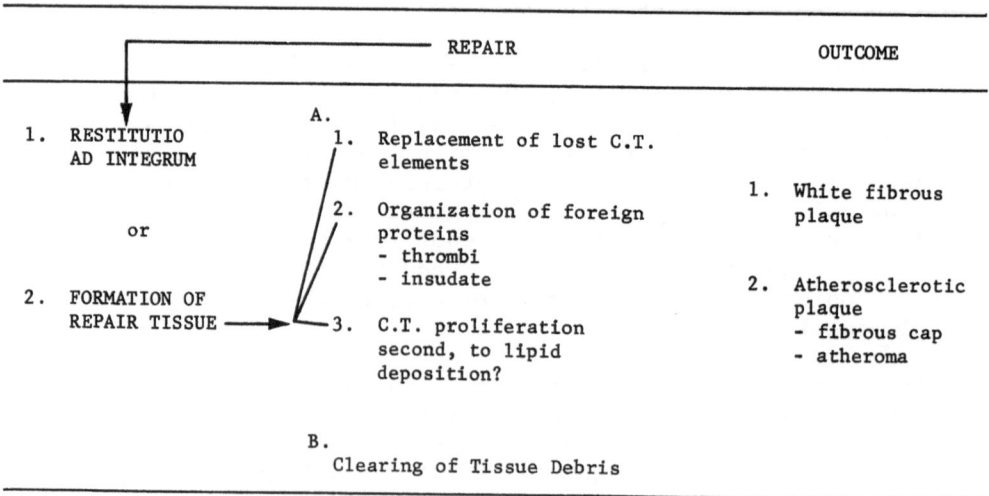

of an increased amount of connective tissues is the a priori factor determining that smooth muscle cells rather than fibroblasts are the cells of choice. These cells were identified by light micros- copy as smooth muscle cells on the basis of special stains and general morphological characteristics (Haust et al., 1957, 1959, 1960; Haust and More, 1958, 1963). The elongated cigar-shaped nucleus, slightly acidophilic slender cytoplasm with ramifying processes, a PAS-positive cytoplasmic envelope, and strongly acidophilic and phosphotungstic acid positive intracytoplasmic fibrils (myofibrils) differentiated these cells clearly from fibroblasts. Since they were the only cell type in areas of organization and thus connective tissue proliferation, the conclu- sion had to be drawn that these cells are the only ones responsible for the elaboration of all connective tissue elements. This interpretation was supported by the observation that the collagen and silver-positive reticulin fibrils and elastic tissue fibers developed in close apposition to these smooth muscle cells. The initial stormy reaction to this heretic representation subsided gradually when electron microscopic studies substantiated the observations that smooth muscle cells are capable of elaborating all extracellular connective tissues in developing, normal, and atherosclerotic arteries (Haust, 1965; Haust et al., 1965; Haust and More, 1966a, 1966b, 1966c, 1967), as well as elsewhere in the body (for details see: Geer and Haust, 1972).

The elaboration of connective tissues in an avascular area by the smooth muscle cells remains peculiar for the artery, while other avascular tissues, e.g., the cornea and cardiac valves do not show this phenomenon.

TABLE IV. PATHOGENESIS OF THE ATHEROSCLEROTIC PLAQUE*

A. FIBROUS COMPONENT	B. FATTY COMPONENT (Atheroma)
- Replacement of lost C.T. - Organization of foreign proteins (from 1,2,3,4) - C.T. proliferation secondary to "irritation" by deposited lipids?	- Local synthesis (e.g., in 3) - Accumulation of luminal lipids in 1,2; secondary to A. - Degeneration of blood proteins from 1,2,3,4. - Degeneration and necrosis of local C.T. in 1,3. - Degeneration and necrosis of RBC's in 2,4.

1. Insudate
2. Mural Thrombi
3. Fatty Dots and Streaks
4. Hemorrhages

*Modified TABLE 17-3 from Haust (1971a)

Some of the stimuli for proliferation of smooth muscle cells in atherosclerotic lesions are probably largely the same as those for other proliferating cells. It is logical to assume that the disintegration of myogenic foam cells (Haust et al., 1962; Balis et al., 1964) stimulates the proliferation of smooth muscle cells merely for replacement. The fat released at the same time from necrotic foam cells may have an "irritating" effect. Beyond the need for replacement of cells lost and the organization of proteins (contained in insudates, mural thrombi) there may be other stimuli. It is believed that certain lipids derived from blood may provide potent stimuli for proliferation above and beyond a simple process of repair. Other factors that may be capable of stimulating the proliferation of smooth muscle cells in atherosclerotic lesions need to be identified (Haust, 1972).

The avascular tissue of repair fulfills the demands of structural and functional adaptation only if present in a small amount. However, an area of repair in the intima is susceptible to subsequent repeated episodes of injury and in time may result in a focal accumulation of avascular connective tissues of considerable thickness. These consist usually of layers, each representing an episode of injury with subsequent repair, and therefore the maturation of the connective tissues varies from layer to layer and increases with the distance from the lumen. No matter how much they may mimic normal intima, large amounts of avascular connective tissues are prone to develop secondarily regressive changes. This may be in part caused by a local hypoxia and insufficient diffusion of nutrients from the lumen, and partly because the transmural transport is hindered by the thickened area; consequently, precipitation of substances derived from blood and local arrest of metabolites follows, adding further to the metabolic difficulties, and evoking tissue reactions and renewed connective tissue proliferation.

The regressive changes most commonly encountered in the atherosclerotic plaque are fatty metamorphosis and necrosis, both contributing to the formation of the centro-basal atheroma of this lesion. The mechanisms responsible for these features were briefly referred to above and are reviewed in detail elsewhere (More and Haust, 1961; Haust, 1970).

The other change, i.e., the atrophy of smooth muscle cells, is observed in aging fibrous components of both types of advanced lesions. This atrophy could in part reflect a simple aging phenomenon of cells, and may be in part the result of impaired nourishment of cells that may not have reached the "old age." Since the connective tissues in these plaques age and hyalinize prematurely, the nutrition of cells through diffusion from the lumen becomes increasingly inadequate. The regressive changes in advanced lesions are in part schematically indicated in Table II.

The success of the repair process in the arterial intima depends upon many local and general factors. Some of the local factors were mentioned; to others a suitable reference was made. Of the general factors, the age, sex, vitamins C and D, pyridoxine, choline, adrenal cortical hormones, and many others may influence the efficacy of the repair process.

DISCUSSION

Returning to the overall theme of this communication and the aims set forth at the beginning, it may be stated that the application of the concept of injury, reaction, and repair to the problem of atherosclerosis, with particular reference to mural arterial factors in man, provides a few points of interest.

The concept of injury applied to atherosclerosis shows the need for identification and elucidation of all factors that may be injurious to the arterial intima of man. This is of course not a simple task, and appropriate studies are not easy to design and to carry out. For example, if platelets cause injury by releasing permeability factors when aggregating and precipitating upon endothelium, is it justifiable to advocate prophylactic continuous intake of acetyl-salicylic acid (or other drugs with similar effects) because it alters the aggregation and some other platelet function? Two major clinical trials with drugs in patients with transient cerebral ischemia, believed to be caused by platelet emboli, are indeed presently in progress (Barnett, 1973).

Two tissue reactions stand out prominently in atherosclerosis and appear to be unique for this disease process. One is a regressive change of intimal smooth muscle cells with lipid accumulation representing fatty metamorphosis. This intracellular fat is in part synthesized by the cells (Zilversmit et al., 1961) and in part it may be taken up possibly by pinocytosis and/or phagocytosis from the extracellular space. No matter what the details of the mechanisms of the intracellular lipid accumulation may be, no such mechamisms operate anywhere else in the body; to put it differently, smooth muscle cells elsewhere in the body are not known to undergo fatty metamorphosis. The question is: Why? To elucidate this peculiar regional difference it would seem of great importance to study, under a variety of circumstances, the normal properties and behaviour of smooth muscle cells of the elastic and muscular arteries on one hand and those at other sites of the body on the other. For instance, one may profitably study the appearance and behaviour of arterial smooth muscle cells in tissue culture by cinematography as was exemplified at the meeting in the short "movie" (unpublished observations). Thus, one could observe an apparent repeated cell division, subsequent fusion of the widely separated two daughter cells to a mononuclear (? original) cell, and finally a (repeated) division of the cell. It is of course only a preliminary observation requiring further detailed exploration and it is even uncertain at this stage whether this is a true feature. However, it poses interesting questions if true, e.g., is it characteristic of only arterial or also of other smooth muscle cells?

The other unusual feature in atherosclerosis is the formation of the repair tissue that is avascular but contains smooth muscle cells which are responsible entirely for the organization and connective tissue elaboration. What may be deduced from the fact that the few other avascular tissues in the body contain fibroblasts rather than smooth muscle cells? Could one study the behaviour of the other avascular tissues, specifically that of fibroblasts, by grafting, for example, the cornea into the aorta in the same animal?

Furthermore, if ultimately the proliferation of connective tissue is detrimental to the integrity of the intima would it be desirable to prevent the development of this tissue? It should be remembered in such deliberations that at least in part the proliferation lies within the realm of the repair process and is therefore beneficial and necessary.

In spite of all the data accumulated over more than a century, we may be just beginning to ask pertinent questions regarding atherosclerosis and perhaps learning to isolate individual factors that may represent forms of injury operating in this complex disease.

ACKNOWLEDGEMENTS

The author wishes to thank Mrs. Pamela Woodward for her patient and efficient typing of the manuscript.

Supported by grants-in-aid of research MT-1037 from the Medical Research Council of Canada and T.3-11 from the Ontario Heart Foundation, Toronto, Canada.

The author is the recipient of a Visiting Scientist Award 1972-1973 from The Medical Research Council of Canada.

REFERENCES

Balis, J.U., Haust, M.D., and More, R.H. (1964). Electron microscopic studies in human atherosclerosis. Cellular elements in aortic fatty streaks. Exp. Mol. Pathol. 3, 511.

Barnett, H.J.M. (1973). Platelets, drugs and cerebral ischemia. Canad. Med. Ass. J. 108, 462.

Billimoria, J.D., Drysdale, J., James, D.C.O., and Maclagan, M.F. (1959). Determination of fibrinolytic activity of whole blood with special reference to the effects of exercise and fat feeding. Lancet 2, 471.

Bruce, T.A., and Bing, R.J. (1965). Atherosclerosis. General factors - somatic: hemodynamics. In "The Heart and Circulation." Vol 1 (Research). (E.C. Andrus and C.H. Maxwell, eds.). Second National Conference on Cardiovascular Diseases, Washington, D.C., 1964. Federation of American Societies for Experimental Biology, Bethesda, Maryland.

Connor, W.E., and Poole, J.C. (1961). The effect of fatty acids on the formation of thrombi. Quart. J. Exp. Physiol. 46, 1.

Duff, G.L. (1935). Experimental cholesterol arteriosclerosis and its relationship to human arteriosclerosis. Arch. Pathol. 20, 81; 259.

Duncan, G.G., and Waldron, J.M. (1949). The effect of ingested fat on blood coagulation. Tr. Ass. Amer. Physicians 62, 179.

Duncan, L.E. (1963). Mechanical factors in the localization of atheroma. In "Evolution of the Atherosclerotic Plaque." (R.J. Jones, ed.). University of Chicago Press, Chicago.

Geer, J.C., and Haust, M.D. (1972). "Smooth Muscle Cells in Atherosclerosis." Monographs in Atherosclerosis. Vol. 2. S. Karger, New York.

Greig, H.B. (1956). Inhibition of fibrinolysis by alimentary lipemia. Lancet 2, 16.

Gross, L., Epstein, E.Z., and Kugel, M.A. (1934). Histology of the coronary arteries and their branches in the human heart. Amer. J. Pathol. 10, 253.

Gutstein, W.H. (1965). Atherosclerosis: hemodynamics. In "The Heart and Circulation." Vol. 1 (Research). (E.C. Andrus and C.H. Maxwell, eds.). Second National Conference on Cardiovascular Diseases, Washington, D.C., 1964. Federation of American Societies for Experimental Biology, Bethesda.

Hamilton, W.J., Boyd, J.D., and Mossman, H.W. (1962). "Human Embryology," 3rd edition. W. Heffer and Sons Limited, Cambridge.

Hass, G.M. (1963). Mesenchymal activation. In "Evolution of the Atherosclerotic Plaque." (R.J. Jones, ed.). University of Chicago Press, Chicago.

Hass, G.M. (1955). Observations on vascular structure in relation to human and experimental arteriosclerosis. In "Symposium on Atherosclerosis." pp. 24-32. Publication 338. National Academy of Sciences - National Research Council, Washington, D.C.

Haust, M.D. (1971a). Arteriosclerosis. In "Concepts of Disease. Textbook of Pathology." (J.G. Brunson and E.A. Gall, eds.). MacMillan, New York.

Haust, M.D. (1971b). Development of aortic wall during fetal life and infancy. The Artery and the Process of Arteriosclerosis: Pathogenesis. Proceedings of the Conference on "Fundamental Data on Reactions of Vascular Tissue in Man," April 19-25, 1970, Lindau, Germany. In "Advances in Experimental Medicine and Biology," Vol. 16A, pp. 11-13 and 30-35. Plenum Press, New York.

Haust, M.D. (1965). Fine fibrils of extracellular space (microfibrils). Their structure and role in connective tissue organization. Amer. J. Pathol. 47, 1113.

Haust, M.D. (1970). Injury and repair in the pathogenesis of atherosclerosis. In "Atherosclerosis" Proceedings of the Second International Symposium, 1969." (R.J. Jones, ed.). pp. 12-20. Springer-Verlag, Chicago and New York.

Haust, M.D. (1971c). The morphogenesis and fate of potential and early atherosclerotic lesions in man. Hum. Pathol. 2, 1.

Haust, M.D. (1972). Regressive and progressive changes of intimal smooth muscle cells in atherosclerosis. Kongress für innere Medizin, Kongressbericht 78, 1124.

Haust, M.D., and More, R.H. (1972). Development of modern theories on the pathogenesis of atherosclerosis. In "The Pathogenesis of Atherosclerosis." (R.W. Wissler and J.C. Geer, eds.). pp. 1-19. Williams and Wilkins, Baltimore.

Haust, M.D., and More, R.H. (1968). Diffuse intimal thickening
    of coronary arteries in children and young adults, and its
    role in atherosclerosis. In "Le role de la paroi arterielle
    dans l'atherogenese." Colloques Internationaux, 169, Paris,
    15-17 Juin, 1967. pp. 75-91. Editions du Centre National
    de la Recherche Scientifique.

Haust, M.D., and More, R.H. (1967). Electron microscopy of
    connective tissues and elastogenesis. International
    Academy of Pathology: The Connective Tissues. pp. 352-
    376. Williams and Wilkins, Baltimore.

Haust, M.D., and More, R.H. (1966a). L'Organisation du tissue
    conjonctif et l'elastogenese. Laval Medical 37, 551.

Haust, M.D., and More, R.H. (1966c). Mechanism of fibrosis in
    white atherosclerotic plaques of human aorta. An electron
    microscopic study. Circulation 34, 14.

Haust, M.D., and More, R.H. (1958). New functional aspects of
    smooth muscle cells. Fed. Proc. 17, 440.

Haust, M.D., and More, R.H. (1966b). The role of differentiating
    smooth muscle cells in the organization of human aorta.
    An electron miscroscopic study. Fed. Proc. 24, 475.

Haust, M.D., and More, R.H. (1963). Significance of the smooth
    muscle cell in atherogenesis. In "Evolution of the
    Atherosclerotic Plaque." (R.J. Jones, ed.). pp. 51-63.
    The University of Chicago Press, Chicago.

Haust, M.D., More, R.H., and Balis, J.U. (1962). Electron
    microscopic study of intimal lipid accumulations in the
    human aorta and their pathogenesis. Circulation 26, 656.

Haust, M.D., More, R.H., Bencosme, S.A., and Balis, J.U. (1965).
    Elastogenesis in human aorta. An electron microscopic study.
    Exp. Mol. Pathol. 4, 508.

Haust, M.D., More, R.H., and Movat, H.Z. (1959). The mechanism of
    fibrosis in arteriosclerosis. Amer. J. Pathol. 35, 265.

Haust, M.D., More, R.H., and Movat, H.Z. (1960). The role of
    smooth muscle cells in the fibrogenesis of arteriosclerosis.
    Amer. J. Pathol. 37, 377.

Haust, M.D., Movat, H.Z., and More, R.H. (1957). Organization by
    smooth muscle cells. Amer. J. Pathol. 33, 626.

Hertwig, O. (1881). Die Colomtheorie. Jena; cited by Hamilton
    et al. (1962). pp. 111, 118.

Hueper, W.C. (1944). Arteriosclerosis. A general review.
    Arch. Pathol. 38, 162; 245; 326; 350; 381.

Jores, L. (1924). Arterien. In Handbuch der Speziellen
    Pathologischen Anatomie und Histologie. Band II,
    "Herz und Gefässe." (F. Henke and O. Lubarsch, eds.).
    pp. 608-786. Julius Springer, Berlin.

Mandel, E.E., Rosenthal, W., and Roth, H. (1958). Lipemia-
    induced acceleration of intravascular clotting. Clin.
    Res. 6, 394.

More, R.H., and Haust, M.D. (1961). Atherogenesis and plasma
    constituents. Amer. J. Pathol. 38, 527.

More, R.H., and Haust, M.D. (1968). Diffuse intimal thickening
    of coronary arteries in children and young adults, and its
    role in atherosclerosis. In "Le role de la paroi arterielle
    dans l'atherogenese." Colloques Internationaux, 169, Paris,
    15-17 Juin, 1967. pp. 75-91. Editions du Centre National
    de la Recherche Scientifique.

Movat, H.Z., Haust, M.D., and More, R.H. (1959). The morphologic
    elements in the early lesions of arteriosclerosis. Amer. J.
    Pathol. 35, 93.

Movat, H.Z., More, R.H., and Haust, M.D. (1958). The diffuse
    intimal thickening of the human aorta with aging. Amer. J.
    Pathol. 34, 1023.

Mustard, J.F. (1967). Recent advances in molecular pathology:
    a review. Platelet aggregation, vascular injury and
    atherosclerosis. Exp. Mol. Pathol. 7, 366.

Paterson, J.C., Mills, J., and Lockwood, C.H. (1960). The role
    of hypertension in progression of atherosclerosis. Canad.
    Med. Ass. J. 82, 65.

Poole, J.C.F., and Robinson, D.S. (1956). Further observations
    on the effects of ethanolamine phosphatide on plasma
    coagulation. Quart. J. Exp. Physiol. 41, 295.

Roberts, J.C., and Straus, R. (eds.). (1965). "Comparative
    Atherosclerosis." Harper and Row, New York.

Taylor, C.B., Baldwin, D., and Hass, G.M. (1950). Localized
    arteriosclerotic lesions induced in aorta of juvenile rabbit
    by freezing. Arch. Pathol. 49, 623.

Wolkoff, K. (1924). Über die Altersveränderungen der Arterien
    bei Tieren. Virchows Arch. Path. Anat. 252, 208.

PROLIFERATION OF ARTERIAL CELLS IN ATHEROSCLEROSIS

H.C. Stary

Department of Pathology, Louisiana State University

School of Medicine, New Orleans, Louisiana

The role of cell proliferation in atherosclerosis has received much attention. It has been suggested for many years that the increase in cells during the formation of intimal lesions may be due to intrinsic proliferation. This hypothesis was based mainly on the observation of mitotic figures in the smooth muscle and foam cells of atherosclerotic plaques, even though mitoses were seen only rarely. On the other hand, it was proposed but never definitely established that migration of cells from the circulation, endothelium or media accounts for the cellular growth of the lesions. Monocytes, endothelial cells, and medial smooth muscle cells thus have been implicated.

This area of atherosclerosis research had a rebirth of interest when thymidine containing the isotopic label ^{3}H (tritium) and high resolution radioautography became generally available in the 1960's. The evidence brought forward by means of tritiated thymidine radioautography of atherosclerotic plaques supports the hypothesis that early intimal lesions do indeed increase in size mainly by intramural multiplication of smooth muscle cells and foam cells. Furthermore, there is indication that in hypercholesterolemia increased arterial cell proliferation is not limited to the intimal lesions.

PROLIFERATION OF MEDIAL SMOOTH MUSCLE CELLS

Tritiated thymidine radioautography shows very low proliferative activity of medial smooth muscle cells in normal arterial media. A pulse of the tracer labels about three medial smooth

muscle cells in a 5 micron section of the complete length of the
aorta of a rabbit (McMillan and Stary, 1968a).

Hypertension induced in rats by desoxycorticosterone causes
an increase in tritiated thymidine labeling of smooth muscle cells
in medium sized and small arteries (Crane and Ingle, 1964). Acute
hypertension induced with hypertensin injections, and chronic
hypertension brought about by unilateral nephrectomy also cause
increased labeling of medial smooth muscle cells (Schmitt et al.,
1970).

Spaet and Lejnieks (1967) applied a hemostat to rabbit aortas,
causing a marked increase in tritiated thymidine labeling of
medial smooth muscle cells within one millimeter of the injury.
In two animals, circulating leukocytes were labeled before clamping
of the aorta. Increased aortic labeling did not occur in these
animals, suggesting that replacement cells were derived from the
arterial wall itself, rather than from a remote pool of proliferating cells.

Murata (1967) studied spontaneous atherosclerotic lesions in
squirrel monkeys and found increased labeling of medial smooth
muscle cells adjacent to labeled intimal foam cell lesions. When
hypercholesterolemia and atherosclerosis are induced experimentally
by feeding atherogenic diets to various animal species, there
appears to be slightly higher proliferative activity of medial
smooth muscle cells generally. A marked increase in the labeling
frequency occurs in the medial smooth muscle cells near the internal
elastic lamina adjoining intimal plaques (McMillan and Stary,
1968a,b; Thomas et al., 1968). Epinephrine given to hypercholesterolemic animals causes scattered but frequent tritiated thymidine
labeling of cells throughout the media in addition to increased
labeling in the immediate vicinity of intimal plaques (Cavallero
et al., 1973). When beta aminoproprionitrile is added to an
atherogenic diet containing cholesterol, an increase in aortic
medial smooth muscle cell labeling becomes apparent within six
days (Wegener, 1973).

The positive action of cholesterol on cell proliferation in
the aortic media has also been shown in tissue culture. Myasnikow
and Block (1965) reported enhanced growth of aortic cells cultured
in hyperlipemic rabbit serum. This finding was associated with
increased degeneration and early death of the explant cells. The
effect of hyperlipemia on the medial smooth muscle cell specifically was confirmed by Kao and co-workers (1968). This team found
that hyperlipemic serum obtained from rhesus monkeys fed coconut
oil or peanut oil induced a significant increase in the proliferation of cultured aortic cells confirmed as smooth muscle when
stained with fluorescein anti-monkey actomyosin globulin. Cells

from aortic medial explants of cholesterol-fed swine continued to synthesize DNA at a high rate when subsequently cultured in a low cholesterol serum supplement (Daoud et al., 1970).

Ross cultured aortic cells that uniformly retained the phenotype of differentiated smooth muscle cells (1971b), and confirmed by tritiated proline and electron microscope radioautography that aortic smooth muscle cells secrete both collagen and elastin (1971a). It is now clear that smooth muscle cells play a role in connective tissue formation as well as in contraction.

PROLIFERATION OF INTIMAL SMOOTH MUSCLE CELLS

Smooth muscle cells are found in human arterial intima at birth. The thickness of the intimal smooth muscle layer increases

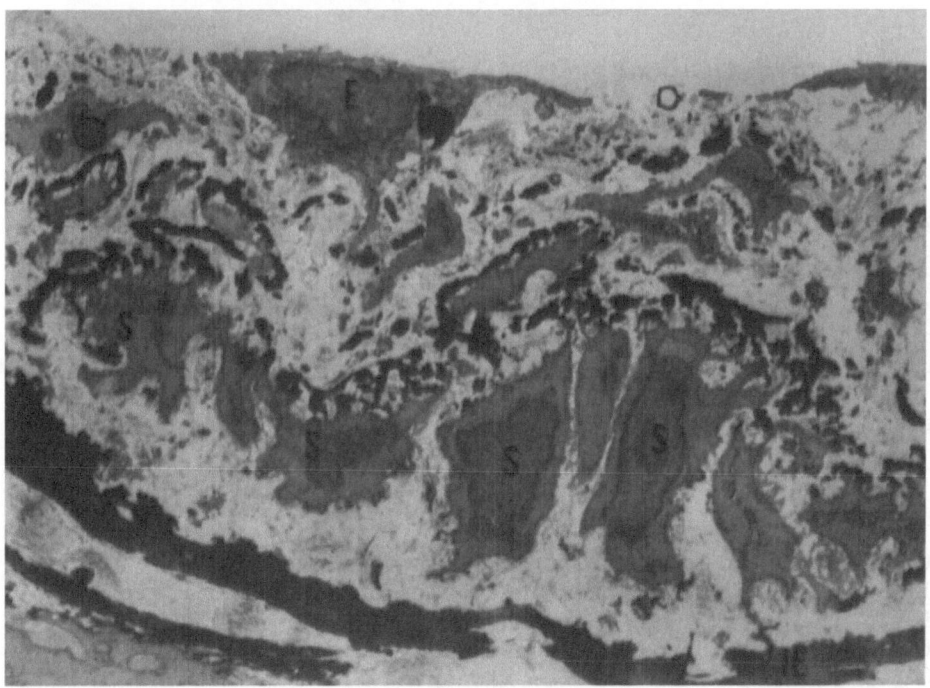

Fig. 1. Intima of the descending thoracic aorta with one layer of smooth muscle cells (S) above a distinct internal elastic lamina (IE). Infrequent lipid inclusions in intimal smooth muscle and endothelial (E) cells. Muscular intimal thickening of this type is seen in much of the normal aorta. This electron micrograph is from an adult monkey on low fat - low cholesterol food with a mean serum cholesterol level of 130 mg/dl. (Rhesus No. 45). (x 8,750).

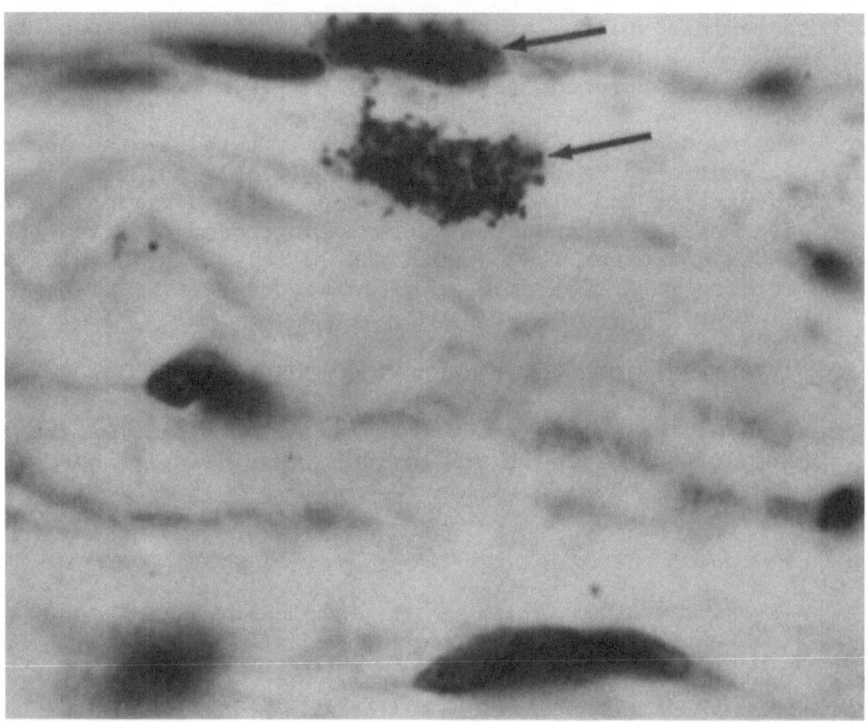

Fig. 2.   Intima of aortic arch midportion with one labeled endothelial cell (arrow) and below one labeled smooth muscle cell
(arrow).   There is no distinct separation between intima and media
in this aortic segment.   Radioautograph from an adult monkey on a
cholesterol and butter supplemented diet for 12 weeks with a mean
serum cholesterol level of 680 mg/dl.   (Rhesus No. 32; 4 injections
of tritiated thymidine i.v. at 6-hour intervals; hematoxylin and
eosin).   (About x 1,250).

with the development of the arteries and with aging. Geer and his
colleagues (1968) have determined that such muscular intimal
thickening is universal in human coronary arteries. Muscular
intimal thickening is also seen in many animal species (French,
1966). We have found it to be widespread in the aorta of normal
rabbits (Stary and McMillan, 1970) and in the coronary arteries
(Stary, 1973) and the aorta (Figure 1) of normocholesterolemic
rhesus monkeys. There is no necessary causal relationship between
muscular intimal thickening and hypercholesterolemia. Nevertheless,
some evidence suggests that hyperlipemia and other factors may
enhance muscular intimal thickening. Atherosclerosis tends to be
more severe at points of pronounced muscular intimal thickening.
This may merely indicate, however, that certain segments of the

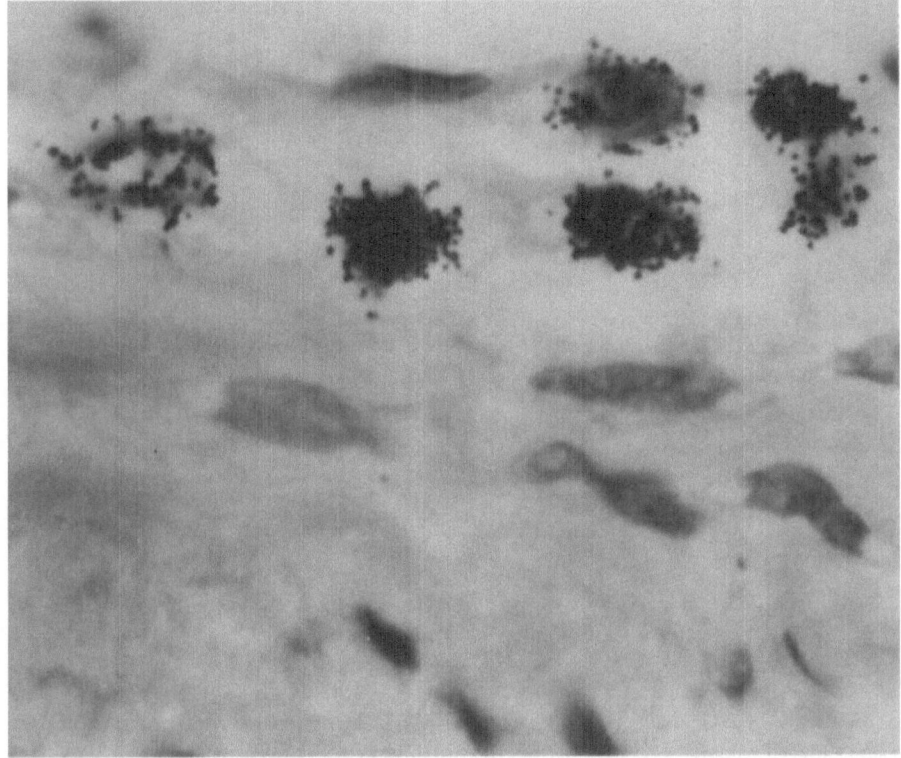

Fig. 3. Incipient intimal lesion in descending aortic arch with
six labeled nuclei resembling smooth muscle cell nuclei. The
intima in this segment normally consists of several strata of
smooth muscle cells. An indistinct internal elastic lamina
separates intima from media in the lower third of the picture.
Radioautograph from a rabbit on a cholesterol and olive oil supplemented diet for 42 days with a serum cholesterol level of 3,340
mg/dl. (Rabbit No. L7; 4 injections of triated thymidine i.v. at
6-hour intervals; hematoxylin and eosin). (About x 1,250).

arterial tree are sites of predilection for insults of varying
etiology.

There is low tritiated thymidine uptake by local intimal
smooth muscle cells under normal conditions, although labeling is
somewhat more frequent in smooth muscle of the prominent cushions
near the ostia of branch vessels (Stary and McMillan, 1970).

Zollinger (1967) demonstrated that a decrease in blood flow
brings about increased proliferation. He induced intimal thickening
by double ligature of the common carotid artery of rabbits and found
numerous mitotic figures in the proliferating intimal cells.

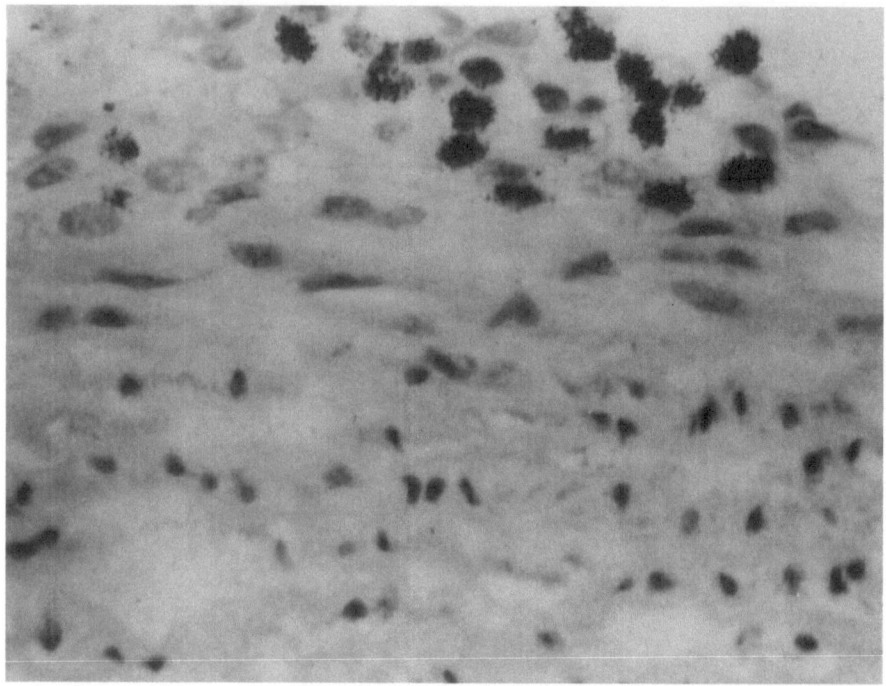

Fig. 4. Margin of a large fatty streak superimposed on muscular
intimal thickening in the ascending part of the aortic arch.
Intimal smooth muscle cells and foam cells are labeled. Radioautograph from the same animal as in Fig. 3. (Hematoxylin and
eosin). (About x 500).

Robertson (1971) caused aortic injury and increased tritiated
thymidine labeling of intimal smooth muscle cells by periodic
immunization of rabbits with heterologous sera.

    Hypercholesterolemia also causes increased proliferation of
intimal smooth muscle cells (Figure 2). Florentin and his colleagues (1969a) used colchicine to study the smooth muscle cells
of the large intimal cushion at the aortic trifurcation of swine.
They found an increased number of mitoses as early as three days
after cholesterol feeding. Tritiated thymidine radioautography
reveals increased labeling of smooth muscle cells in the intimal
cushions of rabbits during hypercholesterolemia (Stary and McMillan,
1970).

    McMillan and Duff (1948), by documenting mitotic figures in
stellate shaped cells, showed that proliferation of intimal smooth
muscle cells takes place in experimental atherosclerotic lesions.

Electron microscopy confirmed the belief that the intimal stellate or spindle cells of light microscopic studies are smooth muscle cells. With tritiated thymidine radioautography there is increased labeling of such cells in the experimental atherosclerotic plaques of rabbits (Figures 3 and 4) (McMillan and Stary, 1968a,b; Cavallero, 1971; Cavallero et al., 1971), swine (Thomas et al., 1968), rhesus monkeys (Figure 5) (Stary, 1969) and baboons (Stary et al., 1968).

Over the years we have made a consistent effort to identify mitotic cells in atherosclerotic lesions with the electron microscope. To date this writer has found one spontaneous mitosis in the fatty streak of an adult rhesus monkey. The cell was poorly characterized as a smooth muscle cell. Serial sections revealed membrane bound lipid inclusions of the homogeneous, moderately electron-dense type, and lipid associated with lamellated bodies. Filaments and pinocytotic vesicles were infrequent (Figure 6).

Investigators differ over the degree to which smooth muscle cells account for the newly formed cells of atherosclerotic lesions. In order to evaluate a possible difference in the proliferative potential of cells with and without smooth muscle characteristics, we have tried to distinguish between these two cell types in radioautographs whenever possible. Since the structural details of labeled cells cannot always be determined by light microscope radioautography, we have processed maraglas-embedded tissue for both light microscope radioautography and for electron microscopy. Comparison of electron micrographs with radioautographs of adjacent thick sections indicates frequent labeling of intimal cells with smooth muscle features and lipid-filled cells without smooth muscle features (foam cells).

There is evidence that different fats may cause one or the other cell type to predominate in atherosclerotic lesions. When corn oil is used as the principal fat in a cholesterol supplemented diet, intimal lesions have many foam cells. The substitution of peanut or coconut oil for corn oil provokes smooth muscle cell proliferation, and there is less intracytoplasmic lipid. (Wissler et al., 1967; Kritchevsky et al., 1971). The type of cell that proliferates also varies with the size of the lesion. While incipient and small fatty streaks are associated with increased labeling mainly of subendothelial smooth muscle cells and a smaller number of foam cells, large fatty streaks show proliferative activity mainly of foam cells (Stary and McMillan, 1970).

Benditt and Benditt (1973) report that all cells within an advanced atherosclerotic plaque are derived from a single smooth muscle cell. Their experiments indicate that smooth muscle cells of normal artery will produce mixed enzyme patterns, while those

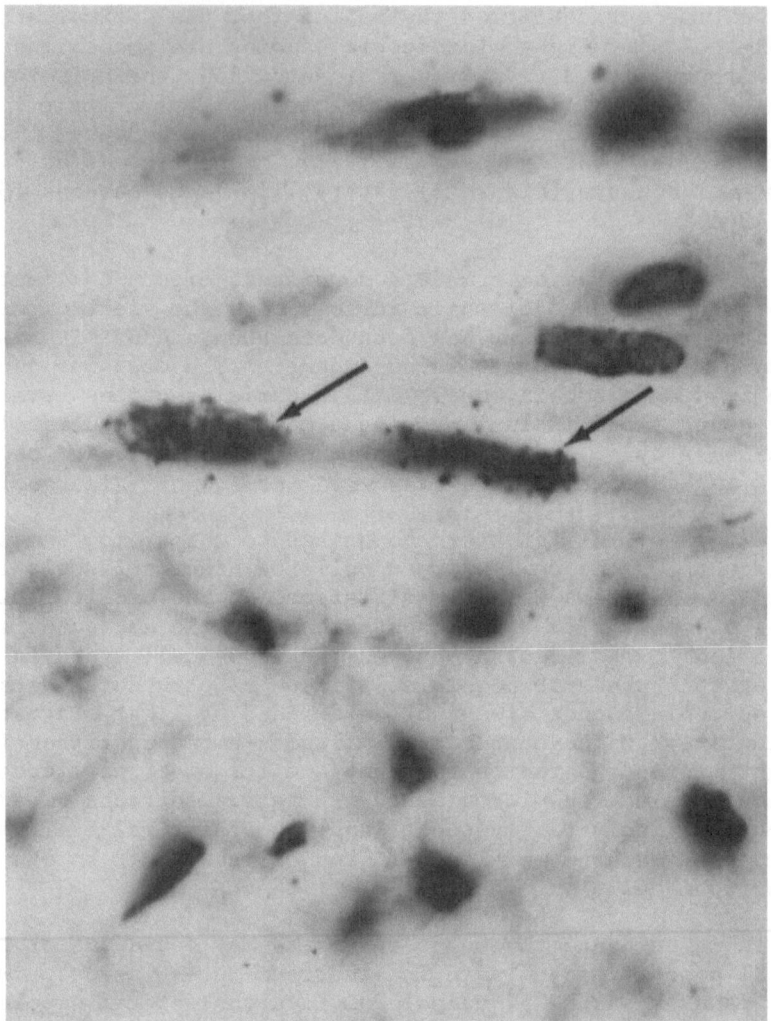

Fig. 5. Intimal fatty streak in the descending thoracic aorta
with two labeled nuclei (arrows) at the base of the lesion,
probably indicating a smooth muscle cell in telophase. Radioautograph from an adult monkey on a cholesterol and butter supplemented diet for 12 weeks with a mean serum cholesterol level of
680 mg/dl. (Rhesus No. 32; 4 injections of tritiated thymidine
i.v. at 6-hour intervals; hematoxylin and eosin). (About x 1,250).

from human fibrous plaques produce a single enzyme, indicating
monoclonal origin. Proliferation of a single cell and its progeny
is best explained by a mutation. The authors note the increased
turnover of smooth muscle cells at sites of predilection for

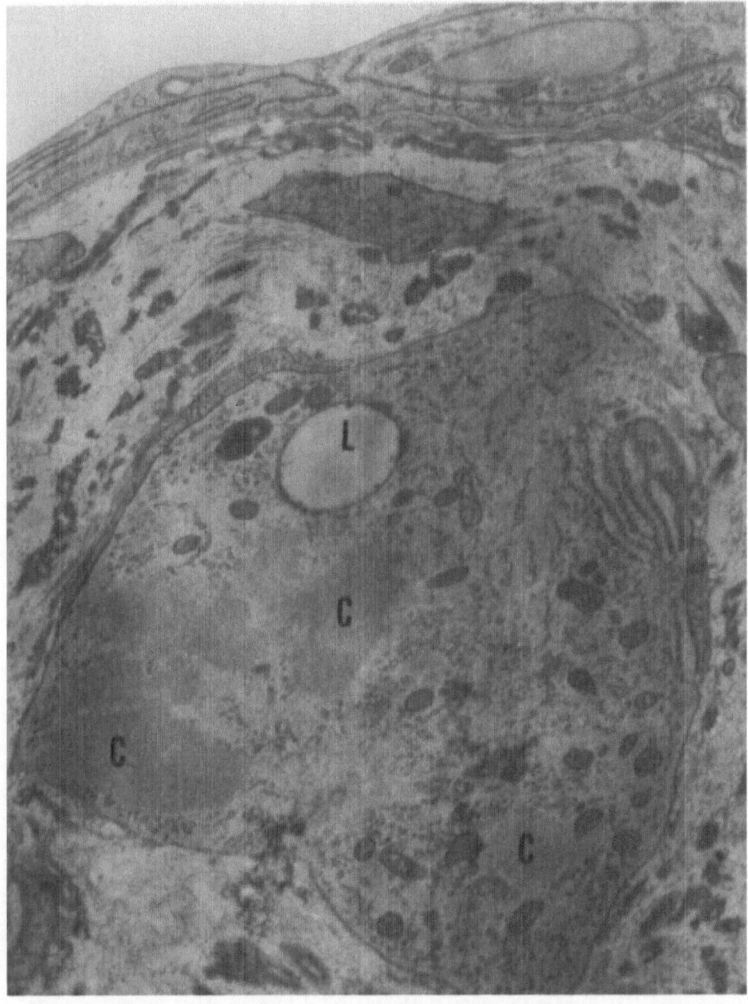

Fig. 6. Fatty streak in the descending thoracic aorta. An intimal cell is in mitosis and shows metaphase chromosomes (C) and membrane-bound lipid inclusions (L). The cell is poorly characterized as a smooth muscle cell having no basement membrane and few pinocytotic vesicles and filaments. Electron micrograph from an adult monkey on a cholesterol and butter supplemented diet for 12 weeks, followed by unsupplemented food for 16 weeks. Mean serum cholesterol level during the cholesterol and butter period was 380 mg/dl. (Rhesus No. 80). (x 16,875).

atherosclerotic plaques. They speculate that this may increase the risk of cell transformation by a virus or a chemical mutagen.

PROLIFERATION OF FOAM CELLS

The foam cells of atherosclerotic lesions are cells with many
lipid inclusions in the cytoplasm, but without special identifying
characteristics. They may evolve from monocytes which have phago-
cytosed lipid or from smooth muscle cells that have lost myofilaments, pinocytotic vesicles,and basement membranes while accumulating lipid. Imai and his associates (1966), using electron
microscopy, and Robertson (1965; 1971) investigating cell cultures
have shown that the usual cytoplasmic features of smooth muscle
can progressively diminish as lipid is accumulated. Monocytes are
thought to convert into foam cells,since they are frequently seen

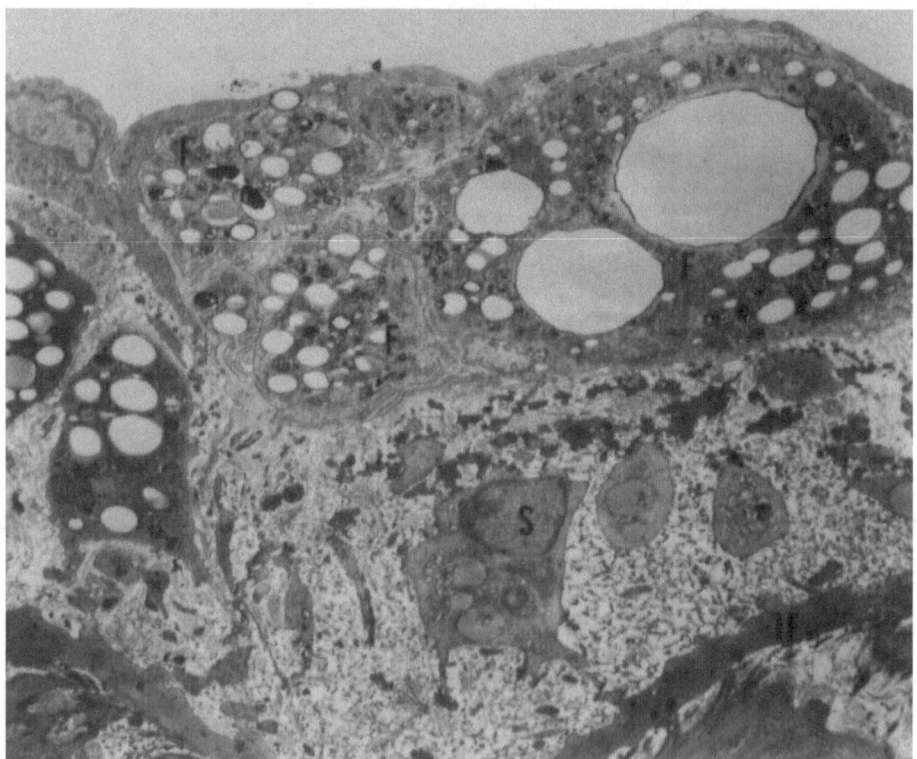

Fig. 7. Fatty streak in the descending thoracic aorta with
several closely joined foam cells (F) in the upper intima, and
smooth muscle cells (S) above the internal elastic lamina (IE).
There are lipid inclusions in all intimal cells except the endothelial cells. The lower half of the intima shows extracellular
lipid. Electron micrograph from an adult monkey on a cholesterol
and butter supplemented diet for 12 weeks with a mean serum cholesterol level of 760 mg/dl. (Rhesus No. 33). (x 6,250).

next to foam cells and because transitional forms between monocytes and foam cells have been observed (Still, 1963; Geer, 1965;
Marshall et al., 1966).

Although usually associated with a high serum cholesterol,
rare isolated foam cells are also found in the aortic and coronary
intima of normocholesterolemic rhesus monkeys (Stary, 1970; Stary
and Strong, in press). These cells, although few and far between,
may be a "normal" component of certain intimal segments. As they
disintegrate, metabolized lipid and necrotic cell debris probably
are completely removed. In hypercholesterolemia increasing numbers
of foam cells accumulate, the physiological equilibrium between
accumulation and removal becomes unbalanced, and intimal fatty
streaks are the result (Figure 7).

Mitoses in the foam cells of atherosclerotic plaques are not
uncommon (Figure 8) and were first documented by McMillan and Duff
(1948). Spraragen and his associates (1962) used tritiated thymidine radioautography to show that foam cells can synthesize DNA.
In 1966 we reported a labeling index of 3.5% for foam cells in
atherosclerotic plaques following pulse labeling of cholesterol-
fed rabbits with tritiated thymidine (McMillan and Stary, 1968a).
Within 24 hours following injection of the tracer the percentage
of labeled foam cells doubles, while grain counts show a reduction
to half the original radioactivity. This indicates that the
labeled foam cells undergo mitosis and that the length of the mitotic cycle is less than 24 hours. Over the course of nine days
there is further loss of grains, indicating that some daughter
cells may divide again (Stary, 1967; Stary and McMillan, 1970).

In certain tissues, cell replication is the function of a
small number of specialized cells. It would be useful to know
whether this is also the case in atherosclerotic lesions. We have
studied this question by injecting rabbits with tritiated thymidine
repeatedly at 6-hour intervals. The technique is likely to have
labeled the great majority of cells proliferating while injections
were being continued. The percentage of labeled cells rose with
each injection (Figures 3 and 4). After 36 hours and six injections, 25 percent of the cells of intimal plaques were labeled.
Although the experiment was not carried far enough to label all
cells, the indication is that there is probably not a large sub-
group of cells that cannot divide. Therefore, mitosis is not a
capacity restricted to only a few cells in intimal lesions (Stary
and McMillan, 1970).

Foam cells also label in rhesus monkeys (Figure 9) and in
baboons. We induced aortic intimal lesions of varying severity
by giving rhesus monkeys a cholesterol and butter supplemented
diet for four, twelve, and forty weeks. Tritiated thymidine

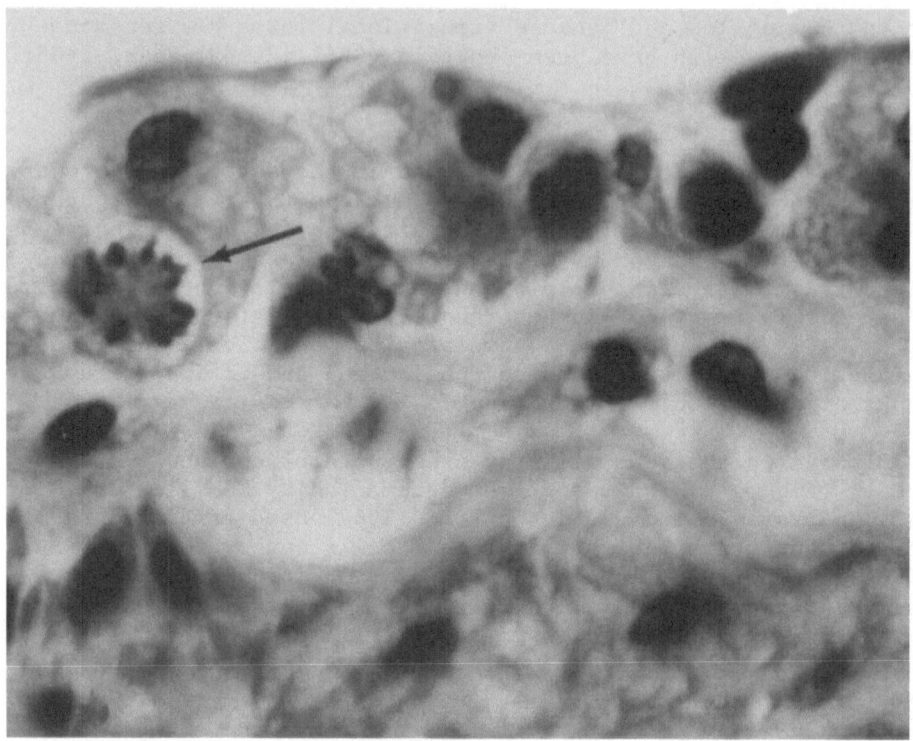

Fig. 8. Fatty streak in the descending thoracic aorta. There are
several foam cells, one of which is in metaphase (arrow). A wavy
internal elastic lamina separates intima from media. Specimen
from an adult monkey on a cholesterol and butter supplemented diet
for 12 weeks, followed by unsupplemented food for three weeks.
Mean serum cholesterol level during cholesterol and butter period
was 500 mg/dl. (Rhesus No. 69; hematoxylin and eosin). (About
x 1,250).

radioautography showed a high rate of labeling in intimal smooth
muscle cells and foam cells at all stages of plaque development
(Stary, 1969). Eggen and Strong (1970) have investigated cholesterol metabolism and intimal lesions in young and old baboons fed
an egg-butter diet for 18 months. We have pulse labeled with
tritiated thymidine one young baboon and one old baboon from this
study. Microscopic sections taken for radioautography from several
regions in the aorta showed no lesions in the young animal. Nevertheless, there was occasional labeling of endothelial cells and
intimal and subintimal smooth muscle cells. The old baboon had
fatty streaks and fibrous plaques largely concentrated in the

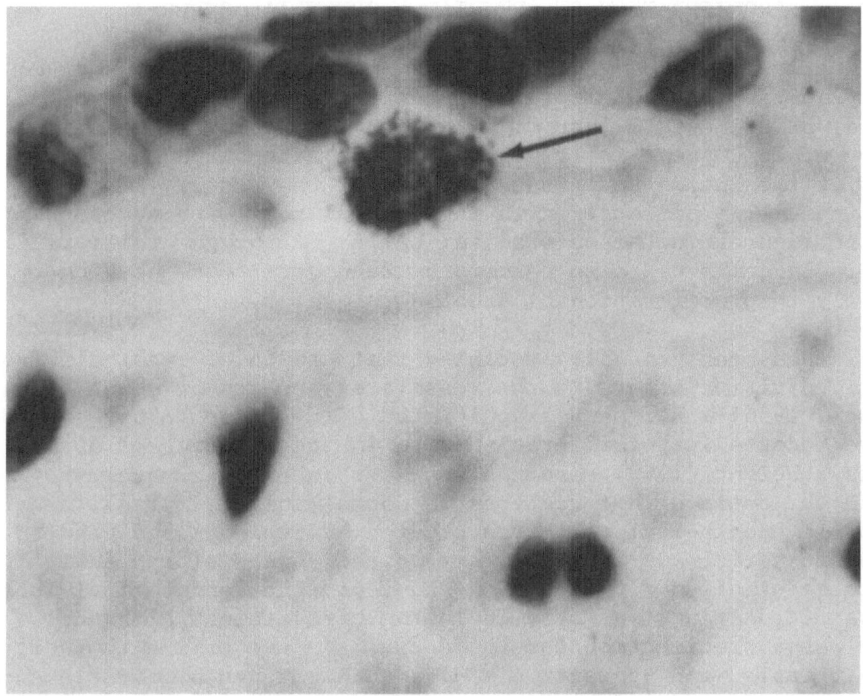

Fig. 9. Fatty streak in the descending thoracic aorta. There
is a layer of foam cells between endothelium and internal elastic
lamina. One cell is labeled (arrow). Radioautograph from an adult
monkey on a cholesterol and butter supplemented diet for 12 weeks
with a mean serum cholesterol level of 540 mg/dl. (Rhesus No. 34;
4 injections of tritiated thymidine i.v. at 6-hour intervals;
hematoxylin and eosin). (About x 1,250).

abdominal aorta. As in the young animal, there was occasional
labeling of endothelial cells and intimal and subintimal smooth
muscle cells. Heavier labeling of smooth muscle cells occurred
in fibrous plaques, and some of the foam cells at the core of the
lesions were labeled also (Stary et al., 1968).

The hypothesis that some of the intimal foam cells may be
derived from blood-borne monocytes receives some support from a
radioautographic study by Spraragen and his associates (1969).
Monocytes labeled in one group of rabbits were transfused into a
recipient group in which intimal lesions had been induced by an
atherogenic diet. A few weakly labeled foam cells were found in
the intimal lesions of the recipient animals after one to two days
and were presumed to be derived from the labeled donor monocytes.

PROLIFERATION OF ARTERIAL ENDOTHELIAL CELLS

Nearly a century ago Zahn (1884) studied intimal and medial injury in rabbits by temporarily constricting one carotid or one femoral artery with a loop of silk thread. He investigated the artery up to 80 days following the trauma with surface prepara- tions of the intima and cross-sections of the vessel. There was striking cell proliferation in the intimal tear with numerous mitotic figures in the endothelial cells. Although proliferation of spindle cells was also described, Zahn attributed healing entirely to proliferation of endothelial cells.

It has been generally accepted that growth of endothelium by mitotic division occurs in the vessels of newborn or young animals (French, 1966). Radioautographic studies by Poole (1964) showed active endothelial proliferation also in the arteries of normal adults. Wright (1968) reported a higher labeling frequency around the ostia of bifurcations in normal animals. Proliferation of aortic endothelial cells was studied by Schwartz and Benditt (1973) in normal adult rats. They coated sheets of the entire aortic endothelium with emulsion and found that endothelial label- ing was in distinct patterns including circumferential bands. There was a predilection for the dorsal surface of the thoracic aorta. Caplan and Schwartz (1973) used Haeutchen preparations to disclose increased endothelial cell labeling in areas of high aortic permeability to Evans Blue dye.

Higher than normal endothelial cell proliferation was demon- strated in atherosclerosis by Duff and his associates (1954) by the discovery of mitotic figures in endothelial cells covering plaques. More recent radioautographic studies show generally greater proliferation of endothelial cells in hypercholesterolemic animals than in controls. The labeling frequency is even higher in endothelial cells overlying intimal lesions. Following pulse labeling, 3.1% of endothelial cells are labeled at the surface of plaques (McMillan and Stary, 1968a). Endothelial cell prolifera- tion may be increased as early as three days after initiation of cholesterol feeding (Florentin et al., 1969b).

Endothelial cells have been implicated in the formation of atherosclerotic lesions, mainly through the observations of Altschul (1950) who regarded them as one source of foam cells. Hassler (1971) has come to the same conclusion by using tritiated thymidine radioautography to study the doubly ligated carotid artery after injecting various atherogenic agents into the lumen. Our data do not support a migration of endothelial cells into plaques as a source of foam cells. If such a translocation occurs, labeled endothelial cells should disappear from the surface and appear in the intima as labeled foam cells. However, the ratio of

labeled endothelial cells over plaques to labeled foam cells
within remains constant when labeled cells are counted at several
intervals over nine days following pulse labeling (Stary and
McMillan, 1970). Electron microscopic studies point to a high
frequency of endothelial cell necrosis, especially in intimal
segments predisposed to lesion formation and particularly during
hypercholesterolemia. It appears likely that endothelial cell
proliferation is a regenerative phenomenon.

CELL PROLIFERATION DURING REGRESSION OF ATHEROSCLEROSIS

Zahn (1884) has observed that intimal thickening induced by
injury consists at first of several cell layers which decrease
progressively until a single layer of surface cells is re-
established.

Kunz and co-workers employed tritiated thymidine radioautography to demonstrate that intimal cell proliferation and labeling
induced by double stenosis of a segment of the abdominal aorta
can be reduced with hydrocortisone (1967) and delayed by alloxan
(1971). Observations pointing to an effect of tissue-specific
inhibiting substances (chalones) on the regulation of cell proliferation were tested in the arterial system by Florentin and his
colleagues (1973). Intraperitoneal injection of aortic tissue
extract reduced the normal proliferative activity of smooth muscle
cells in the carotid artery of young swine. Kramsch and his
associates (1972) gave rabbits an atherogenic diet for eight weeks
with and without colchicine. Serum cholesterol levels in the two
groups were comparable,but foam cell and collagen formation was
inhibited in animals receiving the colchicine.

These studies indicate that arterial cell proliferation can
be influenced by a variety of factors. The question arises as to
whether increased cell proliferation, once induced by hypercholesterolemia, can be returned to normal levels. It is known that
atherosclerotic lesions can lose lipid and diminish in size when
low cholesterol food is substituted for a high cholesterol diet
(Armstrong et al., 1970). Cavallero (1971) has found, however,
some persistent cell proliferation in intimal plaques and the
underlying media as long as five months after the return of hypercholesterolemic rabbits to a normal diet, even after the serum
cholesterol level had returned to normal.

This writer has used tritiated thymidine radioautography to
study early aortic lesions in rhesus monkeys at several intervals
after withdrawal of a butter and cholesterol dietary supplement
(Stary, 1972; Stary, in press). Following induction
of lesions with the atherogenic diet for 12 weeks, the animals

were returned to unsupplemented, low fat - low cholesterol food.
One group of animals was killed three weeks later when serum
cholesterol levels had just returned to normal. Electron microscopy
of intimal lesions showed smooth muscle cells with lipid inclusions
and foam cells. In radioautographs the labeling index of both cell
types was high. A second group of animals was killed 16 weeks
after return to unsupplemented food. The intimal lesions contained necrotic cells, cell debris, and extracellular lipid. While
there was a marked decrease in the number of foam cells, many
intimal smooth muscle cells still had some intracytoplasmic
lipid. The labeling frequency of both cell types was reduced. A
third group of animals was killed 40 weeks after return to unsupplemented food. Cellular intimal lesions had disappeared, although
some extracellular lipid and some intracytoplasmic lipid in smooth
muscle cells persisted in some intimal segments. The labeling
frequency of all types of cells was similar to that seen in normal
control animals.

It is possible that cell proliferation will continue to play
a more persistent role during regression of larger atherosclerotic
lesions and that additional cell types will appear. Fibroblast
activity and an increased number of smooth muscle cells during
lipid removal from advanced lesions have been reported. (Anitschkow,
1928; Prior and Ziegler, 1965).

SUMMARY

Cellular proliferative activity is low in the normal artery;
however, it is normally higher in endothelial cells than in either
intimal or medial smooth muscle cells. Furthermore, there is
increased proliferative activity of endothelial cells and intimal
smooth muscle cells in certain segments of normal arteries,
particularly near the ostia of branch vessels.

Increased arterial cell proliferation occurs in hypercholesterolemia. It predominates in cells related to atherosclerotic
intimal lesions; that is, the intimal smooth muscle cells and foam
cells of lesions, the medial smooth muscle cells near lesions, and
the endothelial cells on the surface of lesions.

Although the present evidence suggests growth of atherosclerotic lesions by in situ division of cells, recruitment of monocytes
from the circulation may be important in some situations.

Increased arterial cell proliferation of hypercholesterolemia
can be reversed when the serum cholesterol is reduced. Return to
normal proliferative activity occurs before extracellular lipid
has disappeared entirely from the intima.

ACKNOWLEDGEMENTS

This work was supported by a grant-in-aid of research by the
Louisiana Heart Association and by United States Public Health
Service Grant HL-08974.

REFERENCES

Altschul, R. (1950). "Selected Studies on Arteriosclerosis."
    1st edition. Charles C Thomas, Springfield, Illinois.

Anitschkow, N. (1928). Über die Rueckbildungsvorgaenge bei der
    experimentellen Atherosklerose. Verh. Deut. Pathol. Ges.
    23, 473. Zentralbl. Allg. Pathol. Pathol. Anat., Suppl.
    43.

Armstrong, M.L., Warner, E.D., and Connor, W.E. (1970).
    Regression of coronary atheromatosis in rhesus monkeys.
    Circ. Res. 27, 59.

Benditt, E.P., and Benditt, J.M. (1973). Evidence for a monoclonal
    origin of human atherosclerotic plaques. Proc. Nat. Acad.
    Sci. U.S.A. 70, 1753.

Caplan, B.A., and Schwartz, C.J. (1973). Increased endothelial
    cell turnover in areas of invivo Evans Blue uptake in the
    pig aorta. Atherosclerosis 17, 401.

Cavallero, C. (1971). The proliferative nature of atherosclerosis.
    In "The Artery and the Process of Arteriosclerosis:
    Pathogenesis." (Stewart Wolf, ed.). Proceedings of the
    Conference on Reactions of Vascular Tissue in Man, Lindau,
    1970. Adv. Exp. Med. Biol. 16A, 225. Plenum Press, New York.

Cavallero, C., DiTondo, U., Mingazzini, P.L., Pesando, P.C., and
    Spagnoli, L.G. (1973). Cell proliferation in the
    atherosclerotic lesions of cholesterol-fed rabbits. Part 2.
    Histological, ultrastructural and radioautographic
    observations on epinephrine-treated rabbits. Atherosclerosis
    17, 49.

Cavallero, C., Turolla, E., and Ricevuti, G. (1971). Cell
    proliferation in the atherosclerotic plaques of cholesterol-
    fed rabbits. Part 1. Colchicine and [^{3}H]thymidine studies.
    Atherosclerosis 13, 9.

Crane, W.A.J., and Ingle, D.J. (1964). Tritiated thymidine uptake in rat hypertension. Arch. Pathol. 78, 209.

Daoud, A.S., Fritz, K.E., and Jarmolych, J. (1970). Increased DNA synthesis in aortic explants from swine fed a high cholesterol diet. Exp. Mol. Pathol. 13, 377.

Duff, G.L., McMillan, G.C., and Lautsch, E.V. (1954). The uptake of colloidal thorium dioxide by the arterial lesions of cholesterol atherosclerosis in the rabbit. Amer. J. Pathol. 30, 941.

Eggen, D.A., and Strong, J.P. (1970). Diet and cholesterol metabolism in young and old baboons. Atherosclerosis 12, 359.

Florentin, R.A., Nam, S.C., Janakidevi, K., Lee, K.T., Reiner, J.M., and Thomas, W.A. (1973). Population dynamics of arterial smooth muscle cells. II. In vivo inhibition of entry into mitosis of swine arterial smooth muscle cells by aortic tissue extracts. Arch. Pathol. 95, 317.

Florentin, R.A., Nam, S.C., Lee, K.T., Lee, K.J., and Thomas, W.A. (1969a). Increased mitotic activity in aortas of swine. Arch. Pathol. 88, 463.

Florentin, R.A., Nam, S.C., Lee, K.T., and Thomas, W.A. (1969b). Increased ^{3}H-thymidine incorporation into endothelial cells of swine fed cholesterol for 3 days. Exp. Mol. Pathol. 10, 250.

French, J.E. (1966). Atherosclerosis in relation to the structure and function of the arterial intima, with special reference to the endothelium. Int. Rev. Exp. Pathol. 5, 253.

Geer, J.C. (1965). Fine structure of canine experimental atherosclerosis. Amer. J. Pathol. 47, 241.

Geer, J.C., McGill, H.C., Jr., Robertson, W.B., and Strong, J.P. (1968). Histologic characteristics of coronary artery fatty streaks. Lab. Invest. 18, 565.

Hassler, O. (1971). Arterial cell renewal under hyperlipidemic conditions. Virchows Arch. Abt. A. 352, 26.

Imai, H., Lee, K.T., Pastori, S., Panlilio, E., Florentin, R., and Thomas, W.A. (1966). Atherosclerosis in rabbits. Architectural and subcellular alterations of smooth muscle cells of aortas in response to hyperlipemia. Exp. Mol. Pathol. 5, 273.

Kao, V.C.Y., Wissler, R.W., and Dzoga, K. (1968). The influence of hyperlipemic serum on the growth of medial smooth muscle cells of rhesus monkey aorta in vitro. Circulation 38 (Suppl. 6), 12.

Kramsch, D.M., Hollander, W., and Franzblau, C. (1972). Suppression of fibrous plaque formation by a connective tissue inhibitor (penicillamine) and by an antimitotic agent (colchicine). Circulation 46 (Suppl. 2), 254.

Kritchevsky, D., Tepper, S.A., Vesselinovitch, D., and Wissler, R.W. (1971). Cholesterol vehicle in experimental atherosclerosis. Part II. Peanut Oil. Atherosclerosis 14, 53.

Kunz, J., Kranz, D., and Keim, O. (1967). Effect of hydrocortisone acetate on cell metabolism in experimental intima proliferation of rat aorta. Virchows Arch. Pathol. Anat. 342, 353.

Kunz, J., Sajkiewicz, K., Kranz, D., Fuhrmann, I., Bausdorf, B., and Keim, U. (1971). Intimal proliferation in the rat aorta in experimental diabetes mellitus. Exp. Pathol. 5, 78.

Marshall, J.R., Adams, J.G., O'Neal, R.M., and DeBakey, M.E. (1966). The ultrastructure of uncomplicated human atheroma in surgically resected aortas. J. Atheroscler. Res. 6, 120.

McMillan, G.C., and Duff, G.L. (1948). Mitotic activity in the aortic lesions of experimental atherosclerosis in rabbits. Arch. Pathol. 46, 179.

McMillan, G.C., and Stary, H.C. (1968a). Preliminary experience with mitotic activity of cellular elements in the atherosclerotic plaques of cholesterol-fed rabbits studied by labeling with tritiated thymidine. Ann. N.Y. Acad. Sci. 149, 699.

McMillan, G.C., and Stary, H.C. (1968b). Radioautographic observations on DNA synthesis in the cells of arteriosclerotic lesions of cholesterol fed rabbits. In "Recent Advances in Atherosclerosis." Proceedings of the International Symposium on Atherosclerosis, Athens, 1966. Progr. Biochem. Pharmacol. 4, 280-281, S. Karger, Basel.

Murata, K. (1967). Tritiated thymidine incorporation into aortic cells in vivo; cell regeneration in spontaneous atherosclerosis in monkeys. Experientia 23, 732.

Myasnikov, A.L., and Block, Y.E. (1965). Influence of some
    factors on lipoidosis and cell proliferation in aorta tissue
    cultures of adult rabbits. J. Atheroscler. Res. 5, 33.

Poole, J.C.F. (1964). Regeneration of aortic tissues in fabric
    grafts of the aorta. In "Cardiovascular Anatomy and Pathology."
    (R.G. Harrison and K.R. Hill, eds.). Symposia of the
    Zoological Society of London, Vol. 11, 131. The London
    Society.

Prior, J.T., and Ziegler, D.D. (1965). Regression of experimental
    atherosclerosis. Arch. Pathol. 80, 50.

Robertson, A.L. (1965). Metabolism and ultrastructure of the
    arterial wall in atherosclerosis. Cleveland Clin. Quart.
    32, 99.

Robertson, A.L. (1971). The proliferative nature of
    atherosclerosis: adaptive and reparative. In "The Artery
    and the Process of Arteriosclerosis: Pathogenesis."
    (Stewart Wolf, ed.). Proceedings of the Conference on
    Reactions of Vascular Tissue in Man, Lindau, 1970. Adv. Exp.
    Med. Biol. 16A, 104-107; 229-238. Plenum Press, New York.

Ross, R. (1971a). The smooth muscle cell. I. In vivo synthesis
    of connective tissue proteins. J. Cell Biol. 50, 159.

Ross, R. (1971b). The smooth muscle cell. II. Growth of smooth
    muscle in culture and formation of elastic fibers. J. Cell
    Biol. 50, 172.

Schmitt, G., Knoche, H., Junge-Huelsing, G., Koch, R., and Hauss,
    W.H. (1970). Über die Reduplikation von Aortenwandzellen
    bei arterieller Hypertonie. Z. Kreislaufforsch. 59, 481.

Schwartz, S.M., and Benditt, E.P. (1973). Cell replication in
    the aortic endothelium; a new method for study of the
    problem. Lab. Invest. 28, 699.

Spaet, T.H., and Lejnieks, I. (1967). Mitotic activity in rabbit
    blood vessels. Proc. Soc. Exp. Biol. Med. 125, 1197.

Spraragen, S.C., Bond, V.P., and Dahl, L.K. (1962). Role of
    hyperplasia in vascular lesions of cholesterol fed rabbits
    studied with thymidine-H^3 autoradiography. Circ. Res. 11,
    329.

Spraragen, S.C., Giordano, A.R., Poon, T.P., and Hamel, H. (1969).
    Participation of circulating mononuclear cells in the genesis
    of atheromata. Circulation 40 (Suppl. 3), 24.

Stary, H.C. (1967). Cell proliferation in the experimental
    atheroma as revealed by radioautography after injection of
    thymidine-H^3. Circulation 36 (Suppl. II), 39.

Stary, H.C. (1970). Electron microscopic observations on the
    progression of aortic atherosclerosis in rhesus monkeys.
    Circulation 42 (Suppl. 3), 9.

Stary, H.C. (1973). Electron microscopic observations on the
    progression of coronary atherosclerosis in rhesus monkeys.
    Amer. J. Pathol. 70, 39a.

Stary, H.C. (1972). Progression and regression of experimental
    atherosclerosis in rhesus monkeys. In "Medical Primatology,
    1972." Proceedings of the 3rd Conference on Experimental
    Medicine and Surgery in Primates, Lyon, 1972. Part III, pp.
    356-367. S. Karger, Basel.

Stary, H.C. (In Press). Cell proliferation and ultrastructural
    changes in regressing atherosclerotic lesions after reduction
    of serum cholesterol. In "Atherosclerosis." Proceedings of
    the 3rd International Symposium, Berlin, 1973. Springer,
    New York.

Stary, H.C. (1969). Radioautographic observations on DNA
    synthesis of aortic cells in rhesus monkeys. Circulation
    40 (Suppl. 3), 25.

Stary, H.C., and McMillan, G.C. (1970). Kinetics of cellular
    proliferation in experimental atherosclerosis. Arch. Pathol.
    89, 173.

Stary, H.C., and Strong, J.P. (In press). Coronary artery fine
    structure in rhesus monkeys: nonatherosclerotic intimal thick-
    ening. In "Atherosclerosis in Primates" (J.P. Strong, ed.).
    Prim. Med., S. Karger, Basel.

Stary, H.C., Strong, J.P., and Eggen, D.A. (1968). (Unpublished
    observations).

Still, W.J.S. (1963). An electron microscope study of cholesterol
    atherosclerosis in the rabbit. Exp. Mol. Pathol. 2, 491.

Thomas, W.A., Florentin, R.A., Nam, S.C., Kim, D.N., Jones, R.M.
    and Lee, K.T. (1968). Preproliferative phase of atheroscler-
    osis in swine fed cholesterol. Arch. Pathol. 86, 621.

Wegener, K. (1973). (Personal Communication).

Wissler, R.W., Vesselinovitch, D., Getz, G.S., and Hughes, R.H.
    (1967). Aortic lesions and blood lipids in rhesus monkeys
    fed three food fats. Fed. Proc. 26, 371.

Wright, H.P. (1968). Endothelial mitosis around aortic branches
    in normal guinea-pigs. Nature (London) 220, 78.

Zahn, F.W. (1884). Untersuchung über die Vernarbung von Querrissen
    der Arterienintima und Media nach vorheriger
    Umschnuerung. Virchows Arch. Pathol. Anat. 96, 1.

Zollinger, H.U. (1967). Adaptive Intimafibrose der Arterien.
    Virchows Arch. Pathol. Anat. 342, 154.

DISCUSSION FOLLOWING THE PRESENTATION BY H.C. STARY

Dr. Haust: Dr. Stary, I have enjoyed your meticulous presentation and would like to ask the following: Did you have a chance
to look at the dividing foam cells with the electron microscope to
see whether they represent smooth muscle cells with features
"beyond return" to normal? In other words, could cells go on
dividing as foam cells after losing all their typical features and
thus, presumably, their characteristic normal function as smooth
muscle cells?

Dr. Stary: Comparison of electron micrographs and radioautographs from lesions consisting largely of foam cells indicate that
cells without smooth muscle features do indeed label and can undergo
mitosis. Absence of myofilaments and presence of intracytoplasmic
lipid is not a deterrent from mitotic division.

Dr. Wissler: I think it is not only good to emphasize the
cell proliferation that takes place in lesions with hypercholesterolemia but also the fact that there is probably increased cell death.
I was particularly pleased when you showed some cells that are
degenerating or necrotic. The abundance of such cells, even in
relatively early lesions, has impressed us. I wonder if you would
care to comment on whether you think some of these degenerated cells
might be furnishing a good deal of the extracellular lipid of the
kind that Dr. Geer has shown. The pattern seems rather similar at
times.

Dr. Stary: Yes, I believe that the extracellular material
visible with the electron microscope in intimal lesions, which we
take to be lipid, is the result of necrosis of lipid-filled cells.
The lipid that often predominates in degenerating and necrotic intimal smooth muscle cells and foam cells is of the very electron-dense
type and appears as crinkled membranes. The abundant extracellular
material seen in lesions with frequent cell necrosis has, although
in the form of small fragments, a very similar appearance.

Dr. Yu: You have said that there are two main cell types in atherosclerotic lesions responsible for growth of the lesion, intimal smooth muscle cells and foam cells. Which of the two types labels more frequently?

Dr. Stary: This may depend on the nature of the lesion. Most of the lesions that we produced were foam cell lesions and labeling of foam cells was more frequent than labeling of clearly recognizable smooth muscle cells. In the earliest lesions, however, increased labeling of intimal smooth muscle cells appeared to predominate. Fibrous plaques, like those found in our old baboons, again showed more frequent labeling of spindle cells.

Dr. Yu: As you mentioned, the foam cells are still dividing but do they still express their specific synthetic activities of the smooth muscle cells, such as the syntheses of mucopolysaccharides, collagen, and elastic fibers or elastic units which have been reported by Haust and More[1] and also by Yu and Lai[2].

Dr. Stary: By definition foam cells have no myofibrils. At this point in time they appear to have no function except phagocytosis. However, cells recognizable as smooth muscle cells because they have myofibrils appear to retain some capacity to synthesize collagen and elastin in spite of variable amounts of intracytoplasmic lipid. Organelles, pinocytotic vesicles, and extracellular collagen and elastica frequently are prominent. Definite proof that fat-filled smooth muscle cells can synthesize collagen and elastin could probably be provided with tritiated proline radioautography.

Dr. Kramsch: I want to say that I agree with Dr. Stary. I have a similar impression that cells filled maximally with lipid may not be able to synthesize collagen or elastin. When we give monkeys or rabbits only cholesterol and produce a foam cell lesion, there is very little connective tissue proliferation. If you add butter fat or peanut oil, then you get a great proliferation of collagen and elastin, but this proliferation does not occur in the area of foam cell proliferation. In other words, in these areas you have a big, huge foam cell cap in which there is hardly any collagen or elastin detectable. Collagen and elastin proliferate in areas of cells which have almost a smooth muscle appearance by light microscopy.

---

[1]Haust, M.D., and More, R.H. (1967). In "The Connective Tissue" (B.M. Wagner and D.E. Smith, eds.). pp. 352-376. Williams and Wilkins, Baltimore, Maryland.
[2]Yu, S.Y., and Lai, S.E. (1970). J. Electron Microscopy 19, 362.

SECTION II

LIPID-CONNECTIVE TISSUE INTERACTIONS

THE MACROMOLECULES OF THE INTERCELLULAR MATRIX OF THE ARTERIAL WALL: COLLAGEN, ELASTIN, PROTEOGLYCANS, AND GLYCOPROTEINS

L. Robert, A. Kadar, and B. Robert

Laboratoire de Biochimie du Tissu Conjonctif Faculté de
    Medeciné, Université Paris-Val de Marne, Créteil
Institute of Pathological Anatomy, II. Medical Faculty
    of the Semmelweis University of Budapest, Hungary
Laboratoire de Biochimie du Tissu Conjonctif Faculté de
    Médecine, Université Paris-Val de Marne, Créteil

The arterial wall can be considered as differentiated connective tissue. Three main cell types have been described and characterized as the normal constituents of major arteries; they are the smooth muscle cells of the media, the endothelial cells limiting the intima toward the blood stream, and the "fibroblasts" in the adventitia of large arteries such as the aorta.

Most probably all three cell types are actively involved in the biosynthesis and secretion of the macromolecules of the intercellular matrix (MMIM). Endothelial cells of rat aorta intima have been shown to possess all the morphological characteristics (rough endoplasmic reticulum, Golgi, microtubules, etc.) usually attributed to actively synthesizing cells (Gerrity and Cliff, 1972). They very probably do synthetize the precursor macromolecules of the internal limiting elastic membrane and possibly other macromolecules (see later).

The intercellular matrix of the media of aorta probably is synthesized by the smooth muscle cells whose morphology in normal and pathological arteries was studied and described in detail by several authors (Knieriem et al., 1968; Wissler, 1967).

Smooth muscle cells are usually the only ones present in the medial layers of large arteries such as aorta. Thus they may be considered as expressing most of the biosynthetic potentialities of differentiated connective tissue cells, as shown by the variety

85

of the macromolecules these cells elaborate during the periods of
embryonic development and active growth. These macromolecules
comprise actin; myosin and other specific proteins of the contractile cells; elastin; collagen; glycoproteins; and several proteoglycans such as hyaluronate, chondroitin 4-sulfate, chondroitin 6-
sulfate, dermatan sulfate, and heparan sulfate. It is interesting
to note in this respect that recent investigations carried out in
several laboratories indicated that these "mediacytes" of aorta may
not be exclusively (if at all) of mesenchymal origin. They could
be derived, at least in the aortic arch of chick embryos, from the
neural crest (Le Lievre and Le Douarin, 1973). The "mesectodermal"
origin may not apply, however, to the whole length of the aorta, and
still has to be demonstrated in higher vertebrates.

The third major cell type demonstrated in vessel wall is the
"fibroblast," described as such mainly in the adventitial tissues
of aorta (Berry et al., 1972). Many cells of this type have been
shown in tissue slices, tissue culture, or cell culture to be able
to synthesize several of the MMIM (Kulonen and Pikkarainen, 1973).

Before closing this brief reminder of the nature of the
cellular elements responsible for the synthesis of the macromolecules to be discussed below, we should remember that these cellular
elements with their protein and glycoprotein content contribute
to an unknown extent to the chemical determinations which are
carried out on aorta extracts in order to characterize the components of the intercellular matrix. This contribution may be
particularly important for the determination of lipidic components
and for some glycoproteins, and should warrant special attention
for the interpretation of the results.

THE MACROMOLECULES OF THE INTERCELLULAR MATRIX

Most chemical studies were carried out using the aortas of
different animal species; only limited information is available
on other arteries or on veins. The intercellular matrix of
arterial wall contains four major types of macromolecules (collagen, proteoglycans, elastin, and glycoproteins). As was mentioned earlier, the smooth muscle cells of the aortic media are
considered as capable of synthesizing and secreting into the intercellular space all four of these macromolecules characteristic
of connective tissues. Very unequal attention has been paid to
these four macromolecules during the last decade. Several
recent reviews discuss the chemical and biological characteristics
of these macromolecules (Balazs, 1970; Robert, 1970; Slavkin, 1972)
and a fair amount of experimental work has accumulated recently

on the chemistry and biosynthesis of elastin (Partridge, 1970; 1972). Several laboratories have studied the composition and biosynthesis of proteoglycans and glycoproteins in normal and pathological arterial wall (Picard et al., 1968; Engel, 1971; Kumar et al., 1967; Moczar and Robert, 1970; Srinivasan et al., 1971); but much less effort has been devoted, until recently, to the isolation and characterization of aortic collagen (Frey, 1969; Frey et al., 1969).

We shall describe here mainly those recent results on elastin and glycoprotein biochemistry of the arterial wall which are related to the process of atherogenesis. Proteoglycans and collagen will be mentioned only briefly; several other reports presented at this colloquium are devoted to aortic mucopolysaccharides. No attempt is made to give a complete coverage of even recent literature. Only a few studies could be related here which appeared particularly relevant to the structure and metabolism of aortic macromolecules in their normal state and in arteriosclerosis. The choice of elastin and glycoproteins for a more detailed description is justified by the recent findings suggesting a direct role of structural glycoproteins in elastogenesis (Robert et al., 1971b) and an important role of elastin and structural glycoproteins in the atherogenetic process (Robert et al., 1970c).

Methodology

The methods used for these investigations can be divided roughly into two classes: (a) those which aim at the extraction of one macromolecular component at a high state of purity for the detailed study of its chemical, physical, or immunological properties and (b) those methods which, by fractional extraction and partial hydrolysis (enzymatic, alkaline, or acid), "solubilize" completely the macromolecules of the arterial wall. Only this last category enables detailed comparative studies of quantitative and qualitative variations between normal and pathological arteries. Several methods of "chemical or enzymatic dissection" of the arterial wall have been described (Robert et al., 1965, 1968; Moschetto and Havez, 1969) and used for the preparation and purification of macromolecular fractions and for the study of incorporation of labeled precursors in the arterial wall (L. Robert et al., in press).

Collagen

Collagen Content of the Arterial Wall. Total collagen and elastin content of normal and pathological arteries were determined by several investigators (Harkness, 1961; Fischer and

Llaurado, 1966, 1967; Wirtschafter and Bentley, 1965; Looker and Berry, 1972). Table I (Fischer and Llaurado, 1967) gives the collagen and elastin content, as well as their ratio determined essentially by the procedure described by Neuman and Logan (1950) in several different arteries of the normal dogs and dogs with renal hypertension. It can be seen that the collagen content varies widely (19.6% in ascending aorta and 47.9% in coronary artery). The collagen/elastin ratio appears to be related to the distensibility of the arterial wall. Since this ratio does not increase in hypertensive dogs, the stiffness of these arteries could not be attributed to an increased relative collagen content and ascribed to "accelerated aging."

TABLE I. COLLAGEN AND ELASTIN CONTENT OF NORMAL AND HYPERTENSIVE
          DOGS AND COLLAGEN-ELASTIN RATIO (C/E) (from Fischer and
          Llaurado, 1967). RESULTS GIVEN AS % OF DRY TISSUE,
          AVERAGE ± SEM FOR 9 HYPERTENSIVE DOGS: NORMAL VALUES
          (from Fischer and Llaurado, 1966).

Artery	Collagen		Elastin		C/E Ratio	
	Hyper-tensive	Normal	Hyper-tensive	Normal	Hyper-tensive	Normal
Coronary*	40.0 ± 2.7	47.9 ± 2.6	15.4 ± 1.8	15.6 ± 0.7	2.76 ± 0.46	3.12 ± 0.21
Aorta, ascending	20.0 ± 1.1	19.6 ± 1.2	36.8 ± 1.8	41.1 ± 2.1	0.56 ± 0.04	0.49 ± 0.04
Carotid	46.7 ± 1.6	50.7 ± 2.1	21.1 ± 1.4	20.1 ± 1.0	2.29 ± 0.16	2.55 ± 0.13
Aorta, abdominal	41.2 ± 1.5	45.5 ± 1.7	32.9 ± 1.6	30.1 ± 1.7	1.29 ± 0.09	1.58 ± 0.15
Cranial mesenteric, proximal	33.1 ± 0.6	38.1 ± 1.7	23.4 ± 2.3	26.5 ± 1.7	1.55 ± 0.18	1.51 ± 0.15
Cranial mesenteric, *distal	33.1 ± 1.3	37.4 ± 1.4	19.2 ± 1.3	22.4 ± 1.5	1.75 ± 0.13	1.72 ± 0.11
Cranial mesenteric, *branches	31.9 ± 2.0	36.1 ± 1.5	25.3 ± 1.6	21.8 ± 0.9	1.26 ± 0.04	1.69 ± 0.10
Renal	35.5 ± 1.8	42.6 ± 1.6	23.1 ± 1.9	18.7 ± 1.8	1.61 ± 0.15	2.46 ± 0.27
Femoral	40.1 ± 0.8	44.5 ± 1.4	28.2 ± 2.0	24.5 ± 1.6	1.48 ± 0.12	1.89 ± 0.14
Popliteal* †	41.8 ± 2.7		28.7 ± 0.9		1.47 ± 0.12	
Aorta, descending †	18.7 ± 0.9		38.7 ± 1.8		0.51 ± 0.04	
Aorta, thoracic †	21.4 ± 0.7		35.9 ± 2.3		0.62 ± 0.05	
Pulmonary artery †	24.3 ± 1.5		29.5 ± 1.9		0.85 ± 0.08	

*Specimens from only four hypertensive dogs were available for this site.
†Values for normal dogs not available.

     The increase of collagen content in rat aorta from birth to about 55 weeks of age was reported recently. Figure 1 shows the age change of collagen content in rat aorta as given by Looker and Berry (1972). The total collagen content of the entire aorta increases during the whole life span, but the relative collagen content (expressed on a fat-free dry weight basis) remains constant after about 15 weeks of age. After this period, active collagen synthesis is related to the further growth of the animal.

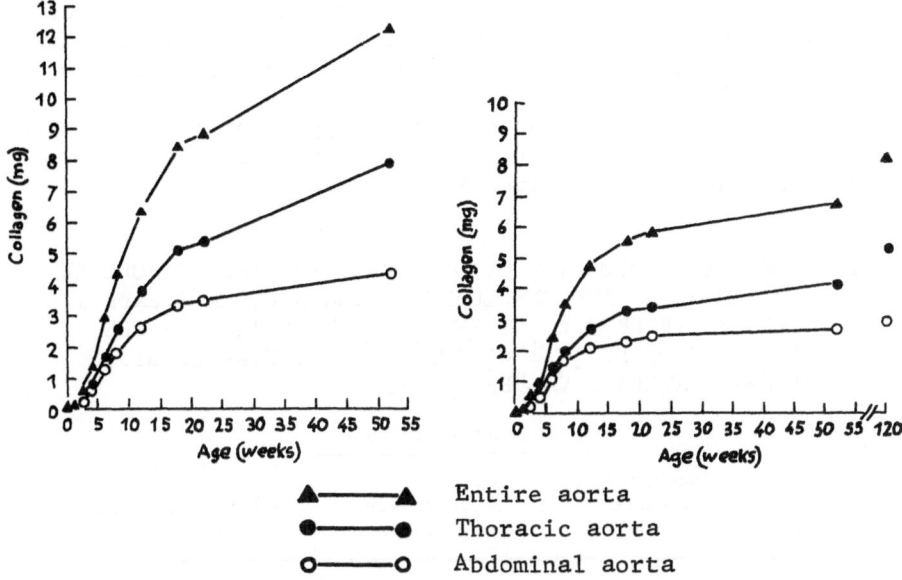

Entire aorta
Thoracic aorta
Abdominal aorta

Fig. 1. Increase in collagen content of the entire thoracic and
abdominal aorta of the male and female rat with age. (Reproduced
with permission from Looker and Berry, 1972).

Only a small fraction of total collagen is extractable with
salt solutions. This salt soluble fraction increases from about
1 mg/g wet weight to 3 to 4 mg/g wet weight in weanling rats
placed on a lathyric diet (Wirtschafter and Bentley, 1965). The
increase in extractable collagen was less dramatic (about 200%) in
similarly treated adult rats.

Injury and repair were shown to increase arterial collagen
synthesis by Lindy et al. (1972), who observed the development of
gross arteriosclerotic lesions parallel to the repair process
following injury (balloon-catheter inflation) of rabbit aorta.
This repair process was characterized by an increase in DNA,
hydroxyproline, and in lactate dehydrogenase (isoenzymes containing
M subunits). This so-called nonspecific response to injury is
similar to that observed by Hauss and co-workers in arterial wall
and other connective tissues following a variety of stress and
stimuli, and demonstrated by the increase of $^{35}SO_4$ incorporation
in proteoglycans (Hauss and Junge-Hulsing, 1963; Hauss, 1973).

Biosynthesis of Aorta Collagen. Frey et al. (1969) devoted some
recent experiments to the metabolism of rabbit aorta collagen as
compared to that of skin and liver. In vitro incorporation of

[^{14}C]proline into collagen proline and hydroxyproline was observed during a two hour incubation period of rabbit aorta slices. When collagen was separated in 0.2 M NaCl-soluble and insoluble fractions, both had incorporated [^{14}C]proline in hydroxyproline. The total radioactivity recovered as hydroxyproline (dpm/g tissue), as well as the specific activity of hydroxyproline in both soluble and insoluble fractions, is given in Table II.

TABLE II.   SPECIFIC RADIOACTIVITY OF HYDROXYPROLINE IN SOLUBLE (0.2 M NaCl) AND INSOLUBLE COLLAGEN OF MALE RABBIT TISSUES AFTER 2 HOURS IN VITRO INCUBATION IN THE PRESENCE OF DL [5-^{14}C]PROLINE (from Frey et al., 1969).   AVERAGE VALUES ± SEM.

Tissue	Numbers of Experiments	Soluble Collagen	
		Total Radioactivity dpm/g Tissue	Specific Activity dpm/μM
Aorta	6	5770 ± 2151	6136 ± 1641
Liver	11	1541 ± 374	23720 ± 5520
Dermis	10	30624 ± 9425	24161 ± 8004
		Insoluble Collagen	
Aorta	9	1567 ± 427	49 ± 12
Liver	9	166 ± 45	82 ± 18
Dermis	9	3986 ± 1110	24 ± 5

The specific activity of 0.2 M NaCl-soluble hydroxyproline was significantly lower in aorta than in skin or liver. The total radioactivity recovered in aorta hydroxyproline (soluble or insoluble) per g tissue was between the values found for skin and liver. Frey compared the ratio of the specific activities of proline and hydroxyproline in the NaCl-soluble and insoluble fractions. A lower ratio of the specific activities of hydroxyproline to proline in the insoluble fractions was found, as compared to the soluble fraction. The specific activity ratio of hydroxyproline to proline (dpm/μg $\frac{OHpro}{pro}$) was found to be 0.71 in the 0.2 M NaCl-soluble collagen fraction of rabbit aorta and 0.53 in the NaCl-insoluble fraction; these ratios were 0.79 and 0.39 for skin collagen. Frey et al. (1969) concluded that there was a selective catabolic elimination of a freshly synthesized fraction

of collagen containing a higher ratio of OHpro/pro than the
limiting value required for "soluble" collagen to be incorporated
in the polymeric stroma. Freshly synthesized collagen with a
lower OHpro/pro ratio than this limit would be preferentially
incorporated into the insoluble stroma. Frey's findings confirm
similar suggestions made by Nimni et al. (1967).

During our studies on the in vitro incorporation of radioactive proline and lysine in rabbit aorta slices, a low but
significant and reproducible incorporation was observed in a
fraction of aorta which remained insoluble after repeated extractions with 1M $CaCl_2$ and was "solubilized" according to Fitch et al.
(1955) by heating it to 90° in 0.15 M trichloracetic acid (TCA)
for 30 minutes (Robert et al., 1968). This TCA-extract, which
contains about 10% hydroxyproline, had a radioactivity of 400 to
500 cpm/mg protein (Table III). A significantly higher incorporation was obtained in the TCA-extract of the precipitate obtained
during the dialysis of the 1M $CaCl_2$-extract of the aorta crude
soluble collagen fraction (CSC), about 7,800 dpm/mg protein
(L. Robert et al., in press). These experiments, although not
specifically designed to study collagen biosynthesis, do suggest,
in agreement with Frey's data, that rabbit aorta slices incubated
in vitro are capable of synthesizing and excreting collagen.

TABLE III. INCORPORATION OF [^{14}C] LYSINE IN THE MACROMOLECULAR
EXTRACTS OF THE INSOLUBLE (1M $CaCl_2$) STROMA OF RABBIT
AORTA DURING FOUR HOURS IN VITRO INCUBATION PERIOD
(from Junqua et al., in preparation; L. Robert et al.,
in press). (For the preparation of extracts see Robert
et al., 1968).

	Specific Activity, dpm/mg Protein		
Rabbit Treated With:	TCA-Extract*	Urea-Mercaptoethanol Extract†	Final Residue‡
Freund adjuvant (complete)	393	6810	631
Immunized with 8M-urea-0.1M-mercaptoethanol extract (structural glycoprotein fraction) of human aorta	538	4870	1773
1% cholesterol-diet fed for 1 month	393	4860	591

*Contains mainly polymeric, insoluble collagen.
†Contains the structural glycoproteins.
‡Contains purified elastin.

The factors regulating the rate of collagen synthesis and degradation in aorta are not yet known. Since fibrous plaques were shown to contain increased amounts of collagen (Robert, 1970), it is to be expected that some of the conditions leading to the development of the arteriosclerotic plaque stimulate collagen synthesis, as well as its incorporation in the insoluble fibrous stroma of the arterial wall. One factor which might be related to such findings is the elevated proline hydroxylase activity observed in rabbits after induction of arteriosclerosis (Crossley et al., 1972).

Another observation which deserves mention in this respect is the recent report by Viidik et al. (1972) concerning the distant effects of local collagen remodeling. If such effects occur in arterial regenerative processes, they might affect the collagen metabolism of parts of the arterial wall distal to the initial fibrotic plaque.

Proteoglycans (Glycosaminoglycans or Acid Mucopolysaccharide-Protein Complexes)

In addition to that previously reviewed by Robert (1970), some new knowledge has accumulated concerning the structure and biosynthesis of aortic glycosaminoglycans (GAGS) (Gardais et al., 1973; Engel, 1971; Kresse et al., 1971). The improvement of the micro-fractionation techniques and the use of a sensitive modification of the cellulose acetate electrophoresis method (Gardais et al., 1969) have made available a relatively reliable determination of the constituent GAGS of the aorta of several animal species.

Distribution of Different GAGS in the Arterial Wall. The distribution of GAGS (in % of total) in the intima-media and adventitia of five animal species is given in Tables IV-A and B. Similar results were reported by Engel (1971), using different techniques. Great variations were found both in total GAGS per mg dry aorta or mg DNA or in the relative distribution of different GAGS. Horse abdominal aorta is reported to have 4 mg uronic acid/mg DNA, and rat aorta has only 0.5 mg/mg DNA. A correlation between proneness to arteriosclerosis and total aorta GAGS was proposed by the data of Mullinger and Manley (1969). The highest values of total uronic acid/g dry aorta were reported for the chicken, pigeon, pig, and rabbit - all four species are known to develop "spontaneous" arteriosclerosis.

TABLE IV-A. DISTRIBUTION OF GLYCOSAMINOGLYCANS IN AORTIC INTIMA-MEDIA OF SEVERAL ANIMAL SPECIES (from Gardais et al., 1973).

	Rat	Rabbit	Hen	Pig		Human	
				Media	Intima	Media	Intima
Hyaluronate	6.8	16.9	16.1	4.6	6.4	6.5	15
Heparan Sulfate	53.0	33.1	16.2	21.5	21.0	26.0	24
Dermatan Sulfate	21.7		48.0			9.5	28
Chondroitin-Sulfate		50.0		73.8	72.4		
Chondroitin-6-Sulfate (A)	18.4		20.7			59.0	33
n	30	15	4	12			

Values are expressed as a percentage of total GAG. The number of samples is indicated at the bottom of each column (n). The analyses on different layers from human aorta are given as an example (man 50 years old, healthy part of aortic cross). Relative proportions of dermatan sulfate and chondroitin sulfate C (A) from rabbit media-intima are, respectively, 20 and 60 percent. Determination of these relative proportions is calculated on the results obtained from less than fifteen samples. Standard deviations, normality test ($Z < 1.96$), are calculated for each GAG ($0.2 < Z < 1.0$).

TABLE IV-B. DISTRIBUTION OF GLYCOSAMINOGLYCANS IN THE ADVENTITIA OF THE AORTA OF SEVERAL SPECIES (from Gardais et al., 1973).

	Rat	Rabbit	Hen	Human
Hyaluronate	17.8	14.7	16.5	6
Heparan Sulfate	26.8	20.7	17.2	17.5
Dermatan Sulfate	41.8	31.7	47.1	15.5
Chondroitin-Sulfate				
Chondroitin-6-Sulfate (A)	13.8	32.2	19.1	61.0
n	30	15	4	-

Mean values are expressed as a percentage of total GAG.

Standard deviations and normality test ($Z = 1.96$) calculated for each GAG ($0.2 < Z < 1$).

The number of samples is indicated at the bottom of each column (n).

Heparan sulfate was found to account for more than 50% of total GAGS in rat aorta and for less than 20% in hen aorta. Dermatan sulfate constitutes about half of the hen aorta GAGS and about 22% of the rat aorta GAGS. Significant differences appear to exist between the hyaluronate contents of the intima and media of human and pig aortas (Table IV-A). The relatively high hyaluronate content of the intima may have some significance with respect to the interactions between aorta macromolecules and blood plasma lipoproteins (Bihari-Varga and Gerö, 1966; Srinivasan et al., 1972; Gerö, 1964; Bihari-Varga and Vegh, 1967; Gerö et al., 1967; Bihari-Varga et al., 1964; Anderson, 1963). This interaction intensively studied at Gerö's Institute, may represent one of the key factors responsible for lipid accumulation in the intima. The studies of Iverius (1968) in T. Laurent's laboratory may furnish the physicochemical basis for this interaction in terms of the excluded volume principle.

Age Changes of Proteoglycans. A complicating factor in the evaluation of these results is the fact that the absolute and relative amount of glycosaminoglycan (GAG) changes with age. A steady decrease of hyaluronate and of $^{35}SO_4$ incorporation was reported in rat and human aorta by Junge-Hülsing and Wagner (1968).

A detailed analysis of normal and atherosclerotic aorta GAGS was carried out by Kumar et al. (1967), Schorah et al. (1968), and others. In accordance with earlier studies by Kaplan and Meyer (1960), a relative decrease of hyaluronate and an increase of heparan sulfate and chondroitin 4-sulfate were found in the first three decades of life in lesion-free aortas, followed by their decrease.

The separate determination of proteoglycans in the intima and media of normal human aortas (Kumar et al., 1967) revealed comparable age changes for some (heparan sulfate) and significantly different profiles for others (chondroitin sulfates). Histochemical studies also suggest differences in the fine distribution of GAGS in the successive layers of the intima and media (Velican, 1966, 1967). These findings complicate the interpretation of the modifications observed in arteriosclerotic lesions. An initial increase followed by a decrease was found by Kumar et al. (1967) as the lesion extended from 10 to 55% of the arterial surface. Ichida and Kalent (1968) found significantly higher sulfated GAG concentrations in fatty streaks of rabbits than in the surrounding normal tissue. Glycoproteins, however, also increased in the aortas of rabbits fed high-cholesterol diets. In rats kept on the same diet, only aorta glycoproteins appeared to increase, GAGS decreased, and there was no significant lipid accumulation. These results were interpreted, on the basis of

$^{35}SO_4$ incorporation data, as the result of an increase of GAG
catabolism in the rat and a stronger increase of GAG synthesis
than removal in the rabbit.

On the contrary, Anastassiades et al. (1972) found in human
sclerotic intima an increase of glycoproteins and collagen, but
no alteration of the GAG content. In Japanese thoracic aortas
Nakamura et al. (1968) found an increase with age in total GAG in
the intima and a decrease in both the intima and media in arteriosclerosis.

Structure of Aorta Proteoglycans. Some recent reports concern
the purification of proteoglycans from aorta. Kresse et al.
(1971) obtained from bovine aorta a purified proteoglycan preparation containing about 80% chondroitin sulfate, and dermatan
sulfate in a ratio of 75:25 with an apparent molecular weight of
about 2×10^6. Light scattering measurements suggested a random
coil configuration. For its structure the authors suggest a
protein core carrying about 80 polysaccharide chains linked by o-
seryl and o-threonyl glycosidic linkages. $^{35}SO_4$ was incorporated
in this compound during a 12 hour in vitro incubation. The specific
radioactivity of the dermatan sulfate chains was found to be about
three times higher than that of the chondroitin sulfate chains,
suggesting a metabolic heterogeneity for this compound.

More recently the possible role of homocysteine and cystathionine synthetase in GAG sulfation and proteoglycan morphology were
studied by McCully (1971, 1972). Cystathionine synthetase-
deficient cells showed an abnormal distribution in culture suggest
ing loss of contact inhibition and imitating neoplastic cells.
This behavior was correlated with the production of "granular"
proteoglycans as distinguished from "fibrillar" proteoglycans
produced by the normal cells. This change of proteoglycan morphology was attributed to increased sulfation. The beneficial effect
of L-cysteine on βamino-propionitril-induced disturbances in the
rat (Lalich and Paik, 1968) might be related to such effects,
although Bentley et al. (1970) found no change of aorta GAG
metabolism in rats fed lathyrogen diet.

Glycoproteins

Aorta macromolecules are relatively rich in carbohydrates
as shown by the hexose and hexosamine content of the extracts
obtained from the polymeric, insoluble (in 1M $CaCl_2$) stroma of
pig aorta (Table V). Glycoproteins have been extracted by several
authors from aortic tissue, and some of these glycoproteins were
purified and characterized (Berenson et al., 1966; Barnes and
Partridge, 1968; Moczar, 1968; Moczar and Robert, 1970).

TABLE V.   CARBOHYDRATE CONTENT OF AORTA MACROMOLECULAR EXTRACT.
           EXTREMES OF SEVERAL DETERMINATIONS (5 to 10) ARE GIVEN.
           (For the preparation of the extracts see Robert et al.
           1968).

Extract	Major Macromolecular Component	Hexose %	Hexosamine%
2.7 Trichloracetic Acid Extract (90°, 30 min)	Polymeric collagen	1.9 - 2.7	1.3 - 3.0
8M-Urea-0.1M-mercapto-ethanol Extract	Structural glycopro-teins	2.1	2.9
Final Residue	Elastin	0.5 - 1.7	0.4

Change with Age and in Atherosclerosis.   Variations of the
relative proportion of glycoproteins to other macromolecules of
the intercellular matrix have been studied by several authors,
with respect to age, pathology, and anatomical location.   Gan and
co-workers (1967) studied the quantitative relationship between
these macromolecules in the normal and cholesterol fed chicken
aortas as a function of age.   They found that glycoproteins, as
well as collagen, increased in the thoracic and abdominal aortas
with age, and that elastin and proteoglycans decreased.   The
relative proportion of glycoproteins to the other macromolecules
was higher in the abdominal aorta, which contained more collagen
and glycoproteins than the thoracic aorta, which is relatively
richer in elastin and proteoglycans.   Figure 2 shows the change
with age of the glycoprotein-bound hexose content in the aortas
of chicken expressed on a dry fat free basis, according to Gan
et al.   (1967).   The steady increase of the hexose content seems
to be sharper in the abdominal than in the thoracic portion of
the aorta.

Nakamura and co-workers (1968) studied the glycoprotein
content (in the intima and in the media) of Japanese human thoracic
aortas.   They found that the total carbohydrate concentration of
the intima decreased until the age of 60 years and increased slightly
thereafter.   Glycoproteins in the media increased progressively with
age; in the intima they found a decrease until 60 years, followed
by an increase.   In atherosclerotic intimas the sialic acid content
seemed to decrease sharply.   Table VI shows the glycoproteins,
hexosamine, hexose, sialic acid, and fucose determinations (for the
intima and media) as a function of age of the normal aorta and of
the plaque (Nakamura et al., 1968).

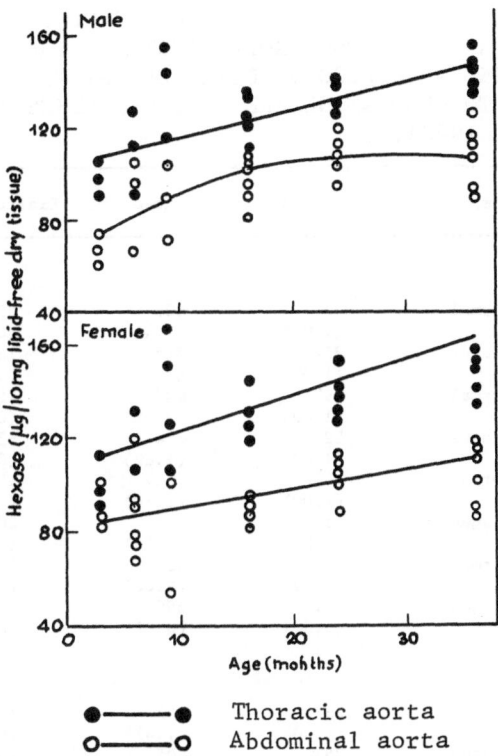

Fig. 2. Change with age of the glycoprotein-bound-hexose values
of chicken aorta (male and female). (Reproduced with permission
from Gan and co-workers, 1967).

It can be seen that the media is significantly poorer on a dry
fat free basis in all these constituents than the intima. This
may be due to the fact that because of the high proportion of
intercellular fibrous components such as collagen and elastin in
the media the intima is relatively richer in cells. Cell membrane
glycoproteins might contribute significantly to the total glycoproteins as stated above. This consideration does not alter
significantly the collagen and elastin determinations reported,
but may interfere to some extent with the proteoglycan determinations and very significantly with the glycoprotein determinations.
Therefore, it is very difficult to give a significant figure for
the intercellular glycoproteins as distinct from the cell membrane
glycoproteins. However, it is currently assumed that intracellular
proteins are poor in carbohydrate. This is certainly not true
for intracellular membranes, which were shown recently to be about
as rich in glycoproteins as the cell membrane itself (Warren, in
press).

L. ROBERT, A. KADAR, AND B. ROBERT

TABLE VI.   CONCENTRATION OF COMPONENT SUGARS OF GLYCOPROTEINS FROM
            NORMAL AND ATHEROSCLEROTIC AORTAS.   THE VALUES ARE
            EXPRESSED AS μg/100 mg DEFATTED DRY TISSUE.   RATIOS OF
            SUGARS TO HEXOSAMINE ARE IN PARENTHESES (from Nakamura
            et al., 1968).

Age	Sex	Sample	Hexosamine	Hexose	Sialic Acid	Fucose
Intima						
25	F	normal	330	805	238	72
			(1.00)	(2.44)	(0.72)	(0.22)
		plaque	314	515	181	39
			(1.00)	(1.74)	(0.58)	(0.12)
53	M	normal	197	497	121	39
			(1.00)	(2.52)	(0.61)	(0.20)
		plaque	227	414	93	49
			(1.00)	(1.82)	(0.19)	(0.22)
59	M	normal	120	204	132	25
			(1.00)	(1.70)	(1.10)	(0.21)
		plaque	151	241	20	27
			(1.00)	(1.59)	(0.13)	(0.18)
70	M	normal	218	437	212	39
			(1.00)	(2.00)	(0.97)	(0.18)
		plaque	441	399	14	39
			(1.00)	(0.91)	(0.32)	(0.09)
Media						
25	F	normal	233	328	132	39
			(1.00)	(1.41)	(0.57)	(0.17)
		plaque	253	405	145	43
			(1.00)	(1.60)	(0.57)	(0.17)
53	M	normal	148	210	5	23
			(1.00)	(1.42)	(0.03	(0.16)
		plaque	139	199	10	23
			(1.00)	(1.43)	(0.07)	(0.16)
59	M	normal	123	165	68	21
			(1.00)	(1.34)	(0.55)	(0.17)
		plaque	115	160	10	18
			(1.00)	(1.39)	(0.09)	(0.15)
70	M	normal	103	158	52	18
			(1.00)	(1.53)	(0.50)	(0.17)
		plaque	117	195	6	19
			(1.00)	(1.67)	(0.05)	(0.16)

An elevated level of glycoproteins was suggested for arteriosclerotic intima by Nakamura's studies, confirming those of
Mullinger and Manley (1969), Schoenebeck et al. (1962), and Parnis
and Clerici (1957).   All these authors reported an increase of
glycoproteins in atherosclerotic aorta.

The interesting reports from Berenson's laboratory over the
last ten years also suggest the presence of tissue specific glycoproteins in several connective tissues, especially the aorta
(Srinivasan et al., 1971).   These authors compared the acrylamide

electrophoretic patterns of glycoproteins isolated by extraction with 0.15 M NaCl and precipitation between 60 and 100% ammonium sulfate, and concluded there were identical patterns in identical twins and different patterns in non-identical twins. The electrophoretic patterns were also different between glycoproteins isolated from different tissues such as skin, spleen, or aorta and were shown to change during development (Fischkin and Spangler, 1968).

These conclusions confirm those of Robert et al. (1970b) who attributed to the structural glycoproteins a tissue specificity which parallels slight but significant differences in amino acid composition and in carbohydrate composition (Robert and Comte, 1968; L. Robert et al., in press).

Structural Glycoproteins of Aorta. Structural glycoproteins were isolated and characterized by Moczar and Robert (1970) and Moczar et al. (1970) from pig and human aortas. Table VII shows the amino acid composition of several structural glycoprotein preparations.

TABLE VII. AMINO ACID COMPOSITION OF STRUCTURAL GLYCOPROTEIN PREPARATIONS FROM SEVERAL CONNECTIVE TISSUES AND OF STREPTOCOCCUS A CELL MEMBRANE (SCM). (From Robert et al., 1972).

Amino Acid	SGP Human Aorta 1	SGP Calf Tendon 2	SGP Calf Skin 3	SGP Calf Cornea 4	SCM 5
ASP	9.8	10.8	7.3	10.2	10.5
GLU	11.3	10.8	7.9	11.3	13.4
THR	4.6	4.7	3.4	5.4	5.0
SER	3.7	4.2	6.2	5.9	4.4
PRO	5.9	5.6	6.9	5.6	3.6
GLY	12.4	8.7	15.8	10.5	8.3
ALA	8.5	7.3	8.9	7.0	13.3
VAL	7.9	9.4	7.9	8.6	5.6
CYS	1.4	1.3	2.7	1.5	1.5
MET	0.4	0.6	-	1.1	1.4
1-LEU	6.2	5.7	5.5	4.7	6.0
LEU	10.9	11.0	9.3	9.6	8.6
TYR	1.4	1.3	-	1.7	1.6
PHE	4.1	4.6	2.4	3.8	3.5
OH-LYS	-	-	-	1.1	-
LYS	4.2	5.6	4.8	4.4	8.5
HIS	2.6	2.7	6.9	1.6	1.5
ARG	4.7	5.9	4.1	6.0	3.5

TABLE VIII.   CARBOHYDRATE COMPOSITION OF THE ELECTROPHORETICALLY
SEPARATED SUBFRACTIONS OF THE GLYCOPEPTIDES OBTAINED
FROM THE INSOLUBLE (1M $CaCl_2$) STROMA OF PIG AORTA BY
COLLAGENASE-PRONASE DIGESTION AND GEL FILTRATION
(Peak No. 5 of Fig. 1 from Moczar et al., 1970).

Fraction No.	Yield (mg)	Molar Ratio of Sugar (Gal = 1)							Hexose/ Hexos- amine ratio	Sial/ fucose ratio
		Gal	Glc	Man	Fuc	Sial	GlcN	GalN		
1	2.20	1	1	1	-	-	-	-		
2	3.98	1	0.6	1.1	0.09	0.2	1.56	-	1.73	2.2
3	3.82	1	0.1	0.8	0.1	0.3	1.25	-	1.52	3.0
4	5.61	1	0.07	1	0.1	0.38	1.43	-	1.5	3.8
5	1.31	1	0.2	1.7	0.15	0.5	1.56	0.26	1.69	3.34
6	4.66	1	0.05	1.2	0.13	0.6	1.39	0.07	1.54	4.62
7	3.92	1	0.6	1	0.09	0.6	1.15	0.23	1.88	6.7

The yields are given in mg of lyophilized material obtained from 41 mg starting material.

Table VIII shows the carbohydrate composition of the glycopeptides
isolated from the structural glycoproteins of pig aorta by pronase
digestion (Moczar et al., 1970).   High voltage electrophoresis
and gel filtration techniques revealed a considerable heterogeneity
of the glycan chains; oligosaccharides with fucose/sialic acid
ratios varying between 2 and 7 could be separated.   As can be seen
by Table VII, the aorta glycoprotein shows a close analogy in its
amino acid composition not only to some other connective tissue
structural glycoproteins but also to the Streptococcus A cell
membrane which Zabriskie isolated and with which it is also immunologically cross-reactive (Robert et al., 1972).   Similar structural
glycoproteins were isolated from elephant aorta.   It was shown
that this preparation gives an immunological cross-reaction with
human aorta structural glycoproteins (McCullagh et al., 1973).
This cross-reaction suggests an organ specific immunochemical
pattern for these substances as shown also by the specificity of
corneal graft rejection obtained by sensitization with the corneal
structural glycoprotein but not with skin structural glycoproteins
(Robert et al., 1970b).

Electron microscopic studies of purified structural glycoprotein preparations obtained by the urea-mercaptoethanol extraction procedure showed a "microfibrillar" pattern (Kadar et al.,
in press).   Figure 3 is an electron micrograph of a structural
glycoprotein preparation obtained from pig aorta.   The typical
microfibrillar arrangement is very similar, if not identical, to
that observed in native unhydrolyzed aortic stroma (Figure 4).
Similar results were obtained with elephant aorta structural glycoproteins (McCullagh et al., 1973).   A beaded subunit pattern can

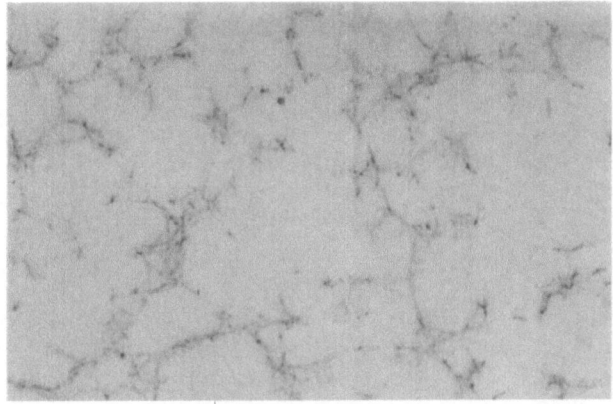

A

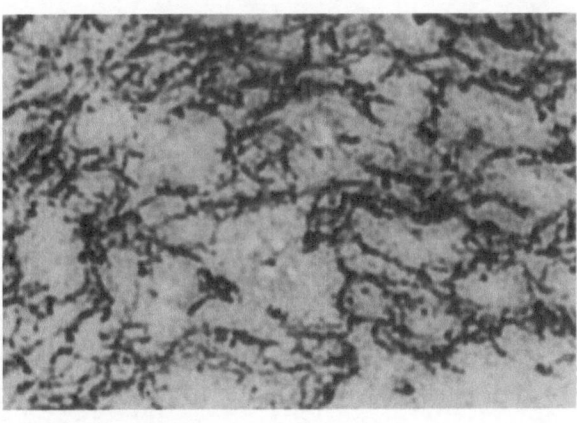

B

Fig. 3. "Microfibrillar" patterns observed on electron microscopy in purified structural glycoprotein preparations of porcine aorta. (Reproduced with permission from B. Robert, A. Kadar, L. Robert, 1973) (A) Purified structural glycoproteins of pig aorta (Ruthenium Red x 57,000). (B) Same preparation as (A), enlarged 150,000 times to show the globular subunit pattern of the structural glycoprotein preparation. (Figure 3 reduced 50% for reproduction).

be detected in these preparations, the globular-shaped subunits having an approximate diameter of 120 Å. In some places subunits of 180 Å diameter can also be seen.

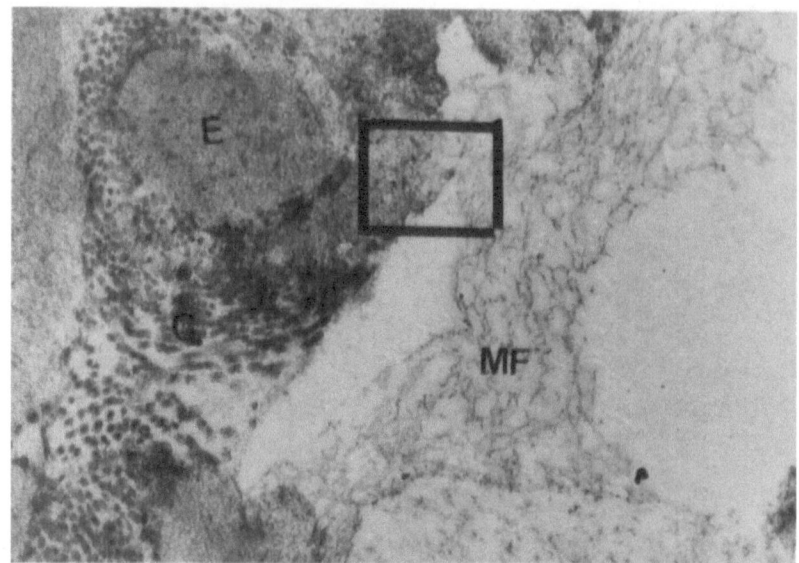

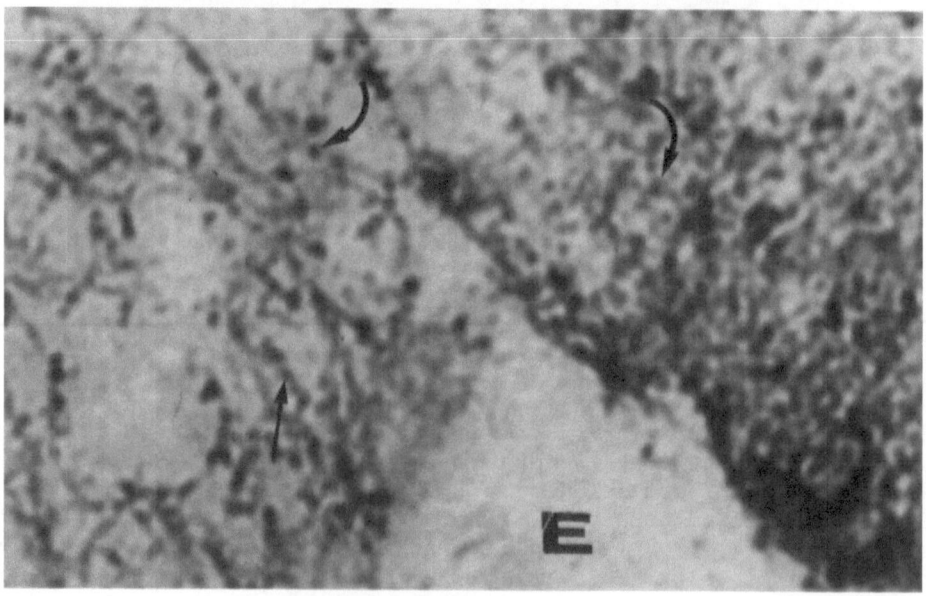

B

Fig. 4. Microfibrillar patterns in elastic tissue of aorta (from
Kadar et al., in press). (A) Stroma of pig aorta with collagen
fibers -C-, elastin -E-, and microfibrils -MF-. (B) Enlargement
of the framed part of A x 350,000 showing the globular subunit
pattern of the native microfibrils (compare with Fig. 3/B).
Subunits of approximately 120 Å diameter (➡) and 180 Å diameter
(⌇) can be seen.

Recent investigations conducted in collaboration with Prunieras and Regnier show that these microfibrillar structures can be recognized in the cell membranes of fibroblasts and extend out of the cell membrane into the intercellular space. These findings, together with those concerning the role of aorta structural glycoproteins in elastogenesis (discussed later), support the proposition we made some time ago that the structural glycoproteins could represent the primitive (phylogenetically) intercellular macromolecular meshwork onto which the more elaborate collagen and elastin fibers are deposited. The isolation of structural glycoproteins from sponge tissues, the lowest metazoa, helps prove this contention (Junqua et al., in preparation).

Biosynthesis of Aorta Glycoproteins. Rabbit aortas incubated in vitro for four hours at 37° incorporated labeled precursors such as lysine, proline, or hexosamine into the structural glycoprotein components (L. Robert et al., in press). Table III shows the specific activities of the aorta extracts of rabbits incubated for four hours with [^{14}C] lysine. It can be seen that the structural glycoprotein fraction (urea-extract) has the highest specific activity with respect to the other macromolecules of the insoluble (1M $CaCl_2$) polymeric stroma. These findings are in agreement with those obtained with other connective tissues such as cornea (Robert and Parlebas, 1965) and show the relatively high metabolic activity (speed of incorporation) of these glycoproteins. Their high rate of labeling is in contrast to their low solubility, which was shown to be due mainly to disulfur and hydrophobic interactions between relatively small subunits of these glycoproteins (about 15,000 daltons appears to be the smallest subunit weight according to recent experiments). The role of these glycoproteins in the formation and biosynthesis of elastic fibers will be discussed later. These results are supported by the investigation of Louisot and co-workers on the presence in aortic tissues of specific transferases such as N-acetyl-glucosaminyl transferase (Guidollet and Louisot, 1973) and mannosyl transferase (Richard et al., 1972). Some of the amino acids were present at a higher concentration in aorta than in blood plasma, suggesting active transport and/or local synthesis (Ebel et al., 1970).

A 25 to 30% decrease of [^{14}C] lysine incorporation in the urea-soluble fraction was found in immuno-atherosclerotic rabbit aortas or in cholesterol-fed rabbit aortas (Table III). A similar decrease of protein synthesis was observed at the ribosomal level in arteriosclerotic rabbit and rat aortas by Henri (1968) and Wortman et al. (1966). No decrease and even a local increase of protein synthesis was reported by Lee et al. (1966) in atherosclerotic monkey aortas. It appears probable that in the same tissue, the synthesis increases for some proteins and decreases for others (Table III). The occurrence of such "shifts" in the ratio of the rate of synthesis of specific proteins may have pathogenetic significance.

Elastin

Composition and Structure.   Elastin is the most specific and conspicuous macromolecular component of the intercellular matrix of large arteries such as aorta. Its structure is now quite well understood (Partridge, 1970, 1972; Banga, 1969). The isolation of proelastin by Carnes (1972) and Sandberg and co-workers (1969), followed by the partial elucidation of the amino acid sequence now renders possible the detailed study of the crosslinking process and desmosine formation.

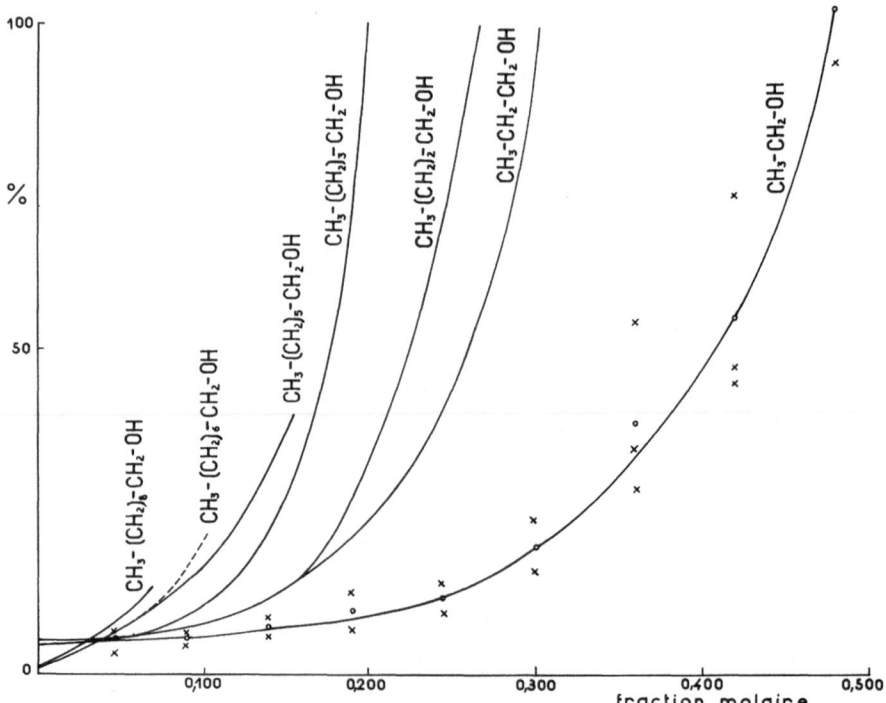

Fig. 5. Rate of "solubilization" of purified elastin of beef ligamentum nuchae in 1M KOH in the presence of organo-alkaline solvents as a function of the chain lengths of alcohols.(Modified with permission from Kornfeld-Poullain and Robert, 1963, and Jacotot et al., 1973). Abscissa: mole fraction of n-alcohol in the ternary mixture. Ordinate: % of total elastin "solubilized."

The amino acid composition of elastin, established some 10
years ago (Partridge, 1963), suggests only one possibility for the
stabilizing forces responsible for its tertiary and quaternary
structure; i.e., hydrophobic interactions (Robert and Poullain,
1963, 1964). These interactions were first studied by the kinetics
of its alkaline hydrolysis in the presence of organic solvents
(Kornfeld-Poullain and Robert, 1968; Poullain and Robert, 1965).
Figure 5 shows the increase of the speed of alkaline hydrolysis
of purified elastin in ternary solvent systems with the increase of
the chain lengths of the added alcohols (Kornfeld-Poullain and
Robert, 1968; Jacotot et al., 1973). The fact that every added
CH_2 unit increased the relative speed of hydrolysis by a constant
amount thus confirmed the importance of hydrophobic interactions
in the stabilization of the elastic fibers. Lipids may play an
analogous role when they accumulate in the arterial wall by
enhancing the unfolding and enzymatic degradation of elastin
through the disorganization of its hydrophobic regions. This
point deserves further investigation (Jacotot et al., 1973). It
has also been suggested, on the basis of these physicochemical
experiments, that the elasticity of elastin could be explained by
the extensive hydrophobic interactions. That is, a lengthening
of the fiber would rupture hydrophobic interactions by increasing

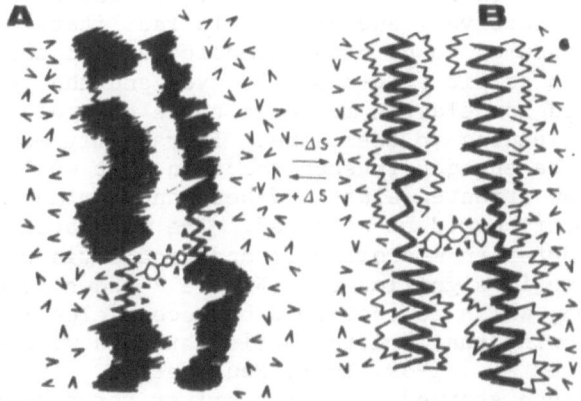

Fig. 6. Schematic representation of the hydrophobic theory of the
elasticity of elastin. (A) In the contracted state the hydrophobic interaction results in a compact conformation excluding water
from the immediate neighborhood of the alkyl side chains of the
elastic molecule. (B) In the extended state, closer contact is
established through transconformation of the molecule, between the
aliphatic side chains and water, leading to a decrease in entropy
of the system. Therefore the return to the original length will be
"spontaneous" because of the increase of the entropy of the system.
(Reproduced with permission from Robert et al., 1964).

the distance between aliphatic side chains. This would establish
a closer contact between aliphatic residues and water molecules, and
lead to a decrease of the entropy of the system. The return of
the fiber to its original length would thus be accompanied by an
increase of the entropy of the system (Robert and Poullain, 1964).
Figure 6 shows the original schematic drawing representing this
hydrophobic hypothesis of elastin elasticity (Robert and Poullain,
1964). All recent findings from several laboratories seem to
confirm this hypothesis (Hoffman, 1971; Mukherjee and Hoffman,
1971).

Formation of Elastic Fibers.   The details of the formation of
desmosine cross-links are understood to some extent (Partridge,
1970). The role of a specific lysine oxidase which would act
specifically on certain lysine residues engaged in specific sequences
in the proelastin molecule seems to be established. Further details
of the enzymatic and non-enzymatic steps of this sequence are not
yet understood. Some time ago we proposed that the positioning of
proelastin molecules on the structural glycoprotein-microfibrils
may be an important step in the oriented biosynthesis of these
desmosine cross-links (Robert et al., 1969). Proelastin rich in
lysine carries a net positive charge and could interact electro-
statically with structural glycoprotein-microfibrils which, due
to their relatively high aspartic and glutamic acid content, carry
a negative charge. This "positioning effect" would enable lysine
oxidase to act selectively and also would facilitate and accelerate
the reactions presumed to be non-enzymatic between the aldehyde
residues of amino adipic acid-semi aldehyde and the lysine residue
of the neighboring proelastin molecule to be engaged in the cross-
linking process leading to desmosine. If randomly moving lysine
residues had to be engaged in such reactions, it would be difficult
to understand how oriented elastic fibers and laminae with exactly
controlled geometry could be obtained. The interaction between
structural glycoprotein-microfibrils and proelastin would, therefore,
have a morphogenetic significance. Figure 7 shows schematically
this proposition, which is confirmed by recent electron microscopic
observations showing that "microfibrils" stained with uranyl acetate
and lead (Kadar et al., 1969, 1971; Haust et al., 1967) and an
amorphous substance stained only with silver tetraphenylporphine
sulfonate (Albert, 1972) appear sequentially and "cooperate" during
elastogenesis. The identification of "microfibrils" as the structural glycoprotein component of elastic tissue (Robert et al., 1971b)
offers now a unified picture of the molecular events of elastogenesis. However, many of its details remain unexplored. It seems
very probable that active elastogenesis is a process continuing
throughout the lifetime; this is shown in Figure 8. Looker and
Berry (1972) noted a continuous formation of interlamellar elastic
fibers during the lifetime of the rat. Only the concentric elastic

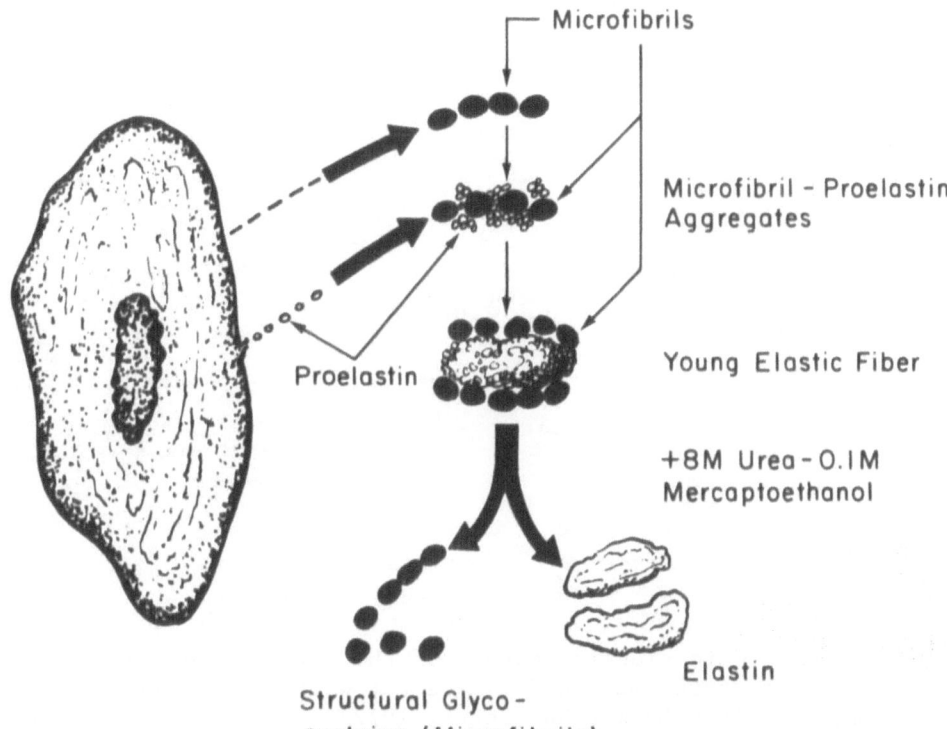

Fig. 7. Schematic representation of the mechanism of oriented
synthesis ("vectorial synthesis") of elastic fibers on a microfibrillar network. Structural glycoprotein-microfibrils are
represented as negatively charged beaded filaments (in black) onto
which positively charged proelastin molecules (in white) aggregate
through electrostatic interactions; following the action of lysine-
oxidase, the "positioned" proelastin molecules are linked together
by desmosine crosslinks. The sterical conditions of this cross-
linking process are defined by the previous formation of the microfibrillar network. Young elastic fibers are still rich in the
"microfibrillar" glycoprotein elements. These can be extracted (as
"structural glycoproteins") from purified elastin by 8M urea-0.1M
mercaptoethanol, leaving "elastin" considered as the proelastin
molecules crosslinked through desmosine residues (Robert et al.,
1971b; Robert et al., 1970).

lamellae were formed early in ontogenesis and active growth; the
interlamellar elastic fibers appeared to be continuously synthesized. Similar observations were made also in diseased human and
animal aortas (Table VII). This continuous synthesis of both
structural glycoprotein-microfibrils and proelastin of the elastic

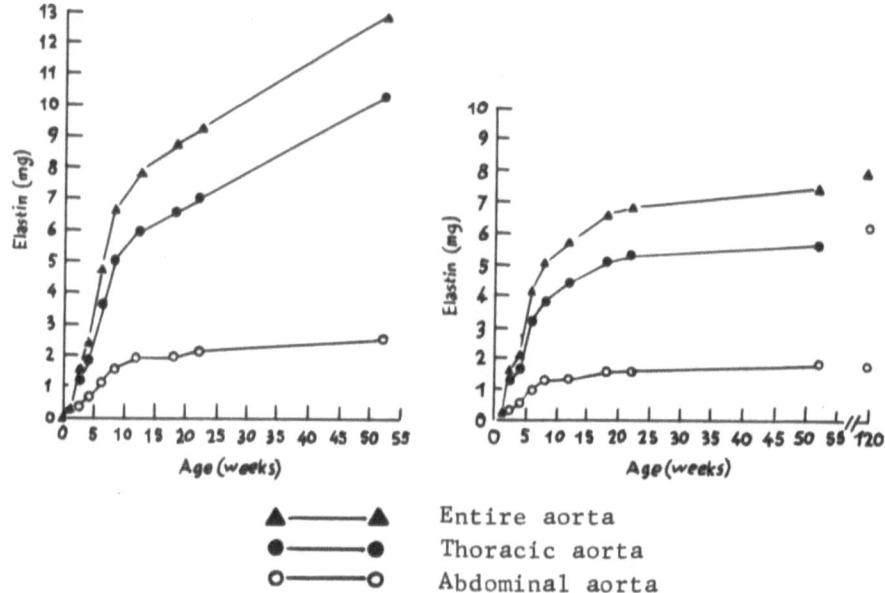

Fig. 8. Increase in elastin content of the entire thoracic and abdominal aorta of the male and female rat with age. (Reproduced with permission from Looker and Berry, 1972).

fibers is necessary, but insufficient conditions may exist for reparative processes in diseased arterial walls, where preexistent elastic laminae are being degraded. The reasons for the absence or inefficacy of the reparative processes of elastic tissue are as yet unknown.

Elastin in Arteriosclerosis. Several investigators report a modified ratio of polar to non-polar amino acids in elastin isolated from atherosclerotic plaques (Lansing, 1966). This finding probably can be attributed to the relative increase in structural glycoprotein-microfibrils in plaque elastin. A similar increase in an "alkali soluble protein" preceding the accumulation of collagen and elastin was reported by Wolinsky (1972) in aortas from hypertensive rats. The microfibrillar component is very difficult to remove completely from purified elastin. We studied systematically the presence of these glycoprotein components in elastins obtained by several different purification procedures (Robert et al., 1971b). Table IX shows the hexose, hexosamine, and sialic acid content of elastin preparations purified by several methods. It can be seen that all contain significant amounts of glycoprotein components, although proelastin and elastin were

TABLE IX.   CARBOHYDRATE CONTENT OF ELASTIN PREPARATIONS OBTAINED
BY SEVERAL DIFFERENT PURIFICATION PROCEDURES FROM CALF
LIGAMENTUM NUCHAE (from Robert et al., 1971b).

Method or Preparation* of Elastin	Water	Ash	Hexoses	Hexosamines	Sialic Acid	Hydroxy-proline
	%	%	%	%	%	%
0.1 N NaOH	9.34	1.33	0.33	0.35	-	1.23
Formic acid 88%	6.47	2.24	0.53	0.51	-	0.97
70% Trichloracetic acid	12.06	1.13	0.97	0.57	0.07	1.15
Autoclaving	11.01	1.03	0.55	0.53	-	0.93
5 M Guanidine-HCl†	9.35	1.66	0.92	0.42	0.04	3.11

*For the details of these purification procedures, see Methods.
†Three extractions with 5 M guanidine-HCl followed by two extractions with 5 M guanidine-HCl-0.1 M 2-mercaptoethanol.

reported not to have carbohydrate components (Grant et al., 1971).
If purified elastin is treated with trypsin, chymotrypsin, or
urea-mercaptoethanol, the glycoprotein component can be removed
completely or nearly so (Robert et al., 1971b).

The composition of the isolated glycoprotein component is
similar or identical to the structural glycoproteins (see above)
and gives immunochemical cross-reaction with them. The electron
microscopic characteristics of this microfibrillar component of
purified elastin are also indistinguishable from those seen in
the intercellular space far from the elastic fibers. Therefore, it
seems probable that during elastogenesis these microfibrillar
structures are entrapped in the elastic fibers and laminae by a
mechanism similar to the one shown schematically in Figure 7.

Electron microscopic studies have shown that the microfibrillar component might be the major site of calcium deposition in
plaque elastin (Shimamura, 1970; Haust and Geer, 1970; Robert et
al., 1971c). On the contrary, no definitive relationship could be
established between GAG content and elastin content (Grant, 1967).
Therefore, the role of proteoglycans in elastogenesis, if any, is
still to be established.

Degradation of Elastin in Arteriosclerosis.   The fragmentation-
degradation of elastic fibers and laminae is one of the most conspicuous findings of the atherosclerotic changes in aortas. It is
observed in the human atherosclerotic plaque and it seems to be
independent of the method used to induce experimental arteriosclerosis. Pancreatic elastase has been suggested by some authors to
be responsible for this degradation. This seems very improbable,
and the role of tissue elastases should be investigated further.

Neutrophil granulocytes (Janoff, 1970) and blood platelets were shown to contain proteases with elastolytic activity (Legrand et al., 1973; Robert et al., 1970a), and it is quite probable that similar enzymes may be isolated from aorta, skin, and other tissues where the degradation of elastin during the atherosclerotic process is demonstrated (Bouissou et al., 1973). Several glycosidases and proteases (cathepsins C and D) have been demonstrated in arterial wall lysosomes (Peters et al., 1972); these enzymes may play an active role in the above mentioned degradative processes (Zemplenyi, 1968).

Regulation of the Biosynthesis of the Macromolecules of the Arterial Wall

The previous succinct description of the macromolecules of the arterial wall shows that all four major types of macromolecules of intercellular matrices are present in various amounts in arterial wall, mainly in aorta. The differentiation and morphogenesis of the arterial wall can be characterized qualitatively and quantitatively by the regulation of the relative rates of synthesis of these macromolecules (Robert and Robert, in press). This ratio changes from one type of vessel to the other and is precisely regulated even in the same vessel wall according to its anatomical location. In pig aorta, for instance, the elastin content falls from 51% of dry weight in the thoracic aorta to 9% in the lower abdominal portion, with a decrease of the elastin/collagen ratio from 3.2 to 0.2 (Grant, 1967). In humans the elastin content falls only from about 38% to approximately 22% with an elastin/collagen ratio of 1.6 to 0.8.

Experiments aimed at understanding the regulatory mechanisms responsible for these changes are currently under way in several laboratories. By using in vitro incorporation methods and organ culture studies, we could show that rabbit aortas can incorporate radioactive precursors such as lysine, proline, and hexosamine into all of the above mentioned macromolecules. Table III shows the specific activities of the successive extracts containing the macromolecules of the insoluble, polymeric stroma of rabbits aorta (L. Robert et al. in press). It can be seen that the incorporation is quite measurable not only in the urea-soluble glycoprotein fraction but also in the elastin of the adult aorta. This finding suggests that the metabolic inertia of elastin was probably overstated by previous authors (see previous section). The probable interpretation of the above findings is that of a continuous synthesis of proelastin, followed by a very slow and very partial incorporation in polymeric elastin.

Relatively high rates of incorporation of these labeled precursors into the structural glycoprotein component (urea-extract, Table III) might be explained by the fact that they are at least partially cell-membrane derived. The relative increase in atherosclerotic plaques could, therefore, be interpreted as a result of the increased synthesis or a replacement of degrading intercellular macromolecules by the medial cells. If no reparation or restitution may not be achieved, this may be due more to the fact that metabolic steps leading from proelastin and structural glycoproteins to oriented and crosslinked elastic tissue are somewhere blocked rather than to absence of the synthesis of the precursors. Further studies along these lines would not only enhance our knowledge on the differentiation and morphogenesis of the arterial wall, but could also suggest new avenues for the therapeutic approach, influencing the metabolic activity and regenerative capacity of the pathological arterial wall.

The Immunochemical Properties of Arterial Wall Macromolecules

In the light of the recent immunological theory of arteriosclerosis (Robert et al., 1964, 1970c; Robert and Robert, 1969; Renais, this publication) it is important to accumulate detailed knowledge on the immunochemical properties of the macromolecules of the arterial wall.

Collagen. As far as we know, very little is known about the immunochemical properties of arterial wall collagen. Detailed knowledge in this field will have to wait the isolation of purified tropocollagen from arterial wall and the comparison of the component chains ($\alpha 1$, $\alpha 2$, etc.) with those of other known connective tissues, as well as detailed sequence studies on cyanogen bromide peptides. However, it is possible that collagen can have tissue specificity and may be involved in the definition of the immunochemical characteristics of a differentiated connective tissue such as that of the arterial wall.

Proteoglycans. Arterial wall proteoglycans very probably do behave in the same manner as the other proteoglycans which were studied immunochemically (Tsiganos and Muir, 1970; B. Robert et al., in press), that is, only the protein part carries antigenic specificity. The polysaccharide chains, similar to those of the other proteoglycans, probably do not contribute to the antigenicity of these macromolecular aggregates.

Glycoproteins.   Some of the glycoproteins isolated from arterial
wall have been shown to be highly antigenic (Srinivasan et al.,
1971; Robert et al., 1971a).   Preliminary evidence was obtained
that the cross-reactions between structural glycoproteins isolated
from different connective tissues parallels, to some extent at
least, the analogy of their amino acid composition, as well as
their cross-reaction with the Streptococcus A cell membrane
(Robert et al., 1972;L. Robert et al.,in press). This can probably
be attributed to conformational specificity determined by slight
variations in sequence. If this is the case, the structural
glycoproteins of connective tissues would have to be considered
as "differentiation antigens."

Elastin.   Elastin,which for a long time was considered as non-
antigenic, has been shown to be definitively antigenic by obtaining
immune sera giving precipitation lines in double diffusion and
passive hemagglutination titers up to several thousand (Robert et
al., 1963; Robert et al., 1971a; Jackson et al., 1966).   Antibodies
to soluble (kappa) elastin were observed in the sera of several
hundred arteriosclerotic and normal human subjects (Stein et al.,
1966).

     Immunoglobulins could also be demonstrated in arteriosclerotic
human elastic tissue by immunofluorescence methods (Robert et al.,
1970c).   These results in addition to the very sclerotic lesions
observed after prolonged immunization of rabbits with purified
elastin, as well as with structural glycoproteins of human and of
porcine aorta (Robert et al., 1971a), gave considerable support
to the immune mechanisms of arteriosclerosis (Robert et al.,
1964).   It should be noted, however, that the efficiency of these
antigens in inducing the calcified lesions appeared to be inversely
proportional to their antigenicity as measured by the titer of
precipitating or hemagglutinating sera obtained (Table X).   This
"anomalous behavior" of arterial wall macromolecules may be in
causal relation with the observation that no lymphocytic infiltrate
can regularly be observed in arteriosclerotic lesions, be they
"spontaneous" human lesions or experimentally induced.   Therefore,
the immune mechanism of the arterial lesion does not seem to be
related directly to the cellular mechanism as observed in graft
rejection.   It is more probable that immunological factors involved
in arteriosclerosis are related to circulating and tissue-fixed
"autoantibodies." The pathogenetic effects of these "autoantibodies"
may be related to their action on the mediacytes or endothelial
cells. Therefore, a purely humoral mechanism leading to metabolic
disturbance of the arterial wall would be a plausible interpretation
for the immunological mechanisms of arteriosclerosis. The findings
of V. and J. L. Beaumont and co-workers favor this contention.
These investigators have described "autoimmune-hyperlipidemias"
in human patients having "autoantibodies" to serum lipoproteins

TABLE X.   ANTIBODY TITER   DETERMINED BY PASSIVE HEMAGGLUTINATION
           AND FREQUENCY OF ARTERIOSCLEROTIC LESIONS OF THE AORTA
           OF RABBITS IMMUNIZED WITH HUMAN AND PORCINE AORTA
           EXTRACTS (from Róbert et al., 1971a).

Immunizing Antigen	Hemag. Titer. 10^{-1}*	% Animals with Aortic Lesions
Unimmunized†	8	0
1M CaCl$_2$-extract of human aorta	$10 - 30.10^3$	12
8M-urea-0.1M mercaptoethanol extract (structural glycoprotein fraction) of pig aorta	1.10^3	50
Elastin from bovine lig. nuchae‡	1.10^2	70

*Most frequent values obtained on 5 to 15 different sera determined at the
   end of the immunization period, using the immunizing antigen as a test
   antigen on red cells.
†Injected with NaCl 0.9% in Freund's adjuvant.
‡Injected as fibrous elastin or as soluble K-elastin.

(Beaumont, 1970), and in rabbits receiving injections either of
complete Freund's adjuvant (Beaumont et al., 1969) or various
antigens (Beaumont and Beaumont, 1968). This post-immunizational
hyperlipidemia was observed in rabbits immunized with purified
protein of the arterial wall such as elastin or structural glycoproteins (Robert et al., 1971a). In these animals, however,
only calcified arterial lesions and no extensive lipid deposition
could be noticed. Whatever the detailed mechanism of this immune
arteriosclerotic lesion may be, it is very probably mediated
through metabolic perturbations (such as shifts in the ratio of
structural proteins synthesized) mediated by humoral immune
factors.

ACKNOWLEDGEMENTS

     The experiments related were carried out under contracts
with D.G.R.S.T. (71.7.2809) I.N.S.E.R.M. (contract 71 4 054) and
the C.N.R.S. (ER No. 53).

     The skillful technical assistance of Miss F. Chavarot and
Mr. J.C. Derouette is acknowledged, as well as a fellowship of
the D.G.R.S.T. for Dr. A. Kadar.

REFERENCES

Albert, E.N. (1972). Amer. J. Pathol. 69, 89.

Anastassiades, T., Anastassiades, P.A., and Denstedt, O.F. (1972).
    Biochim. Biophys. Acta 261, 418.

Anderson, A.J. (1963). Biochem. J. 88, 460.

Balazs, E.A. (1970). "Chemistry and Molecular Biology of the
    Intercellular Matrix," Vols. 1-3. Academic Press, New York.

Banga, I. (1969). In "International Symposium Biochemistry of
    the Vascular Wall, Fribourg, 1968," (M. Comel and L. Laszt,
    eds.). pp. 18-92 (202-276). Karger, Basel.

Barnes, M.J., and Partridge, S.M. (1968). Biochem. J. 109, 883.

Beaumont, J.L. (1970). Eur. J. Clin. Biol. Res. 15, 1037.

Beaumont, J.L., Beaumont, V., and Antonucci, M. (1969). C.R.
    Acad. Sci. (Paris) 268, 1830.

Beaumont, V., and Beaumont, J.L. (1968). Pathol. Biol. 16, 869.

Bentley, J.P., Wuthrich, R.C., and Van Bueren, A.M. (1970).
    Atherosclerosis 12, 159.

Berenson, G.S., Radhakrishnamurthy, B., Fishkin, A.F., Dessauer,
    H., and Arquembourg, P. (1966). J. Atheroscler. Res. 6, 214.

Berry, C.L., Looker, T., and Germain, J. (1972). J. Anat. 113, 1.

Bihari-Varga, M., Gergely, J., and Gero, S. (1964). J. Atheroscler.
    Res. 4, 106.

Bihari-Varga, M., and Gero, S. (1966). Acta Physiol. Acad. Sci.
    Hung. 29, 273.

Bihari-Varga, M., and Vegh, M. (1967). Biochim. Biophys. Acta 144,
    202.

Bouissou, H., Pieraggi, M.T., Julian, M., and Douste, B.L. (1973).
    In "Frontiers in Matrix Biology." Vol. 1. "Aging of Connective
    Tissue Skin." eds. L. Robert and B. Robert. Karger, Basel.

Carnes, W. (1972). In "The Comparative Molecular Biology of
    Extracellular Matrices." (H.C. Slavkin, ed.). p. 400.
    Academic Press, New York.

Crossley, H.L., Johnson, A.R., Mauger, K.K., Wood, N.L., and
    Fuller, G.C. (1972). Life Sci. 11, 869.

Ebel, A., Kempf, E., Bollack, Cl., and Mandel, P. (1970).
    Atherosclerosis 12, 219.

Engel, U.R. (1971). Atherosclerosis 13, 45.

Fischer, G.M., and Llaurado, J.G. (1967). Arch. Pathol. 84, 95.

Fischer, G.M., and Llaurado, J.G. (1966). Circ. Res. 19, 394.

Fishkin, A.F., and Spangler, P.N. (1968). Nature 218, 577.

Fitch, S.M., Harkness, M.L., and Harkness, R.D. (1955). Nature
    176, 163.

Frey, J. (1969). "Contribution à la Connaissance du Métabolisme
    Physiologique du Collagène fondée sur une Etude de la
    Biosynthése de l'Hydroxyproline Protéinique," These Fac. Sci.
    Univ. Lyon.

Frey, J., Farjanel, J., and Crouzet, B. (1969). Bull. Soc. Chim.
    Biol. 51, 471.

Gan, J.C., Narashimha Murthy, P.V., Nichols, C.W., Jr., and
    Chaikoff, I.L. (1967). J. Atheroscler. Res. 7, 629.

Gardais, A., Picard, J., and Hermelin, B. (1973). Comp. Biochem.
    Physiol. 44B, 507.

Gardais, A., Picard, J., and Tarasse, C. (1969). J. Chromatogr.
    42, 396.

Gerö, S. (1964). Symp. Zool. Soc. Lond. 11, 169.

Gerö, S., Virag, S. Bihari-Varga, M., Székely, J., and Fehér, J.
    (1967). Progr. Biochem. Pharmacol. 2, 290.

Gerrity, R.G., and Cliff, W.J. (1972). Exp. Mol. Pathol. 16, 382.

Grant, M.E., Steven, F.S., Jackson, D.S., and Sandberg, L.B.
    (1971). Biochem. J. 121, 197.

Grant, R.A. (1967). J. Atheroscler. Res. 7, 463.

Guidollet, J., and Louisot, P. (1973). Clin. Chim. Acta 43, 157.

Harkness, R.D. (1961). Biol. Rev. 36, 399.

Hauss, W.H., and Junge-Hûlsing, G. (1963). Exp. Ann. Biochim.
Med. 24, 239.

Hauss, W.H. (1973). Arch. Abt. A. Pathol. Anat. 359, 135.

Haust, M.D., and Geer, J.C. (1970). Amer. J. Pathol. 60, 329.

Haust, M.D., More, R.H., Bencosme, S.G., and Balis, J.U. (1967).
Exp. Mol. Pathol. 6, 300.

Henry, J.C. (1968). C.R. Acad. Sci. (Paris) 266, 1449.

Hoffman, A.S. (1971). In "Biomaterials" (A.L. Bement, Jr., ed.).
pp. 285-312. University of Washington Press, Seattle.

Ichida, T., and Kalant, N. (1968). Can. J. Biochem. 46, 249.

Iverius, P.H. (1968). Clin. Chim. Acta 20, 261.

Jackson, D.S., Sandberg, L.B., and Cleary, E.G. (1966).
Nature 210, 195.

Jacotot, B., Beaumont, J.L., Monnier, G., Szigeti, M., Robert, B.,
and Robert, L. (1973). Nutr. Metabol. 15, 46.

Janoff, A. (1970). Ser. Haematol. 3, 96.

Junge-Hulsing, G., and Wagner, H. (1969). In "Aging of Connective
and Skeletal Tissue, 1968." Thule International Symposia,
3rd. (Arthur Engle and Tage Larson, eds.). pp. 213-228.
Nordiska Bokhandelns Forlag, Stockholm.

Junqua, S., Fayolle, J., and Robert, L. (In preparation).

Kadar, A., Gardner, D.L., and Bush, V. (1971). J. Pathol. 104,
253.

Kadar, A., Robert, B., and Robert, L. (In press). Pathol. Biol.

Kadar, A., Veress, B., and Jellinek, H. (1969). Exp. Mol. Pathol.
11, 212.

Kaplan, D., and Meyer, K. (1960). Proc. Soc. Exp. Biol. Med.
105, 78.

Knieriem, H.J., Kap, V.C.Y., and Wissler, R.W. (1968).
J. Atheroscler. Res. 8, 125.

Kornfeld-Poullain, N., and Robert, L. (1968). Bull. Soc. Chim.
Biol. 50, 759.

Kresse, H., Heidel, H., and Buddecke, E. (1971). Eur. J. Biochem.
    22, 557.

Kulonen, E., and Pikkarainen (In press). "Biology of the
    Fibroblast." Academic Press, New York.

Kumar, V., Berenson, G.S., Ruiz, H., Dalferes, E.R., and Strong,
    J.P. (1967). J. Atheroscler. Res. 7: 573, 583.

Lalich, J.J., and Whang Paik, W.C. (1968). Proc. Soc. Exp. Biol.
    Med. 127, 543.

Lansing, A.L. (1966). Arch. Mal. Coeur Vaiss. 8, Suppl. 2, 23.

Lee, K.T., Jones, R., Kim, D.N., Florentin, R., Coulston, F., and
    Thomas, W.A. (1966). Exp. Mol. Pathol. 5, Suppl. 3, 108.

Legrand, Y., Caen, J., Booyse, F.M., Rafelson, M.E., Robert, B.,
    and Robert, L. (1973). Biochim. Biophys. Acta 309, 406.

Le Lievre, C., and Le Douarin, N. (1973). C.R. Acad. Sci. (Paris)
    276, 383.

Lindy, S., Turto, H., Uitto, J., Helin, P., and Lorenzen, I.
    (1972). Circ. Res. 30, 123.

Looker, T., and Berry, C.L. (1972). J. Anat. 113, 17.

McCullagh, K.G., Derouette, S., and Robert L. (1973). Exp. Mol.
    Pathol. 18, 202.

McCully, K.S. (1972). Amer. J. Pathol. 66, 83.

McCully, K.S. (1971). Nature 231, 391.

Moczar, M. (1968). Glycoprotéides de la Trame Fibreuse de la
    Paroi Artérielle, Thèse Fac. Sci. Lille.

Moczar, M., Moczar, E., and Robert L. (1970). Atherosclerosis
    12, 31.

Moczar, M., and Robert, L. (1970). Atherosclerosis 11, 7.

Moschetto, Y., and Havez, R. (1969). Bull. Soc. Chim. Biol. 51,
    1171.

Mukherjee, D.P., and Hoffman, A.S. (1971). In "Biophysical
    Properties of the Skin." (H.R. Elden, ed.). pp. 219-241.
    John Wiley & Sons, New York.

Mullinger, R.N., and Manley, G. (1969). J. Atheroscler. Res.
    9, 108.

Nakamura, T., Tokita, K., Tateno, S., Kotoku, T., and Ohba, T.
    (1968). J. Atheroscler. Res. 8, 891.

Neuman, R.E., Logan, M.A. (1950). J. Biol. Chem. 184,299.

Nimni, M.E., Guia, E., Bavetta, L.A. (1967). Biochem. J. 102, 143.

Partridge, S.M. (1963). Exp. Ann. Biochim. Med. 24, 133.

Partridge, S.M. (1970). In "Chemistry and Molecular Biology of
    the Intercellular Matrix." (E.A. Balazs, ed.). Vol. 1.
    pp. 593-616. Academic Press, New York.

Partridge, S.M. (1972). In "The Comparative Molecular Biology
    of Extracellular Matrices." (H.C. Slavkin, ed.). p. 388.
    Academic Press, New York.

Pernis, B., and Clerici, E. (1957). Experientia 13, 351.

Peters, T.J., Muller, M., and de Duve, C.J. (1972). J. Exp.
    Med. 136, 1117.

Picard, J., Lacord-Bonneau, M., and Gardais, A. (1968). In "Le
    Role de la Paroi Artérielle dans l'Athérogénèse, Paris,
    1967." Centre national de la recherche scientifique, Paris.
    Colloques internationaux, 169. pp. 721-734.

Poullain, N., and Robert, L. (1966). In "Symposium International
    sur la Biochimie et la Physiologie du Tissu Conjonctif,
    Lyons, 1965." (Ph. Comte, ed.). pp. 139-143. Lyon.

Richard, M., Broquet, P., and Louisot, P. (1972). C.R. Acad.
    Sci. (Paris) 274, 1212; J. Mol. Cell. Cardiol. 4, 465.

Robert, A.M., Grosgogeat, Y., Reverdy, V., Robert, B., and
    Robert, L. (1971a). Atherosclerosis 13, 427.

Robert, A.M., Robert, B., and Robert, L. (1969). Arch. Mal. Coeur
    Vaiss. 62, 25.

Robert, B., and Robert, A.M. (1969). Med. Hyg. 27, 822.

Robert, B., Robert, A.M., and Robert, L. (In press). In "Les
    Glycoconjugués." Centre national de la recherche scientifique,
    Paris. Colloques internationaux. (J. Montreuil and G. Spik,
    eds.).

Robert, B., Szigeti, M., Derouette, J.C., Robert, L., Bouissou, H., and Fabre, M.T. (1971b). Eur. J. Biochem. 21, 507.

Robert, B., Szigeti, M., Robert, L., Legrand, Y., Pignaud, G., and Caen, J. (1970a). Nature 227, 1248.

Robert, L. (1970). In "Atherosclerosis. " Proceedings from the Second International Symposium, 1969. (R.J. Jones, ed.). pp. 59-68. Springer-Verlag, Berlin.

Robert, L., and Comte, P. (1968). Life Sci. 7, 493.

Robert, L., Darrell, R.W., and Robert, B. (1970a). In "Chemistry and Molecular Biology of the Intercellular Matrix." (E.A. Balazs, ed.). Vol. 3. pp. 1591-1614. Academic Press, New York.

Robert, L., Grosgogeat, Y., Robert, A.M., and Robert, B. (1971c). Israel J. Med. Sci. 7, 431.

Robert, L., Junqua, S., Robert, A.M., Moczar, M., and Robert, B. (In press). In "Biology of the Fibroblast." (E. Kulonen and J. Pikkarainen, eds.). Academic Press, New York.

Robert, L., and Parlebas, J. (1965). Bull. Soc. Chim. Biol. 47, 1853.

Robert, L., Parlebas, J., Oudea, P., Zweibaum, A., and Robert, B. (1965). In "Structure and Function of Connective and Skeletal Tissue." NATO - Advanced Study Institute, 1964. (S. Fritton Jackson, ed.). pp. 406-412. Butterworth, London.

Robert, L., Parlebas, J., Poullain, N., and Robert, B. (1963). "Protides of Biological Fluids." Vol. 11. pp. 109-113. Elsevier, Amsterdam.

Robert, L., and Poullain, N. (1963). Bull. Soc. Chim. Biol. 45, 1317.

Robert, L., and Poullain, N. In "Enzymologie et Immunologie dans l'athérosclérose." Colloque Bordeaux, 1964. (H. Bricaud, ed.). pp. 123-129. Bailleres, Paris.

Robert, L., and Robert, B. (In press). In "Différenciation des Cellules Eukaryotes en Culture." Colloque INSERM Juin 1973, Créteil.

Robert, L., Robert, B., and Robert, A.M. (1970c). Exp. Gerontol. 5, 339.

Robert, L., Robert, M., Moczar, M., and Moczar, E. (1968).
    In "La Rôle de la Paroi Artérielle dans l'Athérogénèse,
    Paris, 1967." Centre national de la recherche scientifique,
    Paris. Colloques internationaux. pp. 395-424.

Robert, L., Stein, F., Pezess, M.P., and Poullain, N. In
    "Enzymologie et Immunologie dans l'Athérosclérosis."
    Colloque Bordeaux, 1964. (H. Bricaud, ed.). pp. 233-241.
    Brailleres, Paris.

Sandberg, L.B., Weissman, N., and Smith, D.W. (1969).
    Biochemistry 8, 2940.

Schoenebeck, L., Werber, U., and Voigt, K.D. (1962). J.
    Atheroscler. Res. 2, 332.

Schorah, C.J., Lovell, D., and Curran, R.C. (1968). Brit. Exp.
    Pathol. 49, 574.

Shimamura, T. (1970). Exp. Mol. Pathol. 13, 79.

Slavkin, H.C. (1972). In "The Comparative Molecular Biology of
    Extracellular Matrices." Academic Press, New York.

Srinivasan, S.R., Dolan, P., Radhakrishnamurthy, B., and
    Berenson, G.S. (1972). Prep. Biochem. 2, 83;
    Atherosclerosis 16, 95.

Srinivasan, S.R., Radhakrishnamurthy, B., Pargaonkar, P.S., and
    Berenson, G.S. (1971). Nature 229, 58.

Stein, F., Pezess, M.P., Robert, L., and Poullain, N. (1965).
    Nature 207, 312.

Tsiganos, C.P., and Muir, H. (1970). In "Chemistry and Molecular
    Biology of the Intercellular Matrix." (E.A. Balazs, ed.).
    Vol. 2. pp. 859-866. Academic Press, New York.

Velican, C. (1966). Biochim. Biol. Sper. 5, 151.

Velican, C. (1967). J. Atheroscler. Res. 7, 517.

Viidik, A., Holm-Pedersen, P., and Rundgren, A. (1972). Scand.
    J. Plast. Reconstr. Surg. 6, 114.

Warren, L. (In press). "Différenciation des Cellules Eukaryotes
    en Culture, Colloque INSERM Juin 1973, Créteil.

Wirtschafter, Z.T., and Bentley, J.P. (1965). Arch. Pathol. 79, 635.

Wissler, R.W. (1967). Circulation 36, 1.

Wolinsky, H. (1972). Circ. Res. 30, 301.

Wortman, B., Lee, K.T., Kim, D.N., Daoud, A.S., and Thomas, W.A. (1966). Exp. Mol. Pathol., Suppl. 3, 88.

Zemplenyi, T. (1968). "Enzyme Biochemistry of the Arterial Wall." Lloyd-Luke, London.

DISCUSSION FOLLOWING THE PRESENTATION BY L. ROBERT

Dr. Sobel: You make note of the decrease in proteoglycans. In skin we found a decrease with age in hyaluronic acid which was due to a decreased rate of synthesis from glucose. In addition, the molecular weight also decreased with age. Does this happen as well in the aorta?

Dr. Robert: We did not study this problem, but perhaps Dr. Dorfman can tell us.

Dr. Dorfman: The biggest change that occurs in skin occurs early in life. In embryonic skin there is relatively more hyaluronic acid than in adult skin. The change with age is not great. I don't know anything about a change in hyaluronic acid molecular weight in aorta with age.

Dr. Blohm: I would like clarification. Urea treatment liberated cholesterol from the elastin along with the structural glycoprotein; is that correct? In other words, in the cholesterol fed rats, was cholesterol attached to the structural glycoprotein or to the elastin or to both?

Dr. Robert: Here is the method of extraction we used. First we take the tissue and put it through the two cholesterol extraction procedures. Then the remainder is submitted to the extraction procedure shown on the graph; one step is with urea and the final residue is elastin. Then all these solutions are again extracted with chloroform-methanol. The urea extract was always found to contain very significant amounts of lipids, cholesterol as well as phospholipids. A preliminary characterization of this "bound lipid" fraction was described (Atherosclerosis 11, 7-25, 1970). Does this answer your question?

Dr. Blohm: I am not sure. I would like to know whether it was after the urea treatment step that much of the label in the cholesterol fed arteries appeared to be extracted. I would like to know your interpretation of whether the cholesterol was attached to the glycoprotein or to the elastin peptide.

Dr. Robert: Cholesterol is attached with both (see details in the paper and in Connec. Tissue Res. 1, 145-152, 1972). We don't know exactly how cholesterol is associated with the urea extracted glycoproteins, but we have some idea of how it is associated with elastin (see text of L. Robert's contribution and Nutr. Metabol. 15, 46-58, 1973). We recently undertook experiments to study the lipid glycoprotein interaction in order to understand how and why a significant quantity of lipids accompany the structural glyco-proteins in the urea extract (Atherosclerosis 11, 7-25, 1970).

Dr. Fleischmajer: With reference to aging and glycosamino-glycans, we recently published a paper in Biochemical Biophysical Acta (276: 265, 1972) where we used a different approach. We exhaustively extracted human dermis from newborns to age 96 years with 1 M NaCl solution and analyzed the glycosaminoglycans in the extract and residue. There was a significant reduction in glyco-saminoglycans from newborns to infants, with the levels remaining stable through age 60 years and dropping further from age 60 to 99 years. This last reduction referred to both hyaluronic and dermatan sulfate. No significant changes were noted in the residue.

Dr. Gilbert: Given either your model or the Weis-Fogh model of the sphere drop elastomer, how can we reconcile the fact that both the very polar glycoproteins and relatively nonpolar choles-terol esters are both attracted to the elastin?

Dr. Robert: The structural glycoprotein-microfibrils (Europ. J. Biochem. 21, 507-516, 1971), although more polar than elastin, have extensive hydrophobic interactions: they form extensive aggregates even after maleylation and carboxymethylation and physicochemical studies indicate that mainly hydrophobic inter-actions are involved in this self-association process. We assume that similar forces determine the strong elastin-glycoprotein interactions. It should be remembered, however, that the association between structural glycoprotein-microfibrils and elastin takes place first during the early embryonic phases of morphogenesis, that is between microfibrils and proelastin molecules. Proelastin is quite rich in lysine and electrostatic interactions between the positive charges of proelastin and the negative charges of structural glycoproteins (rich in aspartic and glutamic acids; Life Sci. 7, 493-497, 1968) does probably play an important role (for more details see Arch. Mal. du Coeur 62, 25-43, 1969; Exp. Geront. 5, 339-356, 1970). Later when the desmosine-crosslinks are formed and most lysine residues of proelastin "disappear", the glycoprotein-microfibrils are tightly entrapped in the elastin fibers or lamellae. At this stage elastin is predominantly hydrophobic at its surface as was shown by [85]Kr-absorption and microflow colorimetry using alkanols as "probes" (Biochim. Biophys. Acta. 214, 235-237, 1970; Biochim.

Biophys. Acta 251, 370-375, 1971). Therefore, I do not see any
contradiction between the interaction of elastin with the
structural glycoproteins on the one side and with apolar lipids
on the other.

ACID GLYCOSAMINOGLYCAN, COLLAGEN AND ELASTIN CONTENT OF NORMAL

ARTERY, FATTY STREAKS AND PLAQUES

Elspeth B. Smith

Department of Chemical Pathology, University of Aberdeen

Foresterhill, Aberdeen, Scotland

The intimal connective tissue plays a major role in atherosclerosis. It is directly concerned in the proliferative changes
leading to stenosis, and appears to be significantly involved in
lipid accumulation. The purpose of this paper is to relate the
available information on the amounts of acid glycosaminoglycans
(GAG), collagen, and elastin in the human intima to the amounts of
intact intimal lipoprotein and of bound or precipitated lipid. It
is clear that there are major gaps in our knowledge, and that this
is an area in which further work is urgently required.

Plasma constituents which cross the endothelium must come into
direct contact with the extracellular components of the subendothelial connective tissue. The concentrations of low density (LD)
lipoprotein, albumin, and other plasma proteins in the intima can
be measured by electrophoresis directly from the tissue into an
antibody-containing gel (Smith and Slater, 1971, 1972a). In the
average middle-aged subject $1.cm^2$ of lesion-free intima (average
thickness 200 μ) contains LD-lipoprotein equivalent to 10-20μl of
the subject's own plasma. Thus, the overall concentration of LD-
lipoprotein in the intima is virtually the same as the concentration in the plasma, but the intimal concentration of albumin is
only about one-seventh of the plasma concentration.

In lesion-free intima the absolute concentration of LD-
lipoprotein is very highly correlated with the subject's serum
lipid level, but the volume of plasma from which both LD-lipoprotein
and albumin are derived remains rather constant. This suggests
the concept that "whole plasma" may enter the intima, and that the
change in the ratios of the plasma components in intima results
from physical interactions affecting their rates of egress (Smith

and Slater, 1972a, 1973). Recent studies lend support to this idea; there appear to be much tighter cell junctions in arterial than in capillary endothelium, and proteins apparently cross the endothelium in pinocytotic vesicles. Whereas horseradish peroxidase and apo-HDL (molecular weights 40,000 and 16,000) rapidly appear throughout the media, LD- and HD-lipoproteins (molecular weights 2×10^6 and 2×10^5) remain in the sub-endothelial layers (Schwartz and Benditt, 1972; Stein and Stein, 1973).

In large human fibrous or mixed lesions containing a central pool of amorphous "atheroma" lipid it appears that all or most of the cholesterol ester is derived directly from plasma (Smith and Slater, 1972b). In the "gelatinous" lesions which seem to be the precursors of fibrous plaques (Haust, 1971; Geer and Haust, 1972) there is a two to fourfold increase in the overall concentration of intact LD-lipoprotein and a tenfold increase in the deep layers compared with lesion-free intima from the same subject (Smith and Slater, 1973). This retention of lipoprotein appears to be of great significance in lesion development; presumably it reflects interaction with connective tissue elements, and an understanding of the factors involved must increase our understanding of atherogenesis.

CONCENTRATIONS OF CONNECTIVE TISSUE COMPONENTS

The literature on connective tissue components, and on the glycosaminoglycans in particular, is both extensive and confusing; consequently, this review includes only quantitative data on samples of normal intima and intimal lesions from human aorta.

Total Acid Glycosaminoglycan (GAG) Concentration

Total GAG concentrations in normal intima and their change with age are summarized in Table I. Results for three groups lie within the range 2.5-3.5 mg/100 mg defatted dry tissue, but two are lower - the group of Negroes studied by Kumar et al. (1967a), and the group of Japanese studied by Nakamura et al. (1968). There is no consistent change with age, and in quantitative terms the GAG fraction is a very minor intimal component.

The changes in lesions are summarized in Table II where the concentration in the lesion is expressed as a percentage of the concentration in normal intima. Most authors find total GAG concentration slightly increased in fatty streaks, slightly decreased in uncomplicated fibrous plaques, and substantially decreased in advanced plaques. Pernis and Clerici (1957) also found a highly significant reduction in intima + media preparations of "hyaline plaques".

TABLE I.   TOTAL GLYCOSAMINOGLYCAN CONCENTRATION IN NORMAL INTIMA

Age Range and Numbers	Mean mg/100 mg*	Change with Age: mg/decade	Authors
1½ - 80 (20)	3.4 (A)	+0.14 p< 0.001	Bertelsen (1962)
11 - 75 (23)	2.6 (B)	-0.11 NS	Smith (1965)
½ - 64 (5)	2.4 (C)	+0.05	Klynstra et al. (1967)
2 - 17[†] (11)	0.8	+0.40	‡Kumar et al. (1967)
17[†]- 42 (5)	0.9 (C)	-0.16	
0 - 79 (23)	1.0 (C)	+0.04 NS	Nakamura et al. (1968)

*Concentrations were based on different units:
  A = Fat-free, decalcified dry tissue
  B = Total protein
  C = Fat-free dry tissue (not decalcified)
†Contained 5% fatty streaks
‡Estimated from authors' graphs

TABLE II.   CONCENTRATION OF TOTAL GLYCOSAMINOGLYCANS IN ATHERO-
SCLEROTIC LESIONS EXPRESSED AS PERCENTAGE OF THE NORMAL
LEVEL

Fatty Streak or WHO Grade I	Uncomplicated Fibrous Plaques or WHO Grade II	Calcified or Ulcerated Plaques, or WHO Grade III	Authors
-	104 (4)*	95 (6)	Bertelsen (1962)
116 (19)	94 (7)	41 (5)	Smith (1965)
110 (13)	85 (20)	33 (6)	Klynstra et al. (1967)
-	68 (4)	-	Nakamura et al. (1968)
114(31)			Sanwald et al. (1971)
-	99 (10)	85 (9)	Murata and Oshima (1971)

*Number of samples

TABLE III.   MUCOPOLYSACCHARIDE/GLYCOSAMINOGLYCAN NOMENCLATURE

MPS		GAG
Hyaluronic Acid	HA	Same
Heparitin Sulphate	HS	Heparan Sulphate
Chondroitin Sulphate A	CSA-A	Chondroitin 4-sulphate
Chondroitin Sulphate B	CSA-B	Dermatan Sulphate
Chondroitin Sulphate C	CSA-C	Chondroitin 6-sulphate

Distribution of GAG Fractions

The glycosaminoglycans are a heterogeneous group with considerable differences in physicochemical characteristics, including their ability to form complexes with lipoproteins and other large molecules. Consequently, changes in the ratio of the components might have greater significance than changes in overall concentration. Several workers have fractionated the GAG from normal intima using three main methods.

1. Resistance to hyaluronidase digestion followed by measurement of the glucosamine/galactosamine ratio in digested and resistant fractions
2. Fractionation on Dowex 1 resin
3. Electrophoretic separation

Two different nomenclatures are in use (Jeanloz, 1960), and in order to avoid confusion the equivalent names are summarized in Table III.

The percentage distribution found by different workers in normal intima is shown in Table IV. With the exception of hyaluronic acid, which tends to be high in very young children, there seems to be no consistent variation with age, but there are alarming variations between laboratories. Thus, the New Orleans group (Kumar et al., 1967a; Dalferes et al., 1971), using Dowex columns, found more than twice as much HS as the other groups. Nakamura et al. (1968) find two to four times more HA than the other groups, and CSA-B + CSA-C ranges from 48 to 80%. The distribution of these differences suggests that they may arise from the methodology rather than the material.

A comprehensive study on changes in lesions seems to have been published only by Klynstra et al. (1967). In Table V it can

TABLE IV.   PERCENTAGE DISTRIBUTION OF GAG COMPONENTS IN NORMAL INTIMA

Age Range and Numbers		HA	HS	CSA - B	CSA - C	Authors and Method*	
3 - 64	(4)	10.7	21.3	5.8	62.2	Klynstra et al. 1967	(1)
2 - 42	(16)	14	38	19	29 †	Kumar et al. 1967	(2)
0 - 72	(23)	33.3	16.8	←------- 48.6 -------→		Nakamura et al. 1968	(3)
12 - 18	(10)	6	41	←------- 53† -------→		Dalferes et al. 1971	(2)
Unspecified	(31)	4.3	16.5	←------- 79.2 -------→		Sanwald et al. 1971	(3)

*Methods: 1. Hyaluronidase digestion + glucosamine/galactosamine ratio
             2. Dowex 1 columns
             3. Electrophoresis
†Estimated from author's graphs

TABLE V.   PERCENTAGE DISTRIBUTION OF GAG COMPONENTS IN ATHERO-
SCLEROTIC LESIONS

Tissue and No. of Samples		HA	HS	CSA-B	CSA-C	Authors and Method*
Normal	(3)	9.6	20.4	6.5	63.5	Klynstra et al.
Fatty Streaks	(4)	6.7	24.8	4.0	64.5	(1967) (1)
Plaques	(2)	8.8	18.9	5.7	66.6	
Ulcerated Lesions	(2)	8.0	2.8	1.8	87.7	
Normal	(10)	6	42	52†		Dalferes et al.
60% Fatty Streaks	(1)	6	40	54		(1971) (2)
Normal	(31)	4.3	16.5	79.2		Sanwald et al.
Grade I + II Lesions	(31)	3.9	16.1	80.0		(1971) (3)

*Methods: 1. Hyaluronidase digestion + glucosamine/galactosamine ratio.
            2. Dowex 1 columns.
            3. Electrophoresis.
†Estimated from authors' graphs

be seen that there is no marked change in distribution in fatty
streaks or plaques, but in ulcerated plaques there is a striking
fall in HS, and a marked fall in CSA-B, so that CSA-C rises to 88%
of the total GAG; however, the actual concentration of CSA-C is
only half the concentration in normal intima. From the graphs
published by Dalferes et al. (1971) there seemed to be no change
in composition in an intima with 60% involvement with fatty streaks,
and Sanwald et al. (1971) find no difference between normal and
Grade I + II lesions in 31 aortas. The graphs presented by Kumar
et al. (1967b) may indicate an increase in proportion of CSA-B in
fatty streaks. This slender evidence suggests that marked changes
in distribution of GAG components occur only in advanced lesions;
but it is possible that qualitative changes in sulphation, acetyla-
tion, degree of polymerization or protein binding may be of equal
or greater importance in atherogenesis.

Relationship Between the Concentrations of GAG, Intact LD-
Lipoprotein and Deposited Cholesterol

There is a remarkable change in the ratios of plasma constituents between the plasma and intimal compartments (Table VI).
This is the reverse of the change expected from capillary transu-
dates, suggesting, as discussed in the introduction, that it might
arise from uptake of whole plasma followed by preferential retention or retardation in the intima.

Intimal GAG form complexes with LD-lipoproteins (Amenta and
Waters, 1960; Gerö et al., 1961; Bihari-Varga and Vegh, 1967),which
are probably electrostatic and may be highly dependent on their

TABLE VI.   PLASMA CONSTITUENTS IN INTIMA

| | Concentration in Plasma mg/100 ml | Ratios in Plasma and Intima | | |
| | | | Intima | |
		Plasma	Normal	"Gelatinous"
Albumin	4,000	14	2	1
LD-Lipoprotein	300	1	1	1
Fibrinogen	300	1	1/3	1/2

TABLE VII.   CHANGES IN THE CONCENTRATIONS OF INTACT LD-LIPOPROTEIN, CONNECTIVE TISSUE COMPONENTS AND "DEPOSITED" CHOLESTEROL IN EARLY LESIONS

| | Percentage of the Normal Level | | | |
	Fatty Streaks		"Gelatinous" Thickenings	
LD-Lipoprotein	28	(14)*	196	(17)
Total GAG	116	(19)	91	(7)
Collagen	111	(19)	117	(7)
"Deposited" Cholesterol	1319	(14)	138	(17)

*Number of pairs of samples

ionic environment (Srinivasan et al., 1970; Iverius, 1972). Furthermore, the very large LD-lipoprotein molecule may be unable to enter the GAG gel, or it may be retarded within it. It is therefore relevant to examine the measured concentrations of LD-lipoprotein, connective tissue components and deposited cholesterol in early lesions (Table VII).

In normal intima the concentration of total GAG is about 2mg/100mg dry tissue (Table I); the dry weight is about 15% of the wet weight, so the concentration of GAG in the wet intima is about 3mg/ml. This is comparable with the concentrations required to precipitate LD-lipoprotein from plasma in vitro (Bihari-Varga and Vegh, 1967; Srinivasan et al., 1970). In fatty streaks the concentration of intact LD-lipoprotein measured either by electrophoresis directly from the minced intima into an antibody-containing gel (Smith and Slater, 1972a) or in saline extracts (Smith and Slater, 1970) is about a quarter of the normal level (Table VII). Deposited cholesterol is increased five to thirteenfold, but this is mainly intracellular cholesterol with a high proportion of ester which has probably been esterified in situ (Smith et al., 1967). It is difficult to believe that a 16% increase in GAG could increase cellular uptake of cholesterol tenfold. It is also difficult to understand what role it could be playing in the massive reduction in LD-lipoprotein. GAG-LD-lipoprotein complexes are reported to have a high or unchanged electrophoretic mobility in barbiturate buffer at pH 8.6, and the lipoprotein retains its antigenic properties (Gerö et al., 1961; Srinivasan et al., 1970). At pH 8.6 the complex will probably dissociate, but even if it does not, it should be measurable in both the immunoelectrophoretic and immunodiffusion systems. It is difficult to reconcile the finding of Srinivasan et al. (1972) that much more GAG-LD-lipoprotein complex can be extracted from fatty streaks than from normal intima with the results shown in Table VII. Possibly there is confusion in nomenclature, and their "fatty streaks" are not the fat-filled cell lesions which constitute the "fatty streaks" in Table VII. A possible explanation of the low levels in fatty streaks is that LD-lipoprotein is destroyed by the cells which are taking up cholesterol; the slight increase in GAG might be a by-product of their increased metabolic activity.

In the "gelatinous" lesions the concentration of LD-lipoprotein is doubled and there is a slight increase in deposited cholesterol in the form of fine, extracellular perifibrous droplets (Smith and Slater, 1973). The GAG concentration is slightly reduced, so it is difficult to postulate that increased complex formation is responsible for the increase in lipoprotein. It is possible that a reduction in GAG concentration might reduce the steric exclusion of the LD-lipoprotein from the gel, thus allowing it to enter the tissue spaces more readily, but 10% seems a small reduction in gel concentration to cause a 100% increase in the entry of lipoprotein. Clearly, there is no simple relationship between total GAG, intima lipoprotein and deposition of cholesterol.

The Concentration of Collagen in Aortic Intima

Collagen is a major component of intima that has received little attention. The findings in three studies of "normal" intima are summarized in Table VIII - there is disagreement on the extent and significance of the increase of collagen with age. Surprisingly, there appear to be only two studies on intimal collagen in different types of lesion (Table IX). As might be expected, there is a massive increase in advanced fibrous plaques; in the "gelatinous" lesions there is only a small increase in concentration. In this laboratory we have frequently observed "gelatinous" and very early fibrous plaques with thick collagen bundles which seem to be suffused with diffuse sudanophilic material (Smith et al., 1968) and

TABLE VIII.   COLLAGEN CONCENTRATION IN NORMAL INTIMA

Age Range and Numbers	Concentration of Collagen mg/100 mg*			Authors
	Youngest	Oldest	Mean	
11 - 90 (58)	16.5	26.1	19.8 (A)	Levene and Poole (1962)
1½ - 80 (20)	23.2	40.5	31.8 (B)	Bertelson (1962)
	p < 0.001			
11 - 75 (23)	23.1	27.0	24.8 (C)	Smith (1965)
	NS			

*Concentrations were based on different units:
    A = Whole, dry intima (including fat and calcium)
    B = Fat-free, decalcified dry tissue
    C = Total protein

TABLE IX.   THE CONCENTRATION OF COLLAGEN IN DIFFERENT TYPES OF LESION

Type of Lesion and Numbers	Lesion Collagen		Authors
	mg/100 mg*	% of Normal	
"Atheromata"			
Early (21)	38.4	143	Noble et al.
Advanced (25)	46.5	172	(1957)
Fatty Streaks (19)	26.3	111	Smith (1965)
"Gelatinous" (7)	29.0	117	
Fibrous Plaques			
Non-Calcified (7)	41.0	164	
Calcified (5)	60.7	254	

*mg/100 mg total protein

TABLE X.   THE EFFECT OF TISSUE CALCIFICATION ON APPARENT COLLAGEN CONCENTRATION IN ADVANCED LESIONS

Apparent Collagen Concentration		
mg/100 mg Total Protein	mg/100 mg Lipid-Extracted Dry Tissue	
60.7	27.8	Smith (1965)
51.8	24.7	Anastassiades et al. (1972)

are associated with high levels of intact LD-lipoprotein. In some
fibrous lesions which appear macroscopically yellow, the collagen
bundles are densely coated with lipid. It seems probable that collagen is by no means inert in lipid accumulation.

In some studies there is apparently little increase in collagen
in advanced lesions; this is probably an artifact arising from tissue calcification. The effect of tissue calcium is illustrated in
Table X with data from two studies in which the results were presented on the basis of protein and of lipid-extracted dry tissue
weight. Collagen has increased to 50-60% of the total protein, but
on a weight basis it is still within the normal range.

The Concentration of Elastin in Aortic Intima

There is a very large amount of elastin in the aortic media;
thus any changes occurring in the intima will be masked in intima
+ media preparations. There appears to be only one study on elastin
in isolated intima (Kramsch et al., 1971), and the findings are summarized in Table XI. The elastin concentration falls progressively
with aging and with increasing severity of lesions, suggesting that
"elastic hyperplasia" is not playing a significant role in atherogenesis in the human aorta.

Kramsch et al. (1971) describe their samples as comprising "the
entire intima and a small portion of adherent media." The implications of this, and the problem of what is meant by "intima" are illustrated in Figure 1. In children and young adolescents the endothelium lies very close to the internal elastic lamina (IEL). Presumably the "intima" is the very thin layer of endothelium and connective tissue lying on the luminal side of the IEL, and it is clear
that inclusion of even one or two elastic laminae means that a major
part of the tissue sample will be media. In the second decade the
IEL appears to fragment and stain less darkly with Verhoeff's elastic
stain, and adjacent underlying laminae also start to fragment; in
slightly older age groups a deeper lamina seems to take over the
function of "internal elastic lamina." Thus, if the intima is
defined as the zone on the luminal side of the new IEL, it appears
to undergo progressive thickening with age, mainly as a result of
erosion of elastic laminae, leaving cells and collagen fibers in
situ, rather than as a result of hyperplasia. In the 35-40 age
group three "intimal" zones can often be distinguished with the
Verhoeff and van Gieson stains - (1) a luminal zone containing collagen fibers and cells but no stainable elastic tissue; (2) a middle
layer containing pale brown-staining "ghosts" of fragmentary elastic
laminae; and (3) a deep layer containing dark-staining fragmentary
elastic laminae which have a characteristic appearance of an un-
coiling spring (Figure 2). In normal intima perifibrous lipid droplets are particularly associated with the fragmentary elastic

TABLE XI.   CONCENTRATION OF ELASTIN IN NORMAL INTIMA AND LESIONS
            (Kramsch et al., 1971)

Grade of Atherosclerosis	No.	Avg. Age	mg Elastin/100 mg Decalcified Dry Tissue	
			Normal	Lesions
0	5	23	20.3	-
I	5	45	19.7	17.1
II	6	60	18.2	10.0
III	5	65	14.7	6.7

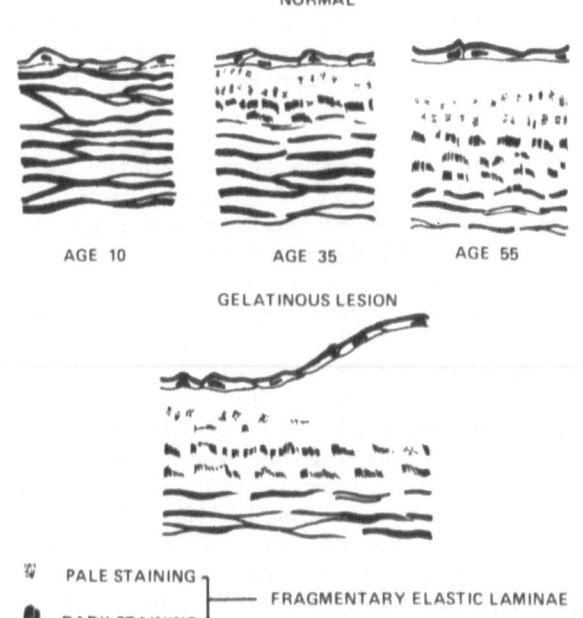

Fig. 1. Diagramatic representation of fragmentary elastic laminae
in thickening intima. The endothelium is at the top. Natural
strip planes can usually be found along the first (nearest the
lumen) dark-staining fragmentary elastic lamina and the first
mainly intact lamina.

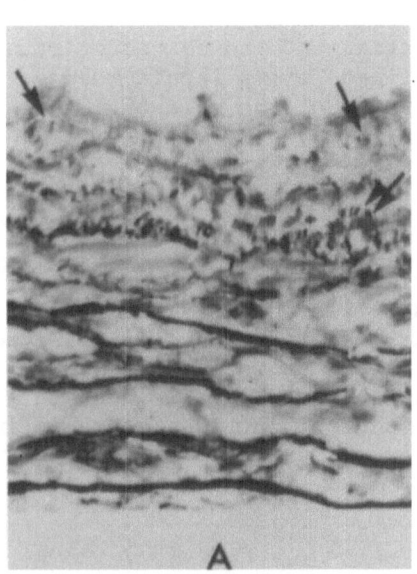
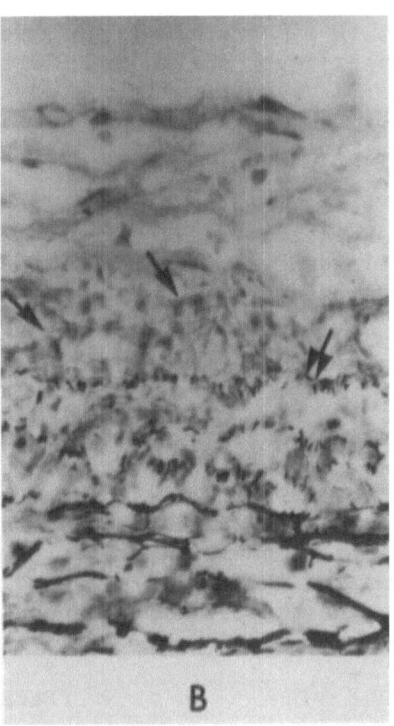

Fig. 2. Photomicrographs of fragmentary elastic laminae in
thickening intima; A. Male aged 37. B. Male aged 58. Pale
brown-staining "ghosts" of fragmentary elastic laminae (arrow).
Dark-staining fragmentary elastic laminae (double arrows).
(Verhoeff/van Gieson: x 600). (Reduced 30% for reproduction).

laminae. These observations closely parallel those of Taylor
(1953); fragmentation of elastic tissue was reviewed by Baló (1963).
In early fibrous lesions a cellular and collagenous hyperplasia
occurs in the luminal zone, and it appears to be only in more
advanced lesions that there is further erosion of elastic laminae.

If the tissue samples analyzed contain one or two intact
elastic laminae there must inevitably be a decrease in apparent
elastin concentration with increase in intimal thickness. But if
an analysis of pure intima is attempted, where should the boundary
be drawn? The first natural strip plane lies along the most superficial dark-staining fragmentary elastic lamina (Smith and Slater,
1972a, 1973), so that the fibers in the upper layer are (histologically) mainly collagen, or a mixture of collagen and "ghosts" of
fragmentary elastic laminae. The second natural strip plane is on
the first intact elastic lamina, so that the lower layer contains
dark-staining fragmentary elastic laminae. Perifibrous lipid droplets are often prominent in this zone, but the concentration of

intact LD-lipoprotein is only about 15% of the concentration in
the upper layer (Smith and Slater, 1973). Thus, either these
fragmentary elastic laminae have a low affinity for LD-lipoprotein
or they have a very high affinity, causing irreversible binding or
destruction. This latter idea would fit the histological findings.

Measurement of both the concentration and the characteristics
of the elastin in these accurately defined layers should make a
valuable contribution to our understanding of the role of elastin
in atherogenesis.

SUMMARY

It is clear that there are major gaps in our basic knowledge
of all the connective tissue elements in lesion-free intima and
in isolated intimal lesions of precisely defined histological type.
This may partly arise because the existing methodology is not
adequate for analysis of very small samples, but until accurate
information is available the role of connective tissue elements in
atherogenesis will remain speculative.

REFERENCES

Amenta, J.S., and Waters, L.L. (1960). Yale J. Biol. Med. 33,
112.

Anastassiades, T., Anastassiades, P. A., and Denstedt, O.F. (1972).
Biochim. Biophys. Acta 261, 418.

Balo, J. (1963). Int. Rev. Connect. Tissue Res. 1, 241.

Bertelsen, S. (1962). J. Gerontol. 17, 24.

Bihari-Varga, M., and Vegh, M. (1967). Biochim. Biophys. Acta
144, 202.

Dalferes, E.R., Ruiz, H., Kumar, V., Radhakrishnamurthy, B., and
Berenson, G.S. (1971). Atherosclersis 13, 121.

Geer, J.C., and Haust, M.D. (1972). "Smooth Muscle Cells in
Atherosclerosis." Monographs on Atherosclerosis, Vol. 2.
S. Karger, Basel.

Gerö, S., Gergely, J., Dévényi, T., Jakab, L., Székely, J., and
Virág, S. (1961). J. Atheroscler. Res. 1, 67.

Haust, M.D. (1971) Hum. Pathol. 2, 1.

Iverius, P.-H. (1972). J. Biol. Chem. 247, 2607.

Jeanloz, R. (1960). Arthritis Rheum. 3, 233.

Klynstra, F.B., Böttcher, C.J.F., Van Melsen, J.A., and Van der Laan, E.J. (1967). J. Atheroscler. Res. 7, 301.

Kramsch, D.M., Franzblau, C., and Hollander, W. (1971). J. Clin. Invest. 50, 1666.

Kumar, V., Berenson, G.S., Ruiz, H., Dalferes, E.R., and Strong, J.P. (1967a). J. Atheroscler. Res. 7, 573.

Kumar, V., Berenson, G.S., Ruiz, H., Dalferes, E.R., and Strong, J.P. (1967b). J. Atheroscler. Res. 7, 583.

Levene, C.I., and Poole, J.C.F. (1962). Brit. J. Exp. Pathol. 43, 469.

Murata, K., and Oshima, Y. (1971). Atherosclerosis 14, 121.

Nakamura, T., Tokita, K., Tateno, S., Kotoku, T., and Ohba, T. (1968). J. Atheroscler. Res. 8, 891.

Noble, N.L., Boucek, R.J., and Kao, K.Y.T. (1957). Circulation 15, 366.

Pernis, B., and Clerici, E. (1957). Experientia 13, 351.

Sanwald, R., Ritz, E., and Wiese, G. (1971). Atherosclerosis 13, 247.

Schwartz, S.M., and Benditt, E.P. (1972). Amer. J. Pathol. 66, 241.

Smith, E.B. (1965). J. Atheroscler. Res. 5, 241.

Smith, E.B., Evans, P.H., and Downham, M.D. (1967). J. Atheroscler. Res. 7, 171.

Smith, E.B., and Slater, R.S. (1970). Atherosclerosis 11, 417.

Smith, E.B., and Slater, R.S. (1971). Biochem. J. 123, 39p. (Abstract).

Smith, E.B., and Slater, R.S. (1972a). Lancet 1, 463.

Smith, E.B., and Slater, R. S. (1972b). Atherosclerosis 15, 37.

Smith, E.B., and Slater, R.S. (1973). In "Atherogenesis: Initiating Factors." (R. Porter and R. Knight, eds.). pp. 39-62. Ciba Foundation Symposium, 12.

Smith, E.B., Slater, R.S., and Chu, P.K. (1968). J. Atheroscler. Res. 8, 399.

Srinivasan, S.R., Dolan, P., Radhakrishnamurthy, B., and Berenson, G.S. (1972). Atherosclerosis 16, 95.

Srinivasan, S.R., Lopez-S., A., Radhakrishnamurthy, B., and Berenson, G.S. (1970). Atherosclerosis 12, 321.

Stein, Y., and Stein, O. (1973). Atherogenesis: Initiating Factors. Ciba Foundation Symposium, 12, 165.

Taylor, H.E. (1953). Amer. J. Pathol. 29, 871.

DISCUSSION FOLLOWING THE PRESENTATION BY ELSPETH B. SMITH

Dr. Kramsch: We have looked at both animal lesions and human lesions and I would suggest that the splitting and fragmentation of elastica which one sees with the light or electron microscope during atherogenesis in vessels might be due to synthesis of new elastic tissue. One can see that there are many new young elastic fibers in lesions which would give the appearance in paraffin sections, such as you showed, of fragmented elastic fibers, where in actual fact they may be new elements.

Dr. Smith: Have you looked at this through a wide age range, because looking through a wide age range it appears as if the media is retreating, rather than laying down new laminae.

Dr. Kramsch: I don't think they are well developed laminae at all. I think they are quite irregularly dispersed elastic fibers. I would agree there. We certainly have not looked at the wide range that you have looked at, but in the human and animal lesions that we have studied there is extensive new elastic fiber formation.

Dr. Bentley: There is a tremendous variation in the concentration of collagen and elastin as you go along the aorta, so that in the area of the renal arteries, for example, there is about twice as much collagen as there is in the arch and there is half as much elastin as there is in the arch. The same thing may hold true for the types and the total amount of mucopolysaccharide. I wondered if you have taken this into account, and are all the analyses that you present, which relate to whether the tissue has fatty streaks, whether the tissue is from a 75 year old or a 20 year old, all from the same location, because if they are not, you have the naturally built-in variation.

Dr. Smith: In most of the published results there is no indication of where the tissue came from. I think a good deal of this variation comes through the differing relationships of intimal thickness and medial thickness in the different regions. If you take abdominal regions, you will find much more collagen and much less elastin because the media is thinner. If you work on stripped intima, wherever your stripping plane, then you do to some extent overcome this difficulty, but this is obviously a very important point. All results from our laboratory report stripped intima from descending thoracic and upper abdominal aorta (above the visceral branches).

Dr. Tracy: Dr. Smith, I am fascinated by your findings that a low concentration of plasma lipoprotein appears to be a normal constituent of healthy arterial ground substance. Do I misstate your findings by interpreting it that way?

Dr. Smith: No, I don't think you are, but of course one can question if the diffusely thickened intima in older age groups is normal. Even if it is not normal it is the arterial lining which is, in fact, found in the 35 to 40 year old human, and it is the lining on which the circulating lipoprotein impinges. We have been trying to get a line on this by looking at young people. In two children aged 8, in one of whom serum cholesterol was known to be 100 mg% I could detect no lipoprotein at all. In two 17 year old children from which I did not get blood samples and one 14 year old with hypercholesterolemia there was only about a tenth of the amount that one would find in a 45 year old; but at age 29 we found the expected concentration so I think this is highly correlated with age up to somewhere around 30. Above age 30 the correlation with serum cholesterol level is so high that this mainly blanks out the age effect. I don't know whether this low concentration in young people results because the endothelium is less leaky or because you need a sort of sponge layer of sub-endothelial connective tissue in which to accumulate lipoprotein.

Dr. Tracy: Possibly another way to get at that same question is to examine ground substance of many different tissues besides artery. I did some tentative work some years back which seemed to imply that low density lipoprotein of plasma may be a normal constituent of ground substance in other tissue besides the aorta. I was wondering if you have given any consideration to that possibility.

Dr. Smith: Well, I haven't actually measured lipoprotein in any other tissue, but I did examine the composition and amount of perifibrous lipid in the sclera of the eye, and it is extremely similar, so I think you are right.

MUCOPOLYSACCHARIDE-LIPOPROTEIN COMPLEXES IN ATHEROSCLEROTIC AORTA

G.S. Berenson, S.R. Srinivasan, B. Radhakrishnamurthy,
    and E.R. Dalferes, Jr.
Departments of Medicine and Biochemistry, Louisiana State
    University School of Medicine, New Orleans,
    Louisiana

The carbohydrate macromolecules present in the arterial wall represent families of complex compounds (Berenson et al., 1971). Although widely distributed throughout the body in all mesenchymal structures, the macromolecules are particularly important to the cardiovascular system. Most studies, including our own, over the past two decades have served largely to describe connective tissue compounds taxonomically, and have not been able to clearly define their function. That connective tissue elements form an integral part of the cardiovascular system is fundamental; still, the task remains to bridge the gap between morphological, biochemical changes of connective tissues, and the functional nature of these changes.

Virchow (1856) suggested that a nonspecific injury to an arterial vessel wall is followed by an inflammatory process exuding "mucous" substances that combine with fatty deposits in the intima. Virchow considered this interaction the early stage of atherosclerosis, and numerous investigations over the past twenty years have not significantly advanced his view. What are these mucous substances and what role do they play in the pathogenesis of atherosclerosis?

Connective tissue has been considered only as an anatomic entity creating an architectural system for structure and support. Now we must advance to the concept that connective tissue is vital, has a dynamic metabolic process, and serves many purposes. Sophisticated chemistry recognizes that carbohydrate macromolecules composing cardiovascular connective tissue represent families of units with different chemical and physical properties, as well as

various biological functions which can be influenced by numerous
basic factors, e.g., hormones or stress. We are just beginning to
slowly unravel the complex nature of the blood vessel chemistry;
our goal is to make sense of the presence of these carbohydrate
macromolecules in atherosclerosis.

EARLY OBSERVATIONS INDICATING IMPORTANCE OF MUCOPOLYSACCHARIDES
IN ATHEROSCLEROSIS

The early histologic studies of fatty streaks suggested that
an accumulation of acid mucopolysaccharides (MPS) at the base of
a lesion was one of the earliest changes of atherosclerosis.
Subsequently, numerous investigators studying variations in MPS
in atherosclerosis by both chemical and histochemical techniques
have produced conflicting reports. Both increases and decreases
in MPS have been reported in natural and experimental atherosclerosis. However, the histochemical observations of Rhinehart (1954),
Taylor (1953), and Bunting and Bunting (1953) clearly indicated
the importance of MPS in the development of the early atheromatous
lesion. Having examined the early lesion of atherosclerosis, the
fatty streak, Gresham and Howard (1961) pointed out the presence
of an admixture of lipid and a considerable amount of sulfated
MPS (the usual consensus). Electron microscopy (Hauss et al.,
1969; Ross and Glomset, 1973) has also supported such findings,
but unfortunately studies by microscopic techniques cannot adequately
specify nor quantitate these individual compounds. The chief
advantage of microscopic techniques, however, is a method for the
localization of changes within the blood vessel wall.

Actually, Mörner isolated MPS from aortic tissue as early as
1895, and Dr. K. Meyer and his co-workers defined the basic chemistry of the MPS during the 1950's (Meyer et al., 1956). The MPS,
all presumably found in the arterial wall, are an interesting

TABLE I.   CLASSIFICATION OF GLYCOSAMINOGLYCANS, ACID MUCOPOLY-
           SACCHARIDES (MPS)

I. NONSULFATED	II. SULFATED
Hyaluronic Acid	Chondroitin 4-Sulfate
Chondroitin	Chondroitin 6-Sulfate
	Dermatan Sulfate
	Heparin
	Heparitin Sulfate
	Keratan Sulfate

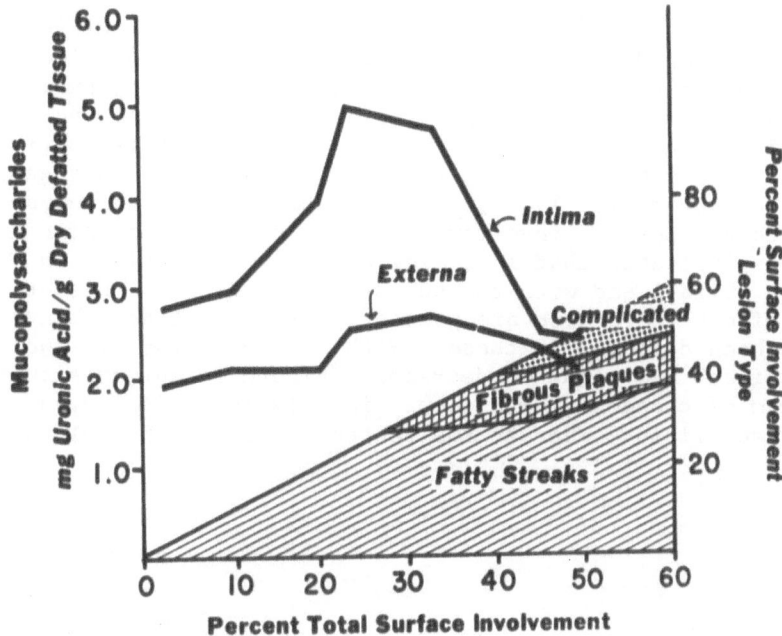

Fig. 1. Acid mucopolysaccharides (MPS) from aorta with varying
types and extent of atherosclerotic involvement. The initial
values are from aortas without significant or grossly visible
lesions. Note the greater content in intimal tissue (intima and
approximately the inner 1/3 of media) compared to the remaining
outer wall, and the greater change of MPS content in the intima
with disease.

group of heteropolysaccharides that consist of repeating units of
hexosamine and hexuronic acid, with acetyl and sulfate groups
occurring in variable amounts. Depending upon the presence,
absence, or low content of sulfate, the compounds can be divided
into the two types shown in Table I. For quantitation of specific
MPS, chemical techniques have been necessary.

Our early efforts to relate changes of MPS to the degree of
atherosclerosis are summarized in Figure 1, which illustrates an
increase in the content of MPS with the early changes of atherosclerotic involvement consistent with most histochemical studies.
These changes occur mainly in the intimal region at the site of
the atherosclerotic disease. Later, the MPS content decreases
with more advanced involvement of the arterial wall. Also, the
concentration of MPS in the intimal region is greater than in the

outer layers of the aorta, and the MPS in the intimal tissue are
largely sulfated MPS (Berenson, 1959). As noted in previous
studies, the content of mucopolysaccharides increases physiolo-
gically as an individual matures (Kumar et al., 1967a), but with
the onset of atherosclerosis a further increase occurs as if the
stage had been set earlier for the development of the disease
process (Kumar et al., 1967b). Quantitation of the different MPS
related to the surface involvement of the aorta by specific types
of lesions indicates that increases occur particularly with
heparitin sulfate and with the chondroitin sulfates. Lesser
amounts of other MPS also are present, but significant changes
have not been detected in these. With advanced disease, the
content of all MPS tends to decrease. Figure 2 indicates that
a spectrum of changes of MPS occurs in relation to collagen,
calcium, and lipid. Whereas the content of collagen, calcium,

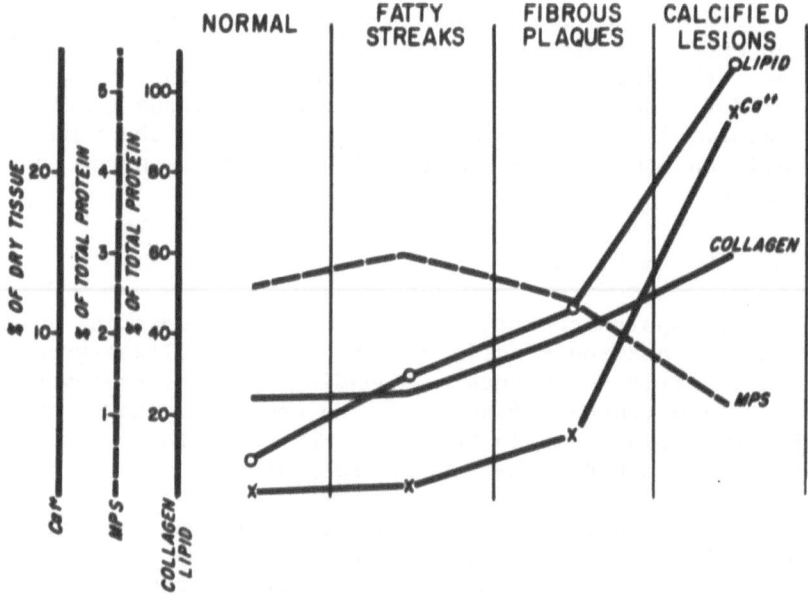

Fig. 2. Comparative changes of lipid, Ca++, collagen, and MPS with
different types and extent of atherosclerotic involvement of the
aorta presented schematically. An interrelationship of the various
components is suggested. Elastin, equally important but more difficult to quantitate, is not shown.

and lipid increases during the transition from normal to fatty
streak to fibrous plaque lesions and finally to complicated and
calcified lesions, the MPS increase in the early lesions (Dalferes
et al., 1971) and perhaps with the fibrous plaque stage, but
ultimately, with more advanced disease, their concentration
decreases. Elastin should also be considered an important fibrous
structure in this scheme because of lipoprotein binding (Kramsch
and Hollander, 1973).

The observations of isotope incorporation reflect the dynamic
nature and complexity of the biochemical changes occurring in the
arterial wall, but do not indicate a role. All these studies are
basic and important, but also frustrating inasmuch as they offer
little toward understanding the functional role of MPS in atherosclerosis.

COMPLEXING OF MUCOPOLYSACCHARIDES AND LIPOPROTEINS

More recently we have been involved in studies which appear
to have bearing on the role of MPS and the pathogenesis of atherosclerotic lesions. For some time it has been known that highly
charged anionic compounds like sulfated polysaccharides, e.g.,
heparin and dextran sulfate, in the presence of divalent cations
will complex with serum lipoproteins. Burstein and Samaille (1955),
Bernfeld et al. (1960), Cornwell and Kruger (1961), Iverius (1972),
and our group (Srinivasan et al., 1970) have studied this complexing. Amenta and Waters (1960-1961), Tracy et al. (1961), and
Bihari-Varga and Vegh (1967) have suggested that similar complexes
might occur in the arterial wall. Investigators have also shown
that lipoproteins are present in the arterial wall and are increased
with the development of fatty streaks (Smith et al., 1967; Smith
et al., 1968).

In an effort to approach this problem, we used as a model the
complexing of MPS with serum lipoproteins and noted that at a low
ionic strength in the presence of Ca^{++} and heparin, serum β and pre-
β lipoproteins can be selectively precipitated from serum (Srinivasan
et al., 1970; Berenson et al., 1972b). During this precipitation
a turbidity results which is quantitative with the amount of
cholesterol precipitated in this system as well as with the concentration of β and pre-β lipoproteins. Analyses using the analytical
ultracentrifuge have shown a close correlation between the precipitation of the β lipoprotein group with quantitation by the ultracentrifuge (Berenson et al., 1972a). In addition, electrophoretic
analysis of isolated serum lipoprotein - Ca^{++}-heparin complexes
indicates the precipitation of the β lipoprotein group exclusive
of α lipoproteins. Similarly, immunoelectrophoretic studies of
these complexes also indicate the specificity of this complexing.

Further studies of the effects of other cations on the interaction
of lipoproteins and heparin to form insoluble complexes indicate
the potential of a variety of ions to complex. These studies
have shown a binding of zinc > copper > cobalt > manganese > iron >
and > magnesium (Srinivasan et al., 1970). However, precipitates
with some of the ions contain proteins in addition to the β and
pre-β lipoproteins. The studies of the different cations suggest
that a particular selectivity of this precipitation of the two
lipoprotein classes occurs with Ca^{++} and Mg^{++}.

Studies of interaction with lecithin isolated from egg yolk
in this system indicate that the binding of MPS and divalent ions
occurs with phospholipids. Further studies on the effects of
varying Ca^{++} and heparin concentrations on the complexing of the
β lipoproteins have shown that at a high concentration of Ca^{++},
maximum precipitation of protein material containing cholesterol
and uronic acid can be obtained. At lower concentrations of Ca^{++}
an incomplete precipitation occurs. At low Ca^{++} levels the complex
material becomes soluble when higher heparin concentrations are
used, and it is suggested that at this point complexing may still
occur, but in a soluble state. Figure 3 illustrates the variations
of concentrations of Ca^{++} and heparin on the precipitation of
serum lipoproteins. It also may be noted that precipitation of
the complex reaches a minimum even with very small quantities of
heparin.

The composition of isolated lipoproteins-MPS was studied
further, using optimum concentrations of Ca^{++} but varying the concentration of heparin. The complex material was analyzed for
calcium, phosphorous, and uronic acid, and expressed as molar
ratios of phosphorous to calcium or phosphorous to uronic acid.
With increasing concentrations of heparin, a decrease in the ratio
of phosphorous to calcium or phosphorous to uronic acid occurred.
Based on these observations, a schematic reaction mechanism of
the β lipoprotein-heparin complexes can be proposed (Figure 4).
At low concentrations of heparin, although calcium might be bound
to the functional binding sites of the lipoproteins, and when not
all of the available sites are complexed with heparin, precipitation can still occur. At higher concentrations the available
sites appear to become bound with approximately 1 mole of lipoprotein and 4 moles of heparin (Srinivasan et al., 1970).

Since heparin is not the major MPS found in the aorta, we
investigated the precipitation of β lipoproteins with other
polysaccharides. Serum lipoproteins precipitated with a number
of the sulfated MPS, but much less than with highly charged heparin. On the other hand, when heparin was N-desulfated, it lost
its ability to complex, indicating the importance of the N-sulfate
group of heparin (Srinivasan et al., 1970). These observations,

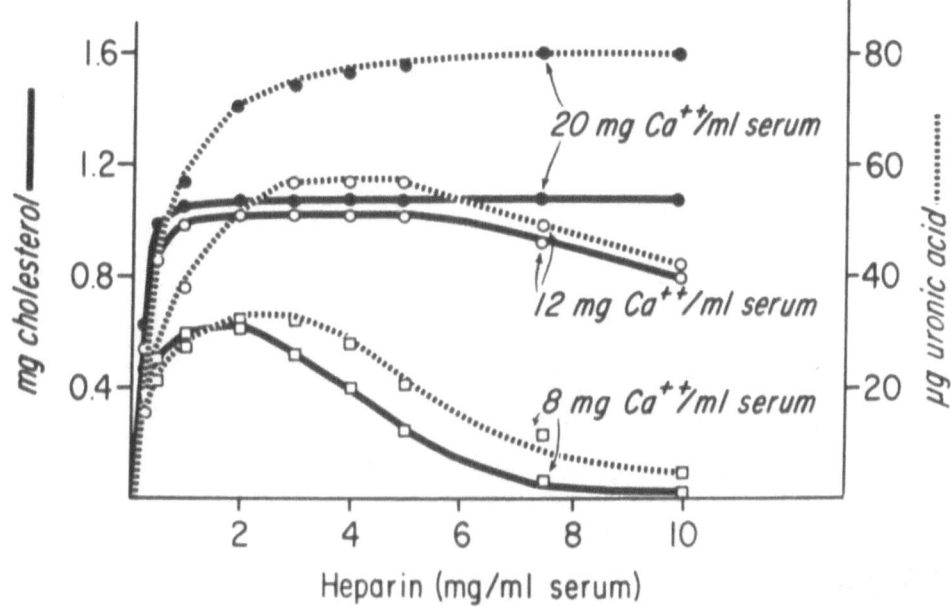

Fig. 3. Effect of Ca^{++} and heparin concentrations on serum β
lipoprotein complexes. Cholesterol is used as a marker for lipoprotein and uronic acid for heparin. At the high concentrations
of Ca^{++}, essentially a complete precipitation of serum β and
pre-β lipoproteins occurs with low concentrations of the polyanion.
At the low concentrations of Ca^{++}, presumably the complexes are
stabilized with the higher concentrations of heparin.

which were made by using an in vitro model, serve as a background
for further studies which might be performed with arterial tissue.
The essential problem is whether or not such complexes actually
exist in the blood vessel wall and take part in the mechanism
developing atherosclerotic lesions. Although lipoprotein-MPS
complexes in the arterial wall have been suggested by a number
of workers, little real evidence has been provided.

COMPLEXING OF MPS WITH LIPOPROTEIN IN THE ARTERIAL WALL

Fatty streaks were obtained from human aortas of varying ages
in an effort to study lipoprotein-MPS complexing in the arterial
wall (Srinivasan et al., 1972). The general outline of the

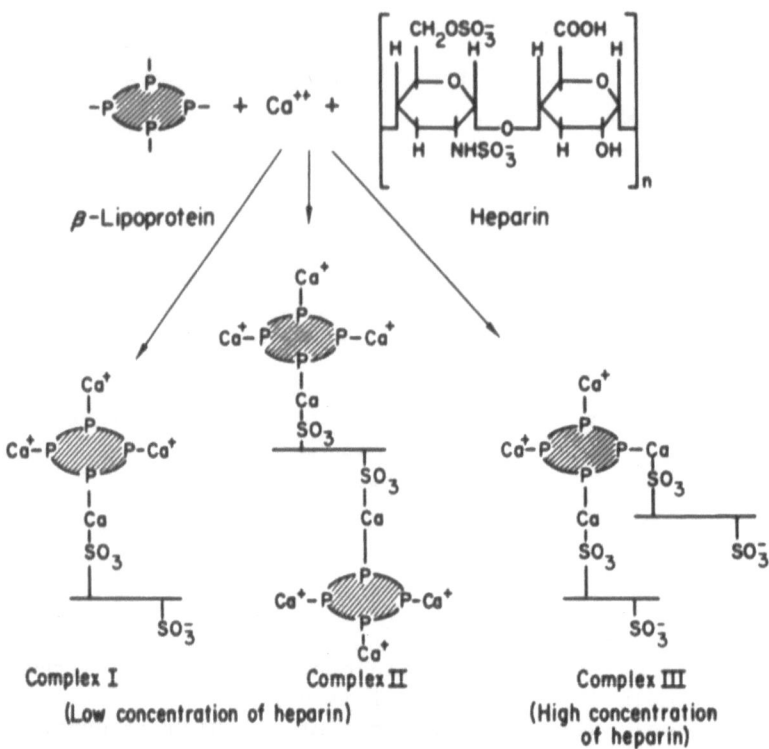

Fig. 4. A schematic reaction mechanism of β lipoprotein-heparin complexes as suggested by observations shown in Fig. 3 and by studies of molar ratios, of phosphorous, calcium, and uronic acid (MPS and lipoprotein concentrations) in precipitates occurring in the presence of different concentrations of Ca++ and heparin.

extraction and isolation of the complexes is shown in Table II. Further attempts were made to separate and characterize materials by chromatography on gels and by ultracentrifugation. In different preparations of fatty streaks varying amounts of material containing uronic acid and cholesterol were obtained, but always in greater concentration than in the uninvolved intimal tissue (Table III). It was also observed that the amount of lipoprotein-MPS material isolated from tissue was reduced when the extracting medium contained Ca++. As noted with serum lipoproteins and heparin interactions, Ca++ enhanced complexing, and presumably stabilized the complex within the tissue, and inhibited extraction.

Gel chromatography was used to fractionate the crude lipid-MPS material. One chromatographic study of material isolated

TABLE II. ISOLATION OF BLOOD VESSEL LIPOPROTEIN-MPS COMPLEXES

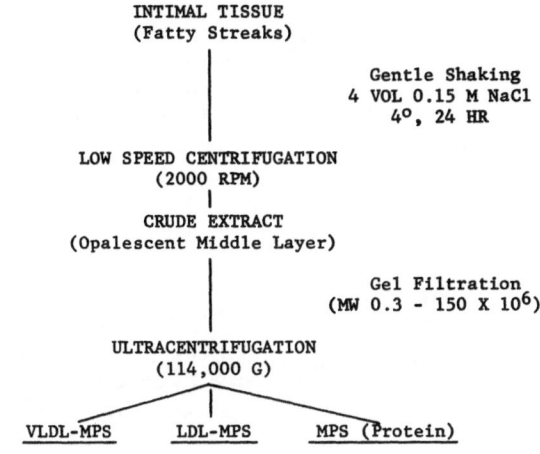

TABLE III. ANALYSES OF EXTRACTS OF FATTY STREAKS AND UNINVOLVED
INTIMA FROM HUMAN AORTA

Sample g/4 ml, 0.15 M NaCl	Uronic Acid μg/ml	Cholesterol mg/ml
Fatty Streaks	46	1.55
Fatty Streaks	56	2.05
Fatty Streaks	193	1.50
Fatty Streaks	212	1.82
Intima (Uninvolved)	15	0.25
Intima (Uninvolved)	12	0.31
Fatty Streaks		
Extracted Without Ca^{++}	100	1.05
Extracted With 0.01M Ca^{++}	73	0.65

from fatty streaks indicated a major peak which contained protein,
cholesterol, and uronic acid, all being eluted simultaneously from
the gel at a molecular weight in excess of 150 million (Figure 5).
Material isolated from gels was then fractionated by ultracentrifugation using the model of the serum lipoproteins and heparin
complexes. At a specific gravity of 1.006, lipoprotein-heparin
complexes were obtained in top and bottom fractions, suggesting
the presence of both very low density lipoproteins (VLDL) and low
density lipoproteins (LDL). Comparable studies of material extracted
from fatty streaks gave similar results (Figure 6). The proportions of VLDL and LDL were approximately the same as those found in
the serum. Since other macromolecules can sediment under these
conditions, i.e. proteoglycans or free MPS, further studies were
needed to establish the presence of LDL complexes.

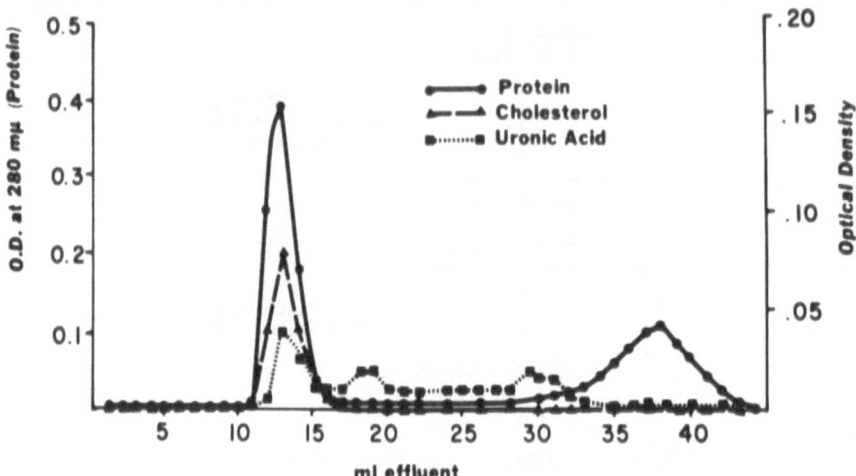

Fig. 5. A gel chromatographic study of lipoprotein-MPS material from aorta fatty streaks. A material was excluded from the gel, indicating a complex containing protein, cholesterol, and uronic acid.

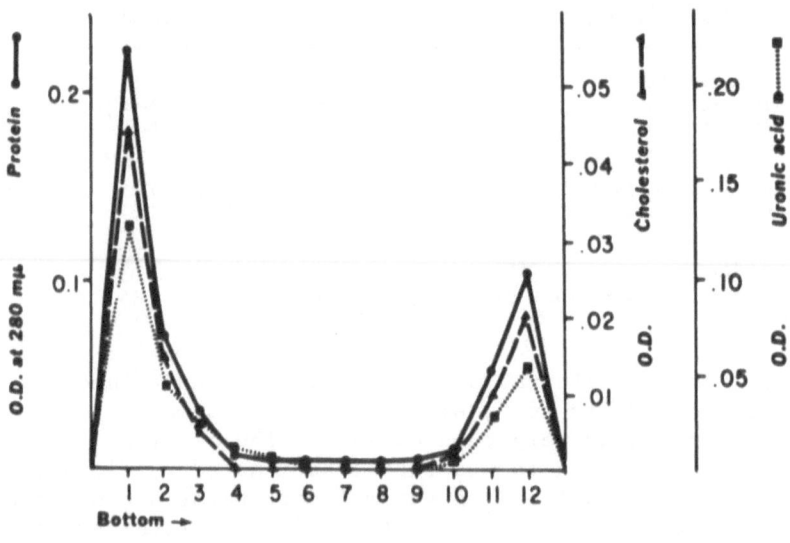

Fig. 6. An ultracentrifuge profile of lipoprotein-MPS material obtained from gels (Fig. 5) at density 1.006 with NaCl, 114,000 g. An indication of material consistent with VLDL (top) and LDL (bottom) complexed with MPS (uronic acid) can be seen.

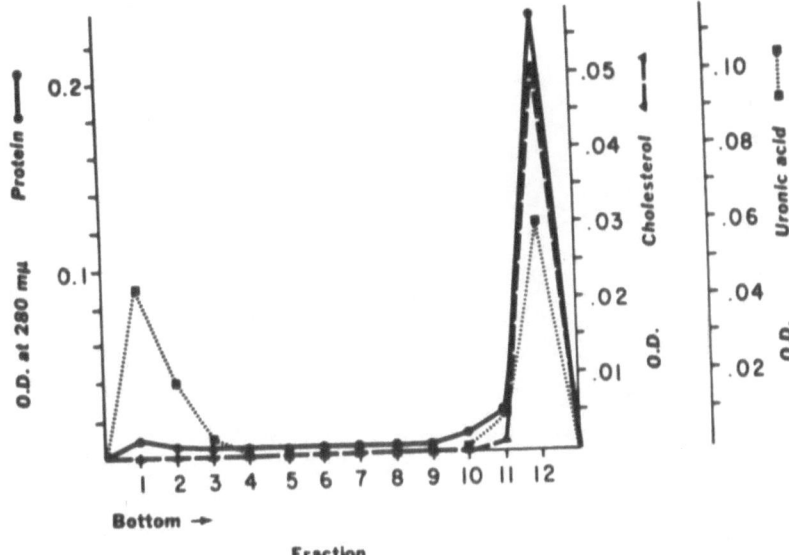

Fig. 7. An ultracentrifuge profile of lipoprotein-MPS complexes
from fatty streaks at density 1.065 using heavy water, 114,000 g.
A complete dissociation of MPS would occur at this density with
salts. Note some uronic acid at the bottom, which could represent
dissociation and/or free MPS also extracted from aorta tissue.
(Refer to text).

        In an artificial model of serum lipoprotein-heparin
complexes studied by ultracentrifugation at 1.065, both lipoprotein materials floated but all of the MPS (heparin) sedimented
to the bottom. These complexes are easily dissociated at high
ionic strength; at high densities where sodium chloride, cesium
chloride, or other ions are used, the complex is broken. To
achieve a higher density, D_2O (heavy water) was used and, as shown
in Figure 7, essentially all lipoprotein material and a large
portion of the MPS were found in the top fraction. Since all of
the MPS is bound as complex, some sedimented to the bottom portion
of the centrifugate. These are tissue extracts, and unbound or
free MPS material could also be present. In an additional study,
again using the model of serum lipoprotein and heparin, some of
the complex also became disrupted under these conditions. However,
a subsequent study indicated that with the addition of Ca^{++} to the
medium the complexes become stabilized, and at a density of 1.065
both VLDL and LDL-heparin complexes float in the top fraction
(Figure 8).

        In order to compare complexes found in other lesions, we
isolated lipoprotein-MPS complexes in raised fibrous plaque
lesions. The fibrous plaques have the advantage of having more

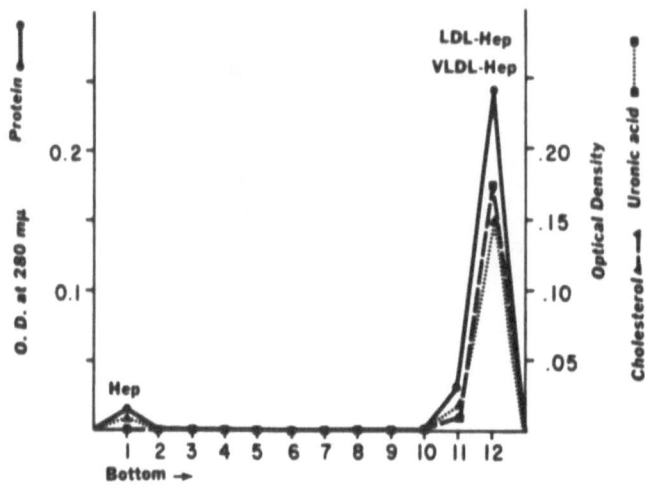

Fig. 8. An ultracentrifuge profile of serum lipoprotein-MPS
complexes using 0.06 M CaCl₂ at density 1.065, 114,000 g. Note
the stabilization of the complexes and the indication of both LDL
and VLDL material. Similar findings were observed with material
from fatty streaks.

available tissue for study than the small fatty streaks. The total
yield of cholesterol-uronic acid material obtained from the fibrous
plaques is greater than that of the fatty streaks, although the
amount of complex that can be extracted under similar conditions
on a weight basis for both types of lesions seems to be comparable
(similar to values shown in Table III). Furthermore, studies of
the molar ratios of phosphorous, calcium, and uronic acid in the
lipoprotein-MPS complexes from the two types of lesions were
similar.

      In a comparative study of gel chromatography of serum lipo-
proteins and the extracts from the fibrous raised plaques, two serum
lipoproteins were separated by the gel, and a high molecular weight
complex containing protein, cholesterol, and uronic acid was
obtained from the fibrous plaque material (Figure 9). The ultracentrifuge profile indicated that fibrous plaque material also
contained MPS complexing with lipoproteins having the characteristics of both VLDL and LDL. As in earlier studies, ultracentrifugation at a higher density using heavy water indicated
the floating of lipoprotein materials in association with uronic
acid. In this instance most of the MPS materials floated with the
top fractions. Perhaps the presence of extractable calcium from
the tissue stabilized the complexes. Thus, it appears that similar
materials were obtained from both fatty streaks and fibrous plaques.

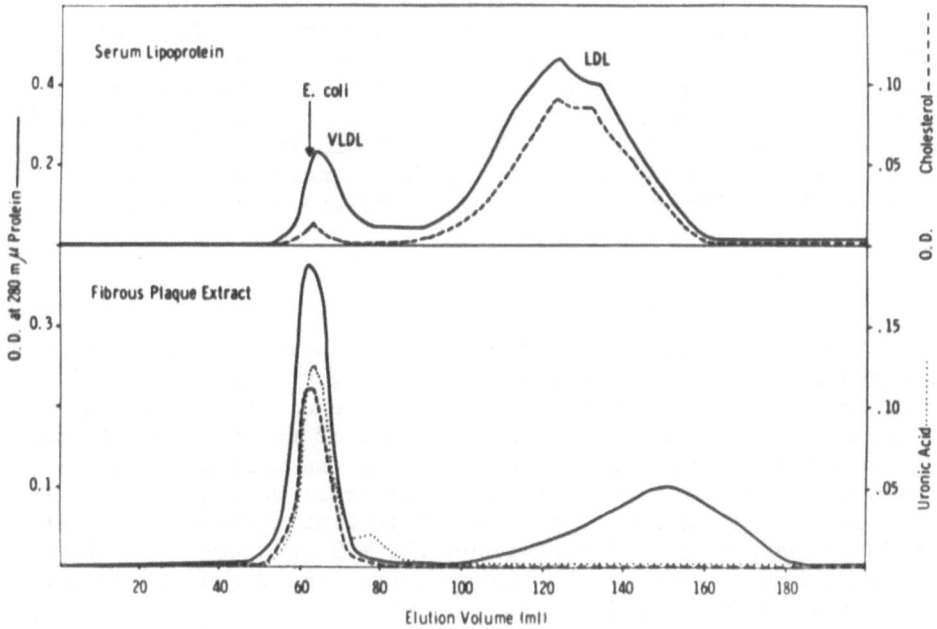

Fig. 9. Comparative gel chromatographic studies of serum lipoproteins and lipoprotein material extracted from fibrous plaques as complexes with uronic acid.

Electrophoretic and enzymatic techniques partly identified the nature of the MPS material obtained in these complexes after isolation from the ultracentrifuge studies. The electrophoretic studies were done on cellulose acetate, using pyridine-formate and calcium acetate buffers. Studies of the LDL material of the fatty streaks were limited essentially to the lipoprotein fraction because of the small amount of material available. The chondroitin sulfates and hyaluronic acid were present in both fatty streaks and fibrous plaque material; in addition, traces of heparin were found in fibrous plaque material. Although heparin was clearly present in the fibrous plaque complexes, it was not observed in the fatty streak material. The electrophoretic studies using calcium acetate buffers indicated the presence of chondroitin sulfate C as the major polysaccharide. Further studies using enzymatic methods aided in the identification. Studies with testicular hyalurondase and the chondroitinases (both chondroitinase ABC and chondroitinase AC) indicated hydrolysis of the MPS. These observations were consistent with the results of the electrophoretic studies.

Several interesting points can be made from the MPS studies of the complexes. Heparitin sulfate was not observed in these preparations while hyaluronic acid was present. The latter compound, which does not bind in vitro, may be present by a co-precipitation or aggregation and not by actual binding. The absence of heparitin sulfate which occurs in high concentration in the intima and is highly charged cannot be explained at this time.

SUMMARY

It is interesting to speculate how the acid mucopolysaccharides and lipoproteins tend to accumulate in the aorta, but the real mechanism for the production of these complexes still needs to be determined. Although no clear explanation of the role of MPS can be given at this time, it is apparent that the carbohydrate-protein macromolecules present in the arterial wall are basic to the structural integrity of the cardiovascular system. It is suggested that under certain conditions the MPS can complex with β and pre-β lipoproteins, not α lipoproteins, and sequester as complexes within the arterial wall.

ACKNOWLEDGEMENTS

The author wishes to acknowledge Barbara S. Lynch, Ph.D., for her assistance in preparation of the manuscript.

Supported by funds from the NHLI of USPHS (HL 02942) and Specialized Center of Research - Arteriosclerosis (HL 15103), and the American Heart Association.

REFERENCES

Amenta, J.S., and Waters, L.L. (1960-1961). The precipitation of serum lipoproteins by mucopolysaccharides extracted from aortic tissue. Yale J. Biol. Med. 33, 112.

Berenson, G.S. (1959). Distribution of acid mucopolysaccharides in inner and outer layers of bovine aorta. Circ. Res. 7, 889.

Berenson, G.S., Radhakrishnamurthy, B., Dalferes, E.R., Jr., and Srinivasan, S.R. (1971). Carbohydrate macromolecules and atherosclerosis. Hum. Pathol. 2, 57.

Berenson, G.S., Srinivasan, S.R., Lopez-S., A., Radhakrishnamurthy, B., Pargaonkar, P.S., and Deupree, R.H. (1972a). Clinical application of an indirect method for quantitating serum lipoproteins. Clin. Chim. Acta 36, 175.

Berenson, G.S., Srinivasan, S.R., Pargaonkar, P.S.,
    Radhakrishnamurthy, B., and Dalferes, E.R., Jr. (1972b).
    A simplified primary screening procedure for the detection
    of hyperlipidemias in "normal" individuals. Clin. Chem.
    18, 1463.

Bernfeld, P., Nisselbaum, J.S., Berkeley, B.J., and Hanson, R.W.
    (1960). The influence of chemical and physiochemical nature
    of macromolecular polyanions on their interaction with
    human serum β-lipoproteins. J. Biol. Chem. 235, 2852.

Bihari-Varga, M., and Vegh, M. (1967). Quantitative studies on
    the complexes formed between aortic mucopolysaccharides and
    serum lipoproteins. Biochim. Biophys. Acta 144, 202.

Bunting, C.H., and Bunting, H. (1953). Acid mucopolysaccharides
    of the aorta. Arch. Pathol. 55, 257.

Burstein, M., and Samaille, J. (1955). Sur la clarification du
    sérum lipemique par l'heparin in vitro. C.R. Acad. Sci.
    (Paris), 241, 664.

Cornwell, D.G., and Kruger, F.A. (1961). Molecular complexes in
    the isolation and characterization of plasma lipoproteins.
    J. Lipid Res. 2, 110.

Dalferes, E.R., Jr., Ruiz, H., Kumar, V., Radhakrishnamurthy, B.,
    and Berenson, G.S. (1971). Mucopolysaccharides of fatty
    streaks in young human male aortas. Atherosclerosis 13, 121.

Gresham, G.A., and Howard, A.N. (1961). The histogenesis of the
    atherosclerotic "fatty streak." J. Atheroscler. Res. 1, 413.

Hauss, W.H., Gerlach, G., Junge-Hülsing, H., Themann, H., and
    Wirth, W. (1969). Studies on the "nonspecific mesenchymal
    reaction" and the "transit zone" in myocardial lesions and
    atherosclerosis. Ann. N.Y. Acad. Sci. 156, 207.

Iverius, P.H. (1972). The interaction between human plasma
    lipoproteins and connective tissue glycosaminoglycans.
    J. Biol. Chem. 247, 2607.

Kramsch, D.M., and Hollander, W. (1973). The interaction of
    serum and arterial intima and its role in the lipid
    accumulation in atherosclerotic plaques. J. Clin. Invest.
    52, 236.

Kumar, V., Berenson, G.S., Ruiz, H., Dalferes, E.R., Jr., Strong,
    J.P. (1967a). Acid mucopolysaccharides of human aorta: II.
    Variations with atherosclerotic involvement. J. Atheroscler.
    Res. 7, 573.

Kumar, V., Berenson, G.S., Ruiz, H., Dalferes, E.R., Jr., Strong, J.P. (1967b). Acid mucopolysaccharides of human aorta: I. Variations with maturation. J. Atheroscler. Res. 7, 573.

Meyer, K., Davidson, E., Linker, A., and Hoffman, P. (1956). Acid mucopolysaccharides of connective tissue. Biochem. Biophys. Acta 21, 506.

Mörner, K.T. (1895). Einige Beobachtungen über die Verbreitung der Chondroitin-Schwefelsäure. Z. Physiol. Chem. 20, 357.

Rinehart, J.F. (1954). Observations on the histogenesis and pathogenesis of arteriosclerosis. In "Connective Tissue in Health and Disease." (G. Asboe-Hansen, ed.), pp. 239-250. Ejnar Munksgaard, Copenhagen.

Ross, R., and Glomset, J.A. (1973). Atherosclerosis and the arterial smooth muscle cell. Science 180, 1332.

Smith, E.B., Evans, P.H., and Downham, M.D. (1967). Lipids in the aortic intima: The correlation of morphological and chemical characteristics. J. Atheroscler. Res. 7, 171.

Smith, E.B., Slater, R.S., and Chu, P.K. (1968). The lipids in raised fatty and fibrous lesions in human aorta: A comparison of the changes at different stages. J. Atheroscler. Res. 8, 399.

Srinivasan, S.R., Dolan, P., Radhakrishnamurthy, B., and Berenson, G.S. (1972). Isolation of lipoprotein acid mucopolysaccharide complexes from fatty streaks of human aortas. Atherosclerosis 16, 95.

Srinivasan, S.R., Lopez-S., A., Radhakrishnamurthy, B., Berenson, G.S. (1970). Complexing of serum β-lipoproteins and acid mucopolysaccharides. Atherosclerosis 12, 321.

Taylor, H.E. (1953). The role of mucopolysaccharides in the pathogenesis of intimal fibrosis and atherosclerosis of the human aorta. Amer. J. Pathol. 29, 871.

Tracy, R.E., Merchant, E.B., and Kao, V.C. (1961). On the antigenic identity of human serum beta and alpha-2 lipoproteins, and their identification in aortic intima. Circ. Res. 9, 472.

Virchow, R. (1856). Gesammelte Abhandlungen zur Wissenschaftlichen Medizin. Meidinger Sohn u. Comp., Frankfurt a.M.

DISCUSSION FOLLOWING THE PRESENTATION BY G. S. BERENSON

UNIDENTIFIED SPEAKER: Can you give us any idea how much of the total intimal cholesterol of plaques was associated with glycoproteins and with mucopolysaccharides?

Dr. Berenson: We did not quantitate glycoproteins but in these extracts we isolated approximately 10% of the total poly-saccharides.

Dr. Yu: Do you have data for the molar ratio of the complex in respect to calcium?

Dr. Berenson: We have molar ratios which were suggested in the schematic diagram. I think the molar ratios obtained by Dr. Srinivasan were 10:7:1 (P, Ca^{++}, uronic acid) at low heparin concentration and 10:11:4 at high heparin concentrations.

Dr. Smith: Were the fibrous plaques the sort with an amorphous lipid central pool and if so, did you examine the pool?

Dr. Berenson: Yes, they were taken as total fibrous plaques.

Dr. Smith: Did they have lipid centers?

Dr. Berenson: Yes

Dr. Smith: I am really very puzzled as to what the relationship is between the lipoproteins we are measuring in the intima and the stuff that you are getting out as a complex, because in our original studies on fatty streaks, we were using really the same methods you were. We were extracting in saline and then ultracentrifuging in salt, and we found much lower concentrations of immunologically intact lipoprotein in fatty streaks than in adjacent normal intima. Presumably, if we were extracting complexes they would dissociate in the high salt concentration so the lipoprotein should behave normally in the immunological assay. I wonder if your "fatty streaks" are in fact the fat-filled cell lesions that we define as fatty streaks. We find exactly the same results with our current immunoelectrophoretic system -- a very low concentration of lipoproteins in the fatty streaks but high concentrations in the early fibrous plaques. In the advanced plaques we find very little in the dense collagen cap and rather a lot in the lipid area.

Dr. Hudson: Do the mucopolysaccharides you have been studying have their protein moiety intact?

Dr. Berenson: I can't give you this answer but we do know that proteoglycans will also complex with lipid.

Dr. Day: I have some data I think that may be germane to the discussions. I have been interested in the control of the inter-action of mucopolysaccharides with lipoproteins. We have studied the lipoproteins from cholesterol fed rabbits with regard to their interaction with different materials. We found that non-ionic surfactants will inhibit almost completely the insoluble formation of lipoprotein precipitates with a number of different mucopoly-saccharides (heparitin sulfate and heparin primarily). Some materials will inhibit complex formation at fairly low concentra-tions of a few micrograms per milliliter of serum, and the non-ionic surfactants are the only materials we have found that will inhibit precipitation in the presence of calcium. A few polyanions will precipitate lipoproteins in the absence of calcium, but if you have calcium in the system, only surfactants such as these will inhibit precipitation. I don't know whether there is any relationship between this and the fact that it has been known for a number of years that non-ionic surfactants are anti-atherogenic, but there is a possibility. We also have looked at the uptake of radio-labeled low density lipoproteins by rabbit aorta. The lipo-proteins had a density of less than 1.063 g/ml. This includes VLDL and LDL in cholesterol fed rabbit serum. We considered these to be the atherogenic proteins, therefore we wanted to see what was happening to the uptake of such atherogenic lipoproteins in arterial tissue. We looked at a number of ways to control this uptake, and in general we found that proteases seemed to increase in vitro uptake of labeled lipoproteins in rabbit aortas. Elastase, papain, and trypsin, all seem to greatly increase incorporation. We were quite surprised that collagenase markedly inhibited uptake. We didn't believe it, and that is the reason we did the experiment so many times, but it always worked the same way. I don't have any explanation for it. You would expect compounds like amylase or ribonuclease to have no effect, and they didn't. We also looked at the uptake of this lipoprotein onto fibrous collagen and elastin from bovine tissues as well as the uptake in the aortic tissue under the influence of different compounds. We found that all of the mucopolysaccharides inhibited the uptake of the radio-labeled lipoproteins by aortic tissue.

Question from the Floor: Could you tell us how the experiments were performed, and how the uptake was determined?

Dr. Day: This was simply an in vitro experiment where we put everything in a flask and incubated it for three hours at 37° C. After three hours we removed the aortic discs and washed them several times in distilled water. We had a total of about 100,000 counts per minute in the system. The uptake in the aortic tissue was about one percent of the total count. Lecithin and phospholipids seemed to inhibit the arterial uptake and again collagenase as well. The substance that we were primarily interested in was succinylated LDL because if you succinylate LDL, it does something magical to it. It increases its stability for one thing so that it can be stored longer than normal LDL. It also completely wipes out any interaction or insoluble precipitate formation with mucopolysaccharides, and it markedly inhibits the uptake by arterial tissue, collagen, and elastin. I am not quite sure what this data means, but I present it for discussion.

SOME ASPECTS OF THE ORGANIZATION AND INTERACTION OF CONNECTIVE

TISSUE PROTEOGLYCANS

K.D. Brandt, T.E. Hardingham, C.P. Tsiganos and
    Helen Muir

Arthritis and Connective Tissue Disease Section,
    University Hospital, Boston, Massachusetts
Laboratory of Biochemistry, University of Patras,
    Patras, Greece
Kennedy Institute of Rheumatology, Bute Gardens,
    London, England

Arterial mesenchyme, because of its micro-architecture and
the variety of macromolecules it contains, is more complex than
other types of connective tissue. In addition to collagen and
elastin, it contains several glycosaminoglycans, including hyaluronic acid, dermatan sulphate, chondroitin-4-sulphate, chondroitin-
6-sulphate and heparan sulphate, as well as glycoproteins that
have yet to be fully characterized. These constituents are not
distributed evenly through the arterial wall, but are localized
in particular regions as shown by histological methods (reviewed
by Muir, 1965). Presumably, therefore, each has a specific
function related to the biomechanical and biochemical properties
of the tissue.

Changes in the overall composition of arterial tissue have
been difficult to correlate with the development of arteriosclerosis. This is not surprising in view of the complexity of connective tissue macromolecules where changes in structure profoundly
alter physicochemical properties without changing the composition
of the tissue. Moreover, new structural constituents formed in
atherosclerotic lesions may not be identical with those in the
original tissue and hence may have somewhat different properties.

Unfortunately, much less is known about the molecular organization and detailed structure of the constituents of arterial
tissue than of other types of connective tissue; nevertheless,
examples from the latter may indicate possible ways in which

constituents of the arterial wall may change. Although largely
speculative, because there is little direct evidence, possible
implications for the function of the structural constituents of
arterial wall will be pointed out in this article.

PROTEOGLYCANS: STRUCTURE AND INTERACTION WITH COLLAGEN

Proteoglycans of connective tissue are very large composite
molecules consisting of a central protein moiety to which a
number of chains of sulphated glycosaminoglycans are attached.
In normal tissue, glycosaminoglycans are not present as free
polysaccharides; arterial mesenchyme is no exception.

The proteoglycans of dermatan sulphate and heparan sulphate
are probably the most important in arterial tissue. In each, the
glycosaminoglycan chains are attached to the protein core by the
same sequence of neutral sugars that form a linkage region as
in the chondroitin sulphate proteoglycans of cartilage (Figure 1).
Rodén (1970) has pointed out that this linkage region provides a
control mechanism for coordinating the biosynthesis of the protein
and carbohydrate moieties of proteoglycans.

Dermatan sulphate (Toole and Lowther, 1968b) and heparan
sulphate (Jansson and Lindahl, 1972) proteoglycans are difficult
to extract from heart valves or aorta - concentrated solutions of
urea are needed to bring them into solution. On the other hand,
chondroitin sulphate proteoglycans may be extracted with salt
solutions (Buddecke and Schubert, 1961; Lowther et al., 1967;
Toole and Lowther, 1968a; Lowther et al., 1970). This difference
suggests that different proteoglycans are not in the same physical
state in the tissue; those that are more difficult to extract
perhaps may be in some form of firm association with the fibrous
proteins of the tissue. Even hot concentrated urea did not extract
all the dermatan sulphate proteoglycan from bovine heart valves
(Toole and Lowther, 1968b). Proteoglycans that are firmly associated with collagen may have some function in modifying the

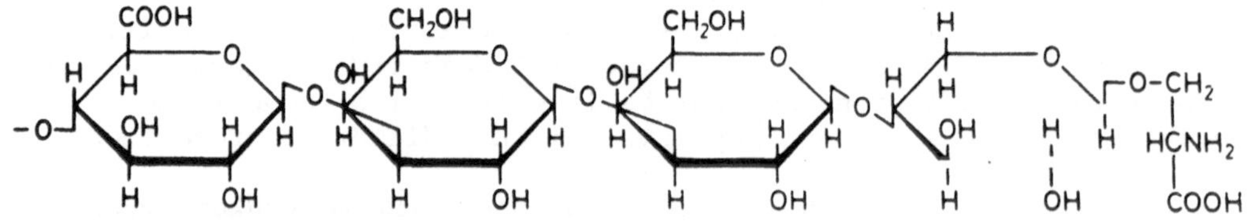

Fig. 1.   Structure of the linkage region of chondroitin sulphate
as established by Rodén (1970).

tensile properties of collagen which may be particularly important
in arteries where pulsatile forces are greatest.

Proteoglycans and glycosaminoglycans interact with skin and
bone collagen by electrostatic forces (Wood, 1960; Toole and
Lowther, 1968a,b; Mathews and Decker, 1968; Öbrink and Wasteson,
1971; Öbrink, 1973). The interaction increases with charge
density and chain length of the glycosaminoglycan, although those
glycosaminoglycans that contain some iduronic acid, namely
dermatan sulphate and heparan sulphate, interact more strongly
than chondroitin sulphates of similar charge density which contain
only glucuronic acid (Öbrink, 1973). It is notable that the
dermatan sulphate proteoglycan extracted from bovine heart valves
had a striking ability to precipitate soluble tropocollagen immediately at 4° C and at physiological ionic strength (Toole and
Lowther, 1968b), whereas the chondroitin sulphate proteoglycan of
heart valves did not interact with collagen (Toole and Lowther,
1968a). It has therefore been suggested that the latter may be
located in the interfiber matrix. Hyaluronic acid and keratan
sulphate also do not interact with collagen (Öbrink, 1973).
Hyaluronic acid may have a function entirely different from that
of other glycosaminoglycans, and there is no conclusive evidence
that keratan sulphate is present in arterial walls. On the other
hand, dermatan sulphate may be principally involved in the formation of collagen fibrils (Toole and Lowther, 1968b). Meyer (1960)
has pointed out that dermatan sulphate is found in those tissues
where there are coarse or thick collagen fibers such as aorta,
tendon and skin, but not in cornea and cartilage where the fibers
are much finer (Maroudas and Bullough, 1968; Muir et al., 1970;
Weiss et al., 1968). Dermatan sulphate appears in scar tissue,
even in cornea where it is not normally found (Anseth and Fransson,
1969). The concentration of dermatan sulphate in fatty streaks of
the arterial intima increases markedly (Kumar et al., 1967b) and
may represent an intimal reaction, analogous to repair in wound
healing. It may underly the appearance of fibrous plaques in more
advanced lesions, even though by this stage dermatan sulphate is
almost absent (Kumar et al., 1967b). It is conceivable that the
intimal increase of dermatan sulphate induces locally the formation of thick collagen fibers which thus resemble the collagen
in scar tissue that is usually not resorbed.

It is also possible that the dermatan sulphate proteoglycan
in fatty streaks may not be the same as that in normal intima.
Dermatan sulphate proteoglycans extracted from different tissues
are not identical and may interact with collagen differently.
The dermatan sulphate proteoglycan isolated from bovine heart
valves was of lower molecular weight, i.e., 2×10^{5} (Preston,
1968) than that extracted from pig skin, which had an average
molecular weight of 2.9×10^{6} (Öbrink, 1972). The protein contents
were similar, namely about 50-60%; nevertheless, the proteoglycan

from skin did not interact with soluble tropocollagen in vitro
in the same manner (Öbrink, 1973) as the dermatan sulphate
proteoglycan from heart valves (Toole and Lowther, 1968b).

The structure of dermatan sulphate proteoglycans may vary in
several ways, such as in the chain length of the glycosaminoglycan
moiety, in the relative proportions of iduronic acid to glucuronic
acid, and in the distribution of each hexuronic acid along the chain.
It has been shown conclusively that dermatan sulphate is a co-
polymer with chondroitin sulphate and has regions with disaccharide
units consisting of glucuronic acid and N-acetylgalactosamine
(Figure 2) characteristic of chondroitin sulphate, interspersed
with repeating disaccharide units consisting of iduronic acid-
N-acetylgalactosamine (Figure 3) (Fransson and Rodén, 1967a,b;
Fransson, 1968,1970). The relative amounts of iduronic acid and
glucuronic acid vary in dermatan sulphate isolated from different
tissues. Iduronic acid comprised about 92% of the total uronic
acid of dermatan sulphate in the proteoglycan from pig skin
(Öbrink, 1972), whereas the L-iduronic:D-glucuronic acid ratio of
dermatan sulphate in horse aorta was only about 1:2 (Fransson and
Havsmark, 1970). In any given tissue there may be considerable
variation in the proportions of the two hexuronic acids in individual chains, as well as in their distribution along the chain,
as is apparent in dermatan sulphate isolated from pig skin after
complete proteolysis (Fransson and Malmström, 1971).

The formation of L-iduronic acid in dermatan sulphate probably
takes place by epimerization of glucuronic acid in the preformed
glycosaminoglycan (Malmström et al., 1972). The formation of
iduronic acid in heparin occurs by such a mechanism (Lindahl
et al., 1972) and it is probable that a similar mechanism operates
in the formation of heparan sulphate. Hence, the actual proportion
of iduronic acid in a given chain could vary, and this in turn
could affect the interaction not only with collagen, but also with
lipoproteins.

In aorta, dermatan sulphate is metabolically heterogenous
(Kresse et al., 1971) and the amount tends to increase with age
(Kaplan and Meyer, 1960; Kumar et al., 1967a). It is therefore

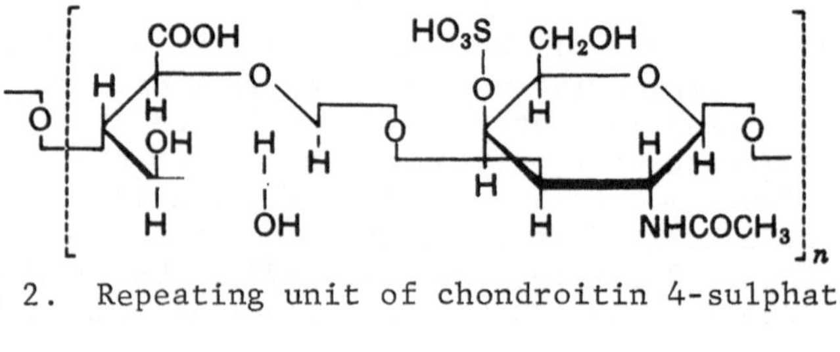

Fig. 2. Repeating unit of chondroitin 4-sulphate.

conceivable that a disturbance in the metabolism of dermatan sulphate during the development of atherosclerosis might induce the production of some varieties at the expense of others.

Heparan sulphate is found in arteries of all sizes (Manley, 1965), and like dermatan sulphate and chondroitin sulphate it occurs as a multichain proteoglycan (Jansson and Lindahl, 1970, 1972). The possibilities of variation in the structure of heparan sulphate are even greater than with dermatan sulphate. The glycosaminoglycan chains may vary in length, in the degree of sulphation, in the proportions of N-sulphate and N-acetyl groups (Cifonelli, 1970), in the relative proportions of iduronic acid and glucuronic acid, and in the distribution of each hexuronic acid along the chain. It may be significant that interaction of heparan sulphate with tropocollagen, as measured by light scattering, was affected by chain length and degree of sulphation (Öbrink, 1973).

The chondroitin sulphate proteoglycans of heart valves show a considerable degree of variation in structure, composition and molecular weight. Salt solutions of comparatively low ionic strength (0.2M) extracted proteoglycans of lower molecular weight containing only 5.5% protein, whereas proteoglycans of higher molecular weight containing much more protein, 32.3%, were extracted with 1M sodium chloride (Lowther et al., 1970). This situation is somewhat similar to that which exists in cartilage (Tsiganos and Muir, 1969a,b.). Similarly, the proteoglycans were polydisperse and did not consist of discrete fractions.

It is possible that the various chondroitin sulphate proteoglycans of arterial mesenchyme may each have different properties as in cartilage. The proteoglycans of cartilage of smaller molecular size contain less protein and have a simpler amino acid composition than those of larger size (Tsiganos and Muir, 1969b; Brandt and Muir, 1971; Tsiganos et al., 1971), while their proportion changes markedly during early development (Simunek and Muir, 1972). They do not appear to be precursors of larger proteoglycans (Hardingham and Muir, 1972a), nor do they appear to be firmly associated with collagen (Simunek and Muir, 1972).

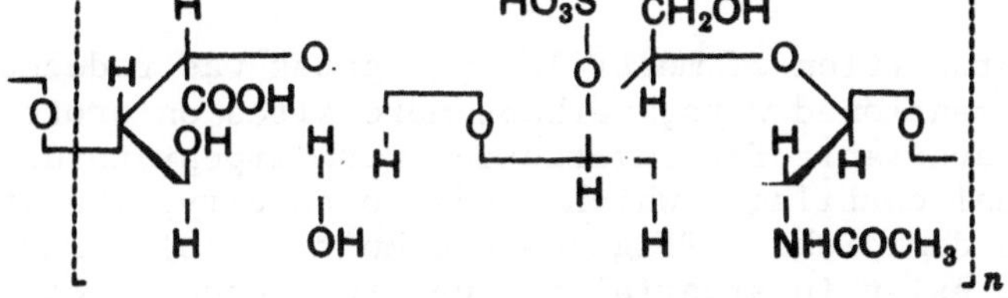

Fig. 3. Repeating unit of dermatan sulphate.

A considerable proportion of the proteoglycans in cartilage exists as aggregates that may be reversibly dissociated in 4M guanidinium chloride (Hascall and Sajdera, 1969), whereas those of smaller molecular size are unable to form aggregates (Hardingham and Muir, 1972a). It has recently been discovered that aggregation depends upon a specific interaction of proteoglycans with hyaluronic acid in which a number of proteoglycan molecules are bound to one molecule of hyaluronic acid (Hardingham and Muir, 1972b). Since there is some hyaluronic acid in arterial walls, it is conceivable that there are aggregates of a similar kind in this tissue. Histochemical studies suggest that hyaluronic acid is not uniformly distributed through the depth of the arterial wall, but is more prevalent in the intima (Muir, 1965). To produce maximum aggregation, only a very small amount of hyaluronic acid is required (Hardingham and Muir, 1972b). If the media, as opposed to the intima, contained only small amounts of hyaluronic acid, it is possible that in the media some of the larger proteoglycan might be present in the form of aggregates. Such aggregates could affect the dynamic properties of the arterial wall because, owing to their very large size, they would be entirely immobilized in the collagen and elastin network and thereby restrict the transient deformation of the network during a pulse wave. The presence of aggregates would thus increase the tensile stiffness of arteries, and because of their large solvent volume they also would prevent the diffusion of all but the smallest solutes from the plasma. If it occurred, the degree of aggregation might be influenced by several factors.

1. The variety of tissue proteoglycans, some of which may not be capable of aggregation, may change.
2. The amount of hyaluronic acid may increase, thereby reducing the proportion of multiple aggregates since each hyaluronic acid molecule would bind fewer proteoglycan molecules. With cartilage proteoglycans there is a marked optimum interaction ratio of hyaluronic acid to proteoglycan of about 1:100 on a weight basis (Hardingham and Muir, 1972b).
3. The chain length of the hyaluronic acid may be reduced so that each molecule would bind fewer proteoglycan molecules.
4. Small oligosaccharides produced by the degradation of hyaluronic acid by hyaluronidase could compete with intact hyaluronic acid for the binding site of proteoglycans (Hardingham and Muir, 1973).

If the proportion of multiple aggregates was reduced in any of the above mentioned ways, perhaps more sites on proteoglycans might become available for interaction with lipoproteins. In aging laryngeal cartilage, which tends to calcify, the proportion of aggregates diminishes (Tsiganos and Muir, 1973). Thus, if aggregates do exist in arterial tissue, the tendency of older

arteries to calcify may be related to the disappearance of
aggregates. All these suggestions, however, are entirely speculative since as yet aggregates have been demonstrated only in
cartilage and nothing is known about their biological function.

INTERACTION OF GLYCOSAMINOGLYCANS WITH HUMAN PLASMA LIPOPROTEINS

The interaction of the various glycosaminoglycans of arterial
mesenchyme with plasma lipoproteins has been studied by a chromatographic procedure in which the glycosaminoglycans were covalently attached to agarose beads (Iverius, 1971). At physiological
pH and ionic strength, low density lipoproteins (LDL) and very
low density lipoproteins (VLDL) but not high density lipoproteins
(HDL) interacted to a significant extent with dermatan sulphate.
At equal charge density, glycosaminoglycans containing L-iduronic
acid interacted more strongly than those containing glucuronic
acid (Iverius, 1972). Heparan sulphate, therefore, interacted
more than would be expected from its relatively low charge density.
This dependence on iduronic acid content of dermatan and heparan
sulphates may be particularly important in view of the variation
in iduronic acid content of dermatan and heparan sulphates and the
variable degree of sulphation. It is possible that iduronic acid
may be more prevalent in the dermatan sulphate of fatty streaks
than in that of normal tissue, where iduronic acid represented
only about one-third of the total uronic acid (Fransson and
Havsmark, 1970). Dermatan sulphate of fatty streaks might,
therefore, bind the lipoproteins more strongly than the dermatan
sulphate of normal tissue. A marked increase has been noted in
the dermatan sulphate content of fatty streaks (Kumar et al.,
1967b) from which complexes of lipoproteins and glycosaminoglycan
have been extracted with solutions of sodium chloride of physiological ionic strength (Srinivasan et al., 1972).

From the studies of interaction _in vitro_, it was calculated
that the minimum binding site of glycosaminoglycans for VLDL or
LDL appeared to be a trisaccharide with three negative charges
(Iverius, 1972). Since iduronic acid and glucuronic acid residues
in dermatan sulphate occur in clusters along the chain (Fransson
and Havsmark, 1970; Fransson and Malmström, 1971), two iduronic
acid residues might sometimes occur in the same trisaccharide.
Hence, the total iduronic acid content would affect not only
binding, but also the distribution of iduronic acid and sulphate
groups. The binding of lipoproteins by heparan sulphate would be
similarly influenced by the amount and distribution of iduronic
acid, by the degree of sulphation, and by the distribution of
sulphate groups along the chain, particularly since N-sulphate
groups are distributed partially at random and are less prevalent
at the linkage region (Cifonelli, 1970; Lindahl, 1970).

The overall chemical analysis of the tissue would not reveal such changes in structure. Moreover, determinations of the glycosaminoglycan composition of arterial tissue might be somewhat misleading because these estimations depend partly upon determinations of the relative proportions of glycosaminoglycans that are resistant to testicular hyaluronidase. It is notable that regions of dermatan sulphate which contain clusters of glucuronic acid residues are susceptible to hyaluronidase (Fransson and Rodén, 1967a,b). In summary, alterations in chain length of glycosaminoglycans affect interaction with collagen, while changes in the proportion of iduronic acid and in the degree of sulphation in dermatan and heparan sulphates affect interaction with both collagen and β-lipoproteins.

PROTEOGLYCANS AND HETEROGENEOUS COLLAGEN

The overall analysis of arterial tissue would not reveal whether there was a change in the type of collagen in the tissue. Recently several types of collagen have been distinguished. The collagen of arteries may be of type III (Miller and Johnson, personal communication), which is found in newborn human skin (Miller et al., 1971). This type of collagen may interact with proteoglycans somewhat differently from the type of collagen (type I) previously used in studies of proteoglycan-collagen interaction or in studies of platelet aggregation. It is possible that the collagen of fibrous plaques may not be the same as the collagen of the original tissue and may interact with proteoglycans and affect platelet aggregation differently. Moreover, the different types of collagen may not be equally susceptible to animal collagenases. Thus, type II collagen of cartilage does not appear to be a substrate for the collagenase that is active against type I collagen of skin and bone (Robertson and Miller, 1972). If the collagen of fibrous plaques differs from that of normal tissue it might not be resorbed because it may not be susceptible to the collagenase produced locally.

Many of the possibilities suggested here are merely speculative. Nevertheless, alterations in the organization of the structural components of arterial mesenchyme could initiate the process that leads to atherosclerosis.

REFERENCES

Anseth, A., and Fransson, L.A. (1969). Exp. Eye Res. 8, 302.

Brandt, K.D., and Muir, H. (1971). Biochem. J. 121, 261.

Buddecke, E., and Schubert, M. (1961). Z. Phys. Chem. 325, 189.

Cifonelli, J.A. (1970). In "The Chemistry and Molecular Biology
    of the Intercellular Matrix" (E.A. Balazs, ed.), Vol. II,
    pp. 961-967. Academic Press, New York.

Fransson, L.A. (1968). J. Biol. Chem. 243, 1504.

Fransson, L.A. (1970). In "The Chemistry and Molecular Biology
    of the Intercellular Matrix" (E.A. Balazs, ed.), Vol. II,
    pp. 823-842. Academic Press, New York.

Fransson, L.A., and Havsmark, B. (1970). J. Biol. Chem. 245, 4470.

Fransson, L.A., and Malmström, A. (1971). Eur. J. Biochem.
    18, 422.

Fransson, L.A., and Rodén, L. (1967a). J. Biol. Chem. 242, 4161.

Fransson, L.A., and Rodén, L. (1967b). J. Biol. Chem. 242, 4170.

Hardingham, T.E., and Muir, H. (1972a). Biochem. J. 126, 791.

Hardingham, T.E., and Muir, H. (1972b). Biochim. Biophys. Acta
    279, 401.

Hardingham, T.E., and Muir, H. (1973). Biochem. J. 135, 905.

Hascall, V.C., and Sajdera, S.W. (1969). J. Biol. Chem. 244,
    2384.

Iverius, P.H. (1971). Biochem. J. 124, 677.

Iverius, P.H. (1972). J. Biol. Chem. 247, 2607.

Jansson, L., and Lindahl, U. (1970). Biochem. J. 117, 699.

Jansson, L., and Lindahl, U. (1972). Scand. J. Clin. Lab. Invest.
    29, Suppl. 123, 19.

Kaplan, D., and Meyer, K. (1960). Proc. Soc. Exp. Biol. Med.
    105, 78.

Kresse, E., Heidel, H., and Buddecke, E. (1971). Eur. J. Biochem.
    22, 557.

Kumar, V., Berenson, G.S., Ruiz, H., Dalferes, E.R., and Strong,
    J.P. (1967a). J. Atheroscler. Res. 7, 573.

Kumar, V., Berenson, G.S., Ruiz, H., Dalferes, E.R., and Strong,
J.P. (1967b). J. Atheroscler. Res. 7, 583.

Lindahl, U. (1970). In "The Chemistry and Molecular Biology of the Intercellular Matrix" (E.A. Balazs, ed.), Vol. II, pp. 943-960. Academic Press, New York.

Lindahl, U., Backstrom, G., Malmström, A., and Fransson, L.A. (1972). Biochem. Biophys. Res. Commun. 46, 985.

Lowther, D.A., Toole, B.P., and Meyer, F.A. (1967). Arch. Biochem. Biophys. 118, 1.

Lowther, D.A., Preston, B.N., and Meyer, F.A. (1970). Biochem. J. 118, 595.

Malmström, A., Fransson, L.A., Hook, M., and Lindahl, U. (1972). Scand. J. Clin. Lab. Invest. 29, Suppl. 123, 23.

Manley, G. (1965). Brit. J. Exp. Pathol. 46, 125.

Maroudas, A., and Bullough, P. (1968). Nature 219, 1260.

Mathews, M.B., and Decker, L. (1968). Biochem. J. 109, 517.

Meyer, K. (1960). In "Molecular Biology" (D. Nachmansohn, ed.), p. 69. Academic Press, New York.

Miller, E.T., Epstein, E.H., and Piez, K.A. (1971). Biochem. Biophys. Res. Commun. 42, 1024.

Muir, H. (1965). In "The Amino Sugars" (E.A. Balazs and R.W. Jeanloz, eds.), Vol. IIa, pp. 311-336. Academic Press, New York.

Muir, H., Bullough, P., and Maroudas, A. (1970). J. Bone Joint Surg. (Br.) 52, 554.

Öbrink, B. (1972). Biochim. Biophys. Acta 264, 354.

Öbrink, B. (1973). Eur. J. Biochem. 33, 387.

Öbrink, B., and Wasteson, A. (1971). Biochem. J. 121, 227.

Preston, B.N. (1968). Arch. Biochem. Biophys. 126, 974.

Robertson, P.B., and Miller, E.J. (1972). Biochim. Biophys. Acta 289, 247.

Rodén, L. (1970). In "Metabolic Conjugation and Metabolic Hydrolysis" (W.H. Fishman, ed.), Vol. II, p. 345. Academic Press, New York.

Simunek, A., and Muir, H. (1972). Biochem. J. 126, 515.

Srinivasan, S.R., Dolan, P., Radhakrishnamurthy, B., and
    Berenson, G.S. (1972). Prep. Biochem. 2, 83.

Toole, B.P., and Lowther, D.A. (1968a). Biochem. J. 109, 857.

Toole, B.P., and Lowther, D.A. (1968b). Arch. Biochem. Biophys.
    128, 567.

Tsiganos, C.P., and Muir, H. (1969a). Biochem. J. 113, 879.

Tsiganos, C.P., and Muir, H. (1969b). Biochem. J. 113, 885.

Tsiganos, C.P., and Hardingham, T.E., and Muir, H. (1971).
    Biochim. Biophys. Acta 229, 529.

Tsiganos, C.P., and Muir, H. (1973). In Workshop Conference
    "Connective Tissue and Ageing," Schloss Reisensburg, 1972.
    Workshop Conference, Hoechst. (H.G. Vogel, ed.), Vol. I,
    p. 132. Excerpta Medica. International Congress Series
    No. 264, Amsterdam.

Weiss, C., Rosenberg, L., and Helfet, A.J. (1968). J. Bone
    Joint Surg. (Am.) 50, 663.

Wood, G.C. (1960). Biochem. J. 75, 605.

DISCUSSION FOLLOWING THE PRESENTATION BY HELEN MUIR

Dr. Nimni: I wonder what role hydrogen bonding may play in
such a phenomenon since it seems that guanidine and temperature
affect dissociation. Doyle and his coworkers[1] have studied the
mechanism by which a glycoprotein, Concanavalin-A, reacts with
polysaccharides using agents and conditions similar to the ones
you have used suggesting that hydrogen bonding may play a
significant role. I think this may also be a reason for the
unusual types of collagen that we see in tissues such as cartilage
and basement membranes. These collagens which are highly
glycosylated and usually found in proteoglycan rich environments
may exhibit a greater capability for hydrogen bonding with

---

[1]Doyle, R.J., Pittz, E.P., and Woodside, E.E. (1968).
Carbohydrate Res. 8, 89.

surrounding polysaccharides and for complexing with divalent cations present in the media. I wonder what you think about this and if you will comment on it.

Dr. Muir: Yes, I am quite sure that hydrogen bonds are involved. Presumably a number of factors have to be taken into account, such as cooperative hydrogen bonds between molecules apposed to each other in the right way. The interaction takes place very rapidly with no gradual precipitation, so that the energy involved must be fairly high.

Dr. Smith: I think some of the things you have brought up might fit into the known lipoprotein pattern in the artery wall. It seems possible that changes in the interactions between glycosaminoglycans and in their interactions with proteins might alter their capacity to complex with lipoproteins in the absence of a change in concentration.

Dr. Dorfman: With reference to the implication of Dr. Muir's work for physiological reactions, it is quite clear that changes in conformation may strikingly affect biological activity. Some years ago Dr. Burton J. Grossman and I showed that dermatan sulfate is strongly antithrombic while chondroitin 4 or 6-sulfate show no such activity; yet they differ in structure only with respect to the configuration at C-5 of the uronic acid. (It is possible that sulfation of L-iduronic acid groups may play some role). The other point that might be worth noting is that at physiological ionic strength, hyaluronic acid is probably highly coiled rather than extended.

AGE RELATED AND ATHEROSCLEROTIC CHANGES IN AORTIC ELASTIN

S.M. Partridge and F.W. Keeley

Agricultural Research Council, Meat Research Institute
    Langford, Bristol, United Kingdom
Research Institute, The Hospital for Sick Children
    Toronto 2, Ontario, Canada

A point we wish to make is the fact that although there has been a great deal of work on dietary fats and their effects on plasma lipids and the effects of these lipids on the development of fatty plaques in the arterial wall, there has been remarkably little effort put into the attempt to find out what components of the arterial connective tissue are damaged at the site of the fatty or calcified plaques, or which of the normal components of the wall are particularly susceptible to fat deposition or calcification. Other questions to be dealt with are how these components of the wall are normally protected and why the damage is so sharply localized.

Our particular interest has been in the protein, elastin, which constitutes the major part of the walls of the largest arteries, particularly the thoracic part of the aorta, a vessel which makes exceptional demands upon its material of construction. According to K.H. Meyer (1950) the elastic coefficient of ox elastin is about 14 kg/cm^2 in the region of 10 to 50% extension where the work diagram is almost linear. In addition to high strength, the wall of the thoracic aorta must display long-range extensibility and, over the period of a lifetime, withstand repeated flexing. In most animals the wall is well capable of doing this with substantially no heat production due to frictional work and no fatigue failures of materials.

According to Harkness et al. (1957), the ratio of elastin to other connective tissue components in adult dogs remains roughly constant at 45 to 55% from the aorta valve to within about 5 cm of the diaphragm. The proportion of elastin then decreases rapidly and remains at about 25 to 30% throughout the abdominal aorta and the iliac and femoral arteries.

Three concentric layers of the arterial wall are usually recognized, but the layer we have been particularly concerned with has been the tunica media. This layer accounts for the greater part of the wall and in chick, bovine, or human aorta it consists mainly of alternating concentric laminae of elastic tissue and cells. We have not always been very successful in stripping off the intima, so that most of our elastin preparations contain material from both of these layers.

In order to remind the non-histologists of what a cross-section of the aorta wall looks like in various animals, we have included photomicrographs of sections stained with Humberstone's, Verhoeff's stains, or Weigert's resorcin fuchsin and counter-stained with green trichrome (Figure 1). These illustrations clearly show concentric laminae that are composed almost entirely of fibrous elastin and, as will be seen later, are highly fene-strated sheets.

However, in spite of its crosslinked structure, elastin is not particularly strong at full stretch and the structure must be reinforced with the long inextensible fibers of collagen. This is arranged in a sort of stockinet-like weave that readily stretches up to a maximum extension, and then resists any further increase in diameter.

It is technically easy to get a good cross-section of the arterial wall; however, a good longitudinal section that reveals the structure of the fenestrations in the concentric membranes offers some problems. The preparation shown in Figure 2(a) was made by using hot alkali to extract the collagen and proteoglycans from a piece of bovine aorta wall and then embedding the lace-like residue of elastin in molten wax. Usually some well-oriented longitudinal sections can be cut from the block, as illustrated. This micrograph shows a particularly highly fenestrated area but it illustrates the point that the structure is almost entirely mem-branous or ribbon-like, although a few fine fibers always seem to maintain the connections between the adjacent concentric laminae. These illustrations may be enough to show that the larger arteries are for the most part composed of elastin and that the properties of this unique protein elastomer have a major influence on the mechanical properties of the walls.

We may now consider what kind of substance elastin is. All elastomers or rubbers are polymers composed of long molecular chains that do not display mutual cohesive forces to any great

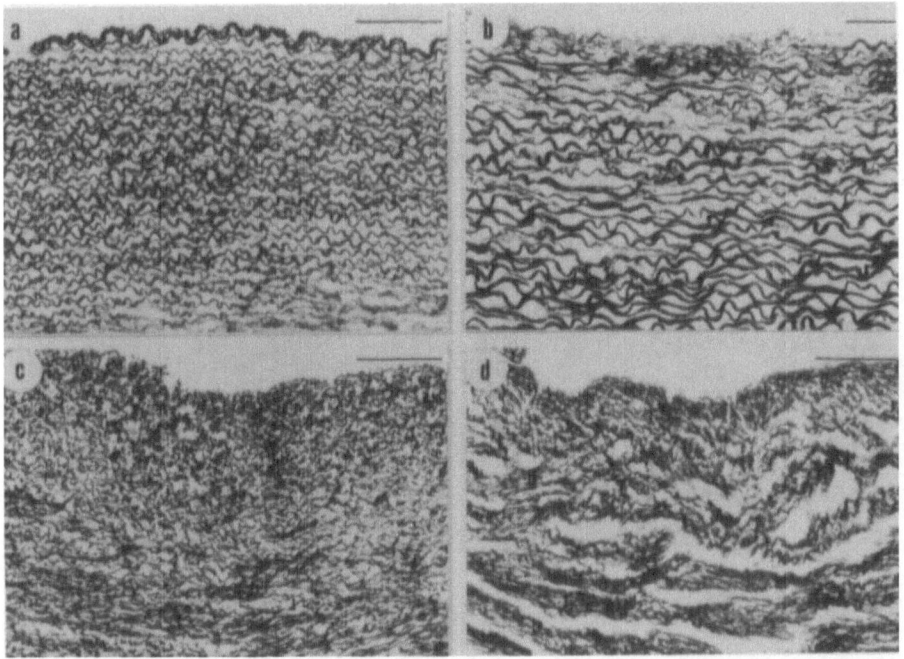

Fig. 1. Transverse sections of the wall of the thoracic aorta in
various animal species. Part of the lumen is visible above each
section. (All magnifications are x 30). (Reduced 33% for reproduction). Bar = 100 μm:

     (a) Bovine foetus: Humberstone's elastica stain with Van
Gieson's picro-acid fuchsin;

     (b) Human thoracic aorta: Verhoeff's elastica stain with
Masson's green trichrome;

     (c) Chick aorta: from a two week old normal chick. Humber-
stone's elastica stain with Van Gieson's picro-acid fuchsin;

     (d) Chick aorta: fed a lathyritic diet containing β-amino
propionitrile (BAPN) from hatching to two weeks of age. Staining
as in (c).

extent, so that they can slide over one another. At the rest-
length of the fibers the molecular chains always occupy a kinked
configuration. When the elastomeric fiber is put under tension,
the kinked chains tend to straighten and on release the snap return
is due to thermal motion which tends to restore the original randomly kinked configuration. It follows that if a weight is hung
on a fiber of elastomer so as to stretch it partially, an increase
in temperature will cause the weight to rise and the elastomer to
shorten in the direction of the stress. Of course the molecular
chains must be cross-linked at intervals by some form of stable
linkage; otherwise there would be nothing to prevent the chains

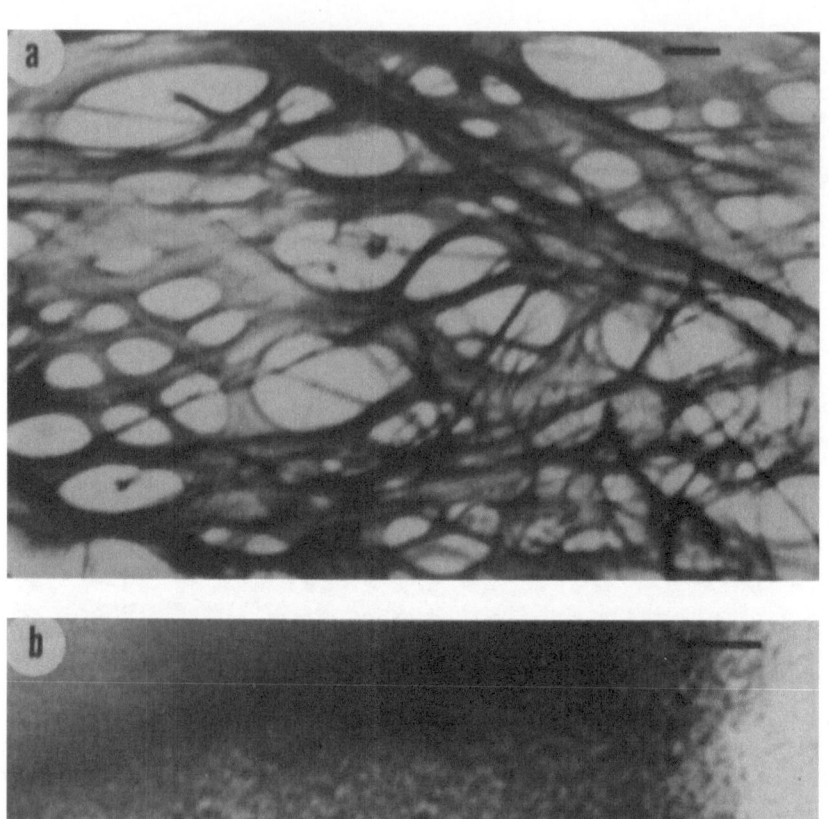

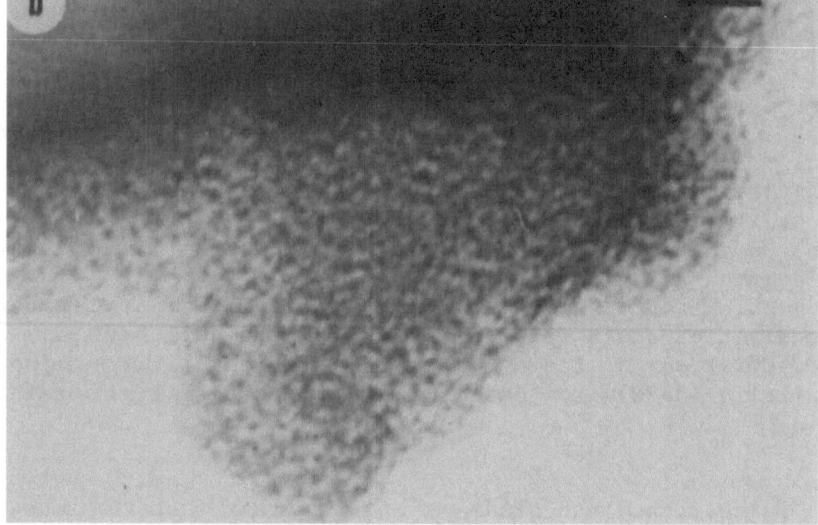

Fig. 2. (a) Longitudinal section of a particle of elastin from
bovine aorta purified by treatment with hot alkali. The section
shows clearly the characteristic pattern of fenestrations that
penetrate an otherwise homogenous membrane of elastin. Stain:
Weigert's resorcin-fuchsin. (x 340). Bar = 10 μm.
　　　　(b) Electron micrograph of the edge of a thin particle
of bovine aorta elastin mordanted with a polyphenol and stained
with uranyl acetate. Drying in high vacuum has caused loss of
structure by shrinkage. Bar = 10 nm.

from slipping over one another as happens with a viscous oil.
With elastin, evidently there are plenty of very stable covalent
cross-links which make this protein the most insoluble of any of
the tissue components.

Historically, such knowledge as we have about the constitution
and composition of elastin was won by starting with the insoluble
protein purified from elastic tissue and trying to break it down
by a process of controlled stepwise degradations. However, to tell
the story this way would take too long. What we would like to do
instead is to try to explain how near we are to an understanding
of the elastomeric protein polymer in the same terms that we
understand man-made elastomers. With synthetic elastomers, of
course, we know about the monomers we use in the synthesis, but we
are obliged to deduce the expected properties of the polymer. This
proposition is not altogether outrageous because already a soluble
protein monomeric precursor of elastin has been isolated from
several animal species; and a reasonably good amino acid analysis,
molecular weight, and other physical properties are available.

Soluble proteins with an elastin-like amino acid composition
were first isolated by Smith et al. (1968) and Sandberg et al.
(1969), but perhaps the purest and best characterized elastin
monomer so far described is the so-called salt soluble elastin
from the aortas of copper deficient pigs. The isolation of this
very pure protein was described by Smith et al. (1972) and has
been achieved by a very simple and mild procedure based on the
known properties of soluble elastin and soluble collagen. Salt
soluble elastin and salt soluble collagen were extracted from the
finely comminuted aortas of copper deficient pigs by 0.5 M NaCl
at pH 7.2 and at 4°C. The soluble collagen was then precipitated
from the crude saline extract by lowering the pH to 4.0 with acetic
acid. After the flocculent precipitate was removed the filtrate
was brought to 1 M in NaCl pH 8.0 and the temperature raised to
37°C. This brought out the soluble elastin as a "coacervate" -
a characteristic property of all soluble elastins.

Table I (Smith et al., 1972) shows the amino acid analyses
of porcine salt soluble elastin. The molecular weight of this
material was shown to be close to 74,000 by equilibrium centrifugation in the presence of 6 M guanidine at 20°C. For this reason
the analytical results in the table are quoted as amino acid
residues per protein molecule of weight 74,000. It will be seen
from Table I that the molecule contains none of the lysine-
derived cross-linking amino acids but contains an excess of about
30 lysine residues above that of the same weight of fibrous
elastin. Otherwise the analyses are extremely close. The small
excess of aspartic acid and serine sometimes found in soluble
elastin may be significant and may be due either to losses of these

TABLE I.   AMINO-ACID COMPOSITION OF SALT-SOLUBLE ELASTIN FROM
           COPPER DEFICIENT PORCINE AORTA   (from Smith et al., 1972)

| Amino Acid | Residues Per Minimal Subunit Weight 74,000 | |
	Salt-Soluble Elastin	Insoluble Porcine Elastin
Hydroxyproline	9	10
Aspartic acid	3	10
Threonine	13	13
Serine	10	12
Glutamic acid	15	21
Proline	92	91
Glycine	287	269
Alanine	203	191
Valine	116	103
Methionine		2
Isoleucine	14	17
Leucine	40	47
Tyrosine	14	15
Phenylalanine	23	27
Desmosine (quarter)		10
Lysine	38	7
Histidine		1
Arginine	4	8

amino acids in the fibrous protein caused by some process involving
glycosylation or to an additional peptide combined in the salt
soluble elastin. We have confirmed minimum weights of the same
order of size, from two other animal species, and also the same
analytical pattern in the soluble elastins both in copper deficiency
and BAPN lathyrism (Sykes and Partridge, 1972).

    There are some differences in the amino acid compositions of
the aortic elastins from different animals - for instance, the
replacement of some phenylalanine by tyrosine in the chick; but
this is understandable and is commonly found when comparing the
same protein between different species. What is more striking is
the close similarity of the general pattern of amino acid composition, physical behavior and the molecular weight of the minimum
kinetic unit in guanidine solution. This uniformity seems to indicate that elastin, like collagen, has a very ancient origin in
evolutionary history. It is also becoming apparent, now that the
repeating unit of the elastomer is known, that elastin can no longer
be regarded as a random network similar to vulcanized rubber.

Evidently, elastin is formed by cross-linking the soluble monomeric units (weight about 74,000) into a three-dimensional biopolymer. We know that this is done by oxidizing some of the ε-amino side-chains of lysine to aldehyde followed by condensation reactions between any aldehydes and amines that find themselves in the correct apposition. A brief summary of the different aspects of covalent crosslinks involving lysine that have been isolated from elastin and characterized up to date is given in Figure 3.

It seems then that we shall not be too much in error if we adopt the view that elastin is built up as a three-dimensional polymer from units of molecular weight about 74,000; but we must remember that the units could be of two or three different kinds as is the case with α1 and α2 sub-units of collagen. Perhaps the most obvious suggestion for the polymerization mechanism is the arrangement shown in Figure 4. Here several points are proposed:

1. The conformation of the precursor monomer is such that it allows exact apposition of lysine and lysine aldehyde residues in order to permit the formation of the known cross-links;

2. The structure of fibrous elastin contains centers of hydrophobic interaction of some size, as well as water spaces of a similar order of size which would be available for the solution of low molecular solutes up to a limiting order of molecular weight of about 1,000 Daltons (Partridge, 1967a,b).

This kind of structure is indeed suggested by x-ray diffraction studies of fibrous elastin which show only the diffuse rings generally obtained with disordered or denatured proteins. The same kind of structure appears from electron microscopy of thin flakes of purified elastin. Figure 2(b) shows an electron micrograph (taken by Dr. Sylvia Fitton Jackson) of the edge of a thin particle of purified elastin which was mordanted with a polyphenol and stained with uranyl acetate. Although drying in high vacuum has caused loss of structure by shrinkage, the micrograph indicates some sort of corpuscular arrangement with interspaces which were originally filled with water. This kind of reticular structure is a notoriously difficult subject for size estimation with the electron microscope, but the arrangement of the particles appears to be isotropic and in the dry preparations the particles appear to be of irregular shape with about 40 to 50 $\overset{o}{A}$ between centers.

3. Lastly, in order to display long-range elasticity the structure must be such that there is freedom of rotation and translation within the hydrophobic corpuscular region, but with thermal motion restricted to the hydrophobic domain.

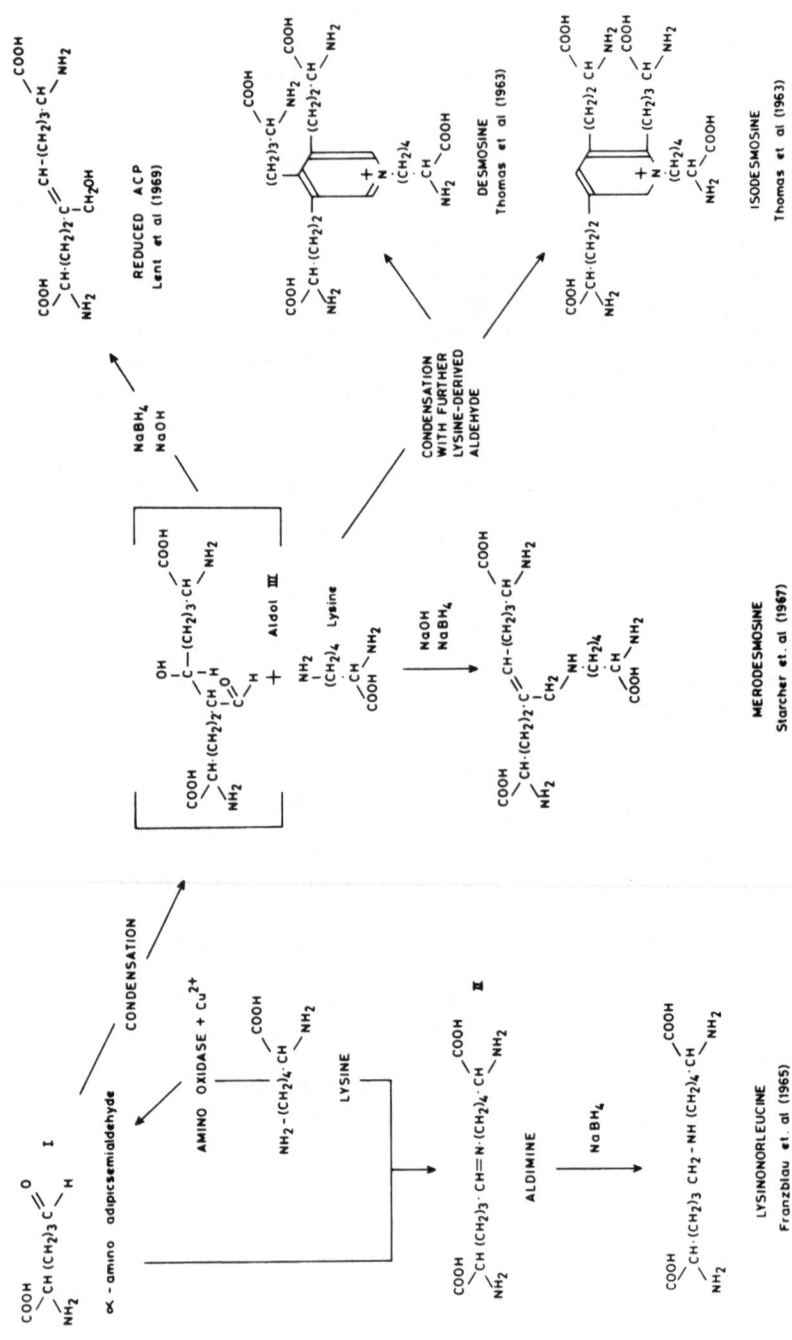

Fig. 3. Proposed route to the desmosine isomers showing steps in their synthesis from three mole-cules of the lysine-derived aldehyde and one of unchanged lysine. The expected combinations of two and three residues of lysine or lysinal now have all been isolated after stabilization by bor-ohydride reduction. The compound in square brackets is the aldol from two molecules of lysinal. It is unstable and can be isolated only after reduction and dehydration; it is regarded as a labile intermediate in the biosynthesis of the permanent cross-linkages.

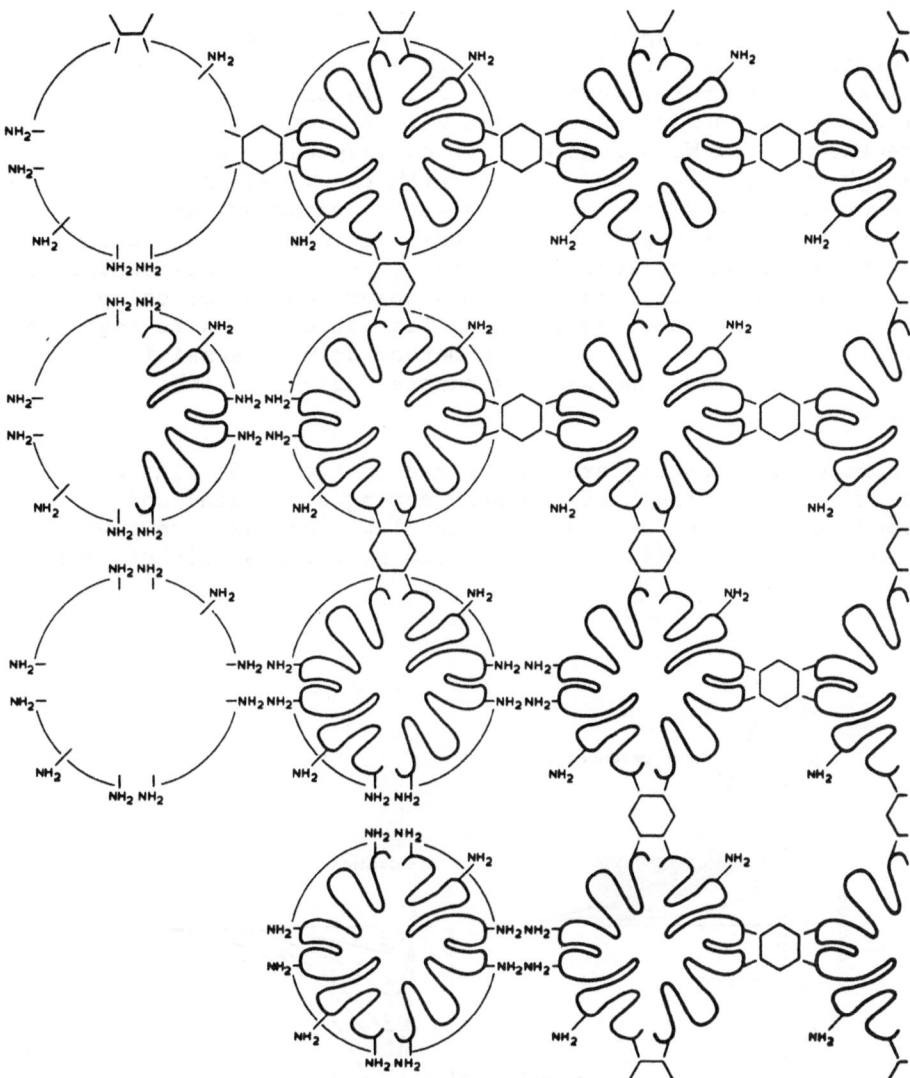

Fig. 4. Two-dimensional representation of the formation of a
space-filling polymer from monomeric units of about 74,000 molecular weight. The units may be identical or there may be a small
number of different kinds of basic repeating units. It is assumed
that cross-linkages form where the required number of lysine or
lysinal residues are presented in apposition, to allow development
of a three-dimensional network. (Reproduced with permission from
Partridge, 1966,and the American Chemical Society).

A considerable part of the work carried out in our laboratories over the last five or six years has consisted of attempts to devise biophysical methods capable of making a clear distinction between the uniformly wetted gel and a structure composed of hydrophobic micelles and free water spaces. An example of the type of structural study that can be carried out with intact elastin fibers is the recent work of Weis-Fogh and his colleagues at Cambridge. Weis-Fogh and Anderson (1970) began with the viewpoint indicated here, that cross-linking of the soluble elastin precursor must give rise to a very hydrophobic polymeric protein gel which is known experimentally to contain at least 66% water (v/v) after full swelling. The standard theory for anhydrous elastomers could not be applied to such a system without questioning its validity. Weis-Fogh and his colleagues set out to devise a method using a sensitive calorimeter for measuring the heat exchanges during stretching and relaxation.

Some of the results are summarized in Figure 5. The curves in the figure show the heat produced during stretching and absorbed again during relaxation. The lower curves were given when the water of swelling was replaced by various solvents that

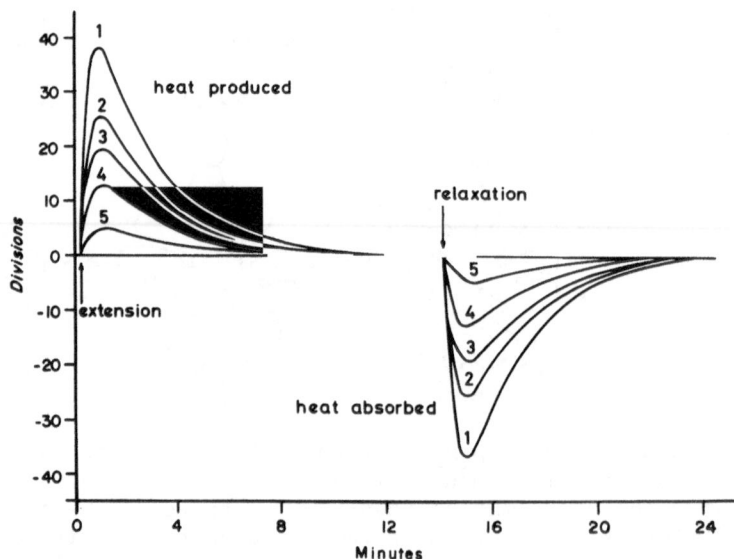

Fig. 5. Heat produced and absorbed when a fiber is extended or relaxed at room temperature in various solvents (1) in water, (2) in 2 M methanol,(3) in 2 M ethanol, (4) in 2 M n-propanol, (5) in pure formamide. (Reproduced with permission from Weis-Fogh and Anderson, 1970. Nature 227, 718).

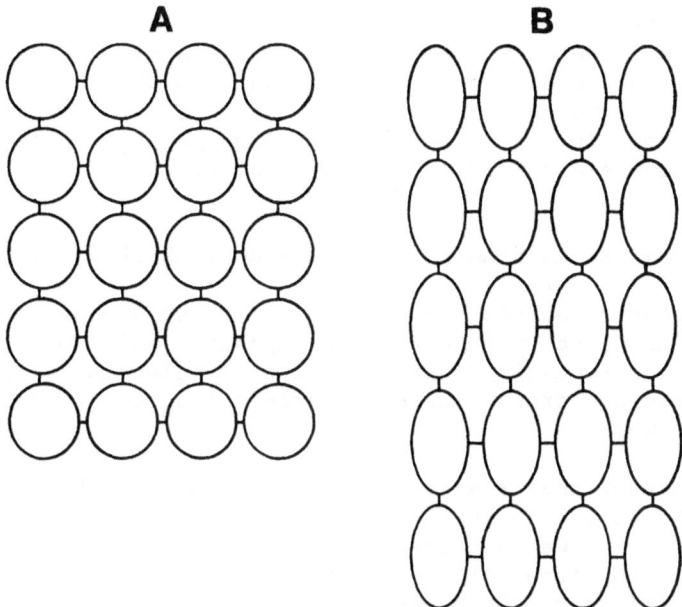

Fig. 6. Structure of elastin as an "oil droplet elastomer."
Corpuscular units which have a hydrophobic interior and carry
hydrophilic groups on the surface are suspended in the water-
phase and are interlinked by covalent bonds. A, relaxed and B,
stretched by 35%. (Reproduced with permission from Weis-Fogh and
Anderson, 1970. Nature 227, 718).

progressively reduced the energy associated with the water interface. The final curve (curve 5) is for a fiber swollen in a
formamide-water mixture which reduced ΔH to nearly zero. This
behavior could not readily be explained on the basis of the
standard theory of rubber-like elasticity, and a preliminary study
led Weis-Fogh and Anderson to propose the scheme in Figure 6.
This theoretical development amounts to the discovery of a new
type of elastomer for which the term "oil droplet elastomer" was
proposed.

The thermodynamic considerations have since been reanalyzed
at much greater length by J.M. Gosline (personal communication)
working in the same laboratory in Cambridge. The conclusions
remain substantially the same, and it is now clear that hydrophobic interactions cause the elastin polymer chain to condense
into a compact protein globule. Gosline's analyses throw a great
deal more light on the nature of the changes that take place as
elastin is stretched and hydrophobic parts of the chain are transferred from the interior to the lipid-water interface. It is now
apparent that the polymer itself becomes less ordered as the sample
is stretched - just the opposite of what is expected for a rubbery

material. This means that the elastic energy is stored as a
change in the structure of water which becomes more ordered as it
is exposed to new hydrophobic side chains from the interior.
Because the elastic energy is stored as a change in the structure
of solvent (that is, water) it seems appropriate to apply the term
"solvent active elastomer" to this type of elastic mechanism.

AGE CHANGES IN RELATION TO THE STRUCTURE OF ELASTIN

Other considerations, in addition to those we have mentioned,
all lead to the idea that there is a repeating unit, or a group of
closely similar repeating units, all with a molecular weight near
74,000. These are cross-linked in three-dimensions to form an
isotropic network.

We also know that the water, which amounts to about two-
thirds of the volume in normal, mature elastin, is grouped in a
system of water spaces and channels in such a way that it is
available for the free solution of solutes with molecular weights up
to 1,000. Similarly, the hydrophobic parts of the molecular
chains are grouped together in hydrophobic domains, probably with
weights of the same order as the molecular weights of the repeating
units.

In these hydrophobic regions the molecular chains are free to
move over one another, and have at various temperatures a "most
probable conformation" rather than a single unique conformation
stabilized by hydrogen bonds, as is the case with collagen and
most other native proteins.

The mechanical properties of elastin depend on the deformation in shape of the hydrophobic regions in response to stretching
and thus are dependent upon the degree of freedom in these regions.
The hydrophobic regions are of course bounded by an interfacial
layer in contact with the water spaces. This boundary layer will
contain the side chains of any hydrophilic amino acids and will
be readily penetrated by any surface active substance that can
diffuse within the system of water spaces. Thus certain surface
active substances of molecular weight of 1,000 or less can certainly be expected to damage elastic fibers and membranes if they
are successful in penetrating the barriers of proteoglycans and
ground substance polyanionic chains. Since we have found remarkably little evidence of such penetration with material from young,
healthy animals there must certainly be barriers which prevent the
entry from the blood of such substances as lipid degradation
products, prostaglandins, bile salts, and sterols. A pathological
situation would be one in which the integrity of these barriers
was disturbed.

CALCIFICATION

Calcification of the walls of arteries occurs progressively throughout life in human subjects. While localized forms of this calcification are seen in the calcified plaques that usually arise from earlier fatty plaques, the otherwise healthy parts of the wall also increase in ash content.

To explain this better, we should return to the original theme - synthetic polymers with elastomeric properties. There has been a trend in recent years to introduce desirable modification in the properties of synthetic elastomers, not so much by altering the degree of covalent cross-linking, but instead by introducing controlled numbers of ionic bonds at points along the covalent backbone. As early as 1953, H.P. Brown first made use of the possibility of producing ionic bonding via pendant carboxylic residues deliberately introduced into synthetic rubber. One such commercial product, Hycar 1072, is a co-polymer of butadiene, acrylonitrile, and methacrylic acid. Normally the salt linkage is formed with a divalent ion such as Zn^{2+} or Ca^{2+}. Bivalent zinc seems to have a particularly favorable place in the formation of ionic bonds in proteins, probably because its ionic radius (0.74 Å) is very small compared with calcium ion (0.99 Å); on the other hand, not much seems to be known about the degree to which chelation and coordination valency is involved in this type of bond.

A great many such examples may be quoted to show that ionic bonds involving calcium, zinc, and other divalent metals are readily formed in proteins and that in elastomers these bonds usually result in stiffening and loss of extensibility. Chelation of calcium ions by specific parts of an elastic network has also been identified (Weis-Fogh and Amos, 1972) as the mechanism of an unusual type of reversible contraction occurring in the contractile organelle or spasmoneme in vorticella, a small fresh-water organism. The organelle is a rod-shaped proteinaceous body containing 20 to 30% dry weight and the mechanism of the rapid non-muscular contraction appears to be a conformational change brought about by release of calcium ions from the calcium pump mechanism (Molinari-Tosatti et al., 1968; Urry, 1971).

With these ideas in mind, two years ago we began a study of individual human aortas regarding changes in the polar amino acid composition of elastin from plaque and non-plaque areas of the same organ (Keeley and Partridge, in preparation). We soon confirmed that ash content, even in the non-plaque areas, rises steadily with age, beginning early in the second decade. The deposition of calcium salts was shown to be closely associated with elastic fibers and, in large part, to penetrate their structure.

Also, either the amino acid composition of elastin itself changes as a function of age and calcification, or else a protein impurity with a very different composition from that of elastin is added to its structure in such a way that it is very hard to remove.

The amino acid analyses of elastin from old subjects show a progressive increase in aspartic and glutamic acid and other polar amino acids, and an increasing loss of glycine, alanine, and valine. Additionally, elastin purified from the areas of calcified plaques contains more polar amino acid residues than does the plaque-free areas.

Examination of material from plaque and non-plaque areas seems to indicate a direct relationship between the degree of calcification and the degree of contamination with non-elastin protein. We should point out that Hall (1959) observed and reported this relationship some years ago.

This kind of situation suggests that the non-elastin protein that seems to be closely associated with the elastic laminae may owe its association to ionic bonding through calcium ions in the way we have suggested for the synthetic elastomers. Accordingly, we attempted de-ashing of some autoclaved aorta elastin from aged subjects that contained the polar protein impurity. Decalcification was done with sodium EDTA and continued until no measurable ash remained.

In both plaque and non-plaque material which were first decalcified with EDTA and subsequently treated with hot alkali, all of the contaminating protein was removed, leaving a residue with an analysis virtually indistinguishable from that of pure elastin. These results seem to indicate rather clearly the involvement of a number of polar and, possibly, chelate bonds attaching a second protein to the backbone network of elastin; and, by inference the work suggests that the stiffening and loss of long-range elasticity of aged elastin may also be due, in part, to such bonds.

Many workers seem to have been surprised that collagen (as measured by hydroxyproline determination) is more difficult to remove from old elastica. In fact, this is simply due to the aging and stabilization of the cross-links in collagen. Old collagen is almost as insoluble in hot water as is elastin.

Perhaps we can summarize with a little speculation. At the present time we view these extremely local calcified lesions that penetrate deeply into the media as a result of a series of different defensive barriers that only yield to assault when all are penetrated successively at some particular point of attack.

Certainly, penetration of the proteoglycan barrier by low molecular weight lipids, as in fatty plaques, may be as harmful to the attacked part of the elastic membrane as mineral oil is for rubber. Flexing such damaged membranes soon would produce breakdown. Also, in the first stage of a repair process, catheptic enzymes are released. These make a bigger hole in the proteoglycan barrier and result in local breakdown of the defenses against mineralization, causing the abnormal situation to be propagated.

It would be interesting to know what component of hard fats, if any, is causally related to the formation of fatty plaques in the large arteries. The local penetration of specific lipids or other surface active substances into the hydrophobic regions contained in the cross-linked network would be expected to have many identifiable consequences.

Any such penetration would be expected to bring new hydrophobic parts of the molecule to the water interface and this would change both the antigenic properties of that part of the fiber and its resistance to proteolytic enzymes. Together this would open up a gamut of pathologically important consequences possibly including the development of a local auto-immune response, inflammation, release of catheptic enzymes, and finally ulceration.

REFERENCES

Brown, H.P. (1953). U.S. Patent 2662874.

Franzblau, C., Sinex, M., Faris, B., and Lampidis, R. (1965). Biochim. Biophys. Res. Commun. 21, 572.

Gosline, J.M. (1973). (Personal communication).

Hall, D.A. (1959). Int. Rev. Cytol. 8, 211.

Harkness, M.L.R., Harkness, R.D., and McDonald, D.A. (1957). Proc. Roy. Soc., Ser. B. 146, 541.

Keeley, F.W., and Partridge, S.M. (1973). (In preparation).

Lent, R.W., Smith, B., Salcado, L.L., Faris, B., and Franzblau, C. (1969). Biochemistry 8, 2837.

Meyer, R.H. (1950). "Natural and Synthetic High Polymers." 2nd ed. Interscience Publ., New York.

Molinari-Tosatti, M.P., Galzigna, L., Moret, V., and Gotte, L. (1968). Calcif. Tissue Res. 2, (Suppl.), 88.

Partridge, S.M. (1966). Fed. Proc. 25, 1023.

Partridge, S.M. (1967a). Biochim. Biophys. Acta 140, 132.

Partridge, S.M. (1967b). Nature 213, 1123.

Sandberg, L.B., Weissman, N., and Smith, D.W. (1969).
    Biochemistry 8, 2940.

Smith, D.W., Brown, D.M., and Carnes, W.H. (1972). J. Biol.
    Chem. 247, 2427.

Smith, D.W., Weissman, N., and Carnes, W.H. (1968). Biochem.
    Biophys. Res. Commun. 31, 309.

Starcher, B.C., Partridge, S.M., and Elsden, D.F. (1967).
    Biochemistry 6, 2425.

Sykes, B.C., and Partridge, S.M. (1972). Biochem. J. 130, 1171.

Thomas, J., Elsden, D.F., and Partridge, S.M. (1963). Nature 200,
    651.

Urry, D.W. (1971). Proc. Nat. Acad. Sci. U.S.A. 68, 810.

Weis-Fogh, T., and Amos, W.B. (1972). Nature 236, 301.

Weis-Fogh, T., and Anderson, S.O. (1970). Nature 227, 718.

DISCUSSION FOLLOWING THE PRESENTATION BY S. M. PARTRIDGE

    Dr. Yu: Since there are at least four kinds of cross-
linking compounds which are formed from the lysine moiety and
the aldehyde of the polypeptides through an aldol condensation
reaction, which is a chemical reaction and is capable of taking
place without requirement of a specific structural configuration
on the precursor peptides, I would like to ask how these
condensation reactions take place in a nice order and form a
compact protein as you have described. Furthermore, regarding
this reaction, which is by the lysine moieties or their derivatives
in proelastin and which concerns more than 36 residues per mole of
the proelastin molecule, is it possible that the precursor
peptides react randomly since there are no enzymes to control this
type of condensation reaction?   The second question is whether
it is possible for condensation to occur between heterogenous
proteins and microfibrillar protein or collagen and elastic fiber,
since these proteins also contain lysine.

Dr. Partridge: In reply to Dr. Shiu Yeh Yu's first question, I would say that all we know at the present time is that in lathyrism or copper deficiency, a soluble protein precursor of elastin is found in the extracellular space which has a composition almost identical with mature elastin except that it has no cross-linking amino acids, but instead it has an excess of at least thirty lysine residues if the molecular weight of the elastin monomer is taken as 74,000. At the present time no one has grown elastin-producing cells in pure cell culture, nor has anyone isolated soluble elastin from the cell itself. When someone has succeeded in doing this perhaps he will find that, like collagen, there are transport forms of elastin containing extra peptides. However this may be, it is evident that any such peptides, if they exist, are removed at some point near the cell surface. In my opinion the most likely site for the oxidative deamination step is also at some specific organelle occupying part of the cell surface, and I imagine that the enzymes that do this would be membrane-bound. Certainly, what we know about the soluble elastin precursor is that it has a very labile tertiary structure but in any kind of aqueous environment, most of the lysine residues must be at the surface of the molecule and presented outwards. In this way it could be readily understood that the molecular surface could have imprinted on it a rather specific array of aldehydes and unchanged lysine residues resulting from the activity of the membrane-bound lysine oxidase. It is this array that would be expected to pre-determine the type of crosslinkages later to be found, and of course the pattern of crosslinkages would pre-determine the three-dimensional structure of the polymeric network eventually formed from the monomer.

Regarding Dr. Shiu Yeh Yu's second question, we have never had any indication that under physiological conditions elastin can become copolymerized with either collagen or glycoprotein. True enough, these substances are often very hard to remove, particularly from the aorta elastin of very young or very old humans or other animals. However, in the end it is always possible to isolate elastin of constant composition from any source, provided appropriate steps are taken. Analytical results, which take into account the usual chemical criterion of constant composition, are being very well confirmed by the rapidly increasing information about sequences in elastin. Thus, as an example, the small content of hydroxyproline always found in purified preparations of elastin is also found by the isolation of typical elastin sequences containing this amino acid. This is evidence that it is a genuine part of the structure.

Dr. Martin: Did I see a recent report from your laboratory suggesting that the molecular weight of tropoelastin is 40,000? I have seen many reports of 68,000 as the size of tropoelastin.

Dr. Partridge: Yes. In fact a molecular weight of 40,000-
50,000 was estimated for a sample of tropoelastin isolated from the
aortas of chicks made lathyritic with BAPN and labelled with ^{125}I.[1]
However, this soluble elastin was isolated by a rather complicated
procedure involving extraction with dilute formic acid at pH 2.80
and solubilization in organic solvents at acid pH, and we now
believe that this brought about some degradation. Our latest
preparations of soluble elastin from lathyritic chick aorta have
been prepared without prolonged exposure to acid conditions by a
procedure based on that of Smith et al.[2] This material appears
to be substantially homogenous, and its molecular weight was
estimated by various methods to be between 68,000 and 75,000.

Dr. Gilbert: I would like to inquire as to whether you
have used a microcalorimeter to look at the heats of solution of
elastin with various solvents rather than just looking at the heat
liberated by stretching.[3] Secondly, I am curious to know whether
you have carried out any stretching experiments in any hydrogen
bond breaking agents like 6 M guanidine HCl or urea. Experiments
in our laboratory show that these agents actually make elastin a
more perfect entropic rubber; the internal energy components of
the stretched fiber approaches zero rather than the usual 10-15%.[4]
Hydrogen bonding may, indeed, play an important role in the
conformation of what has been considered an amorphous protein.[5]

Dr. Partridge: In reply to Dr. Gilbert's first question,
I should say that I have done no microcalorimetry myself, and in
my paper I reviewed the recent work of Weis-Fogh and his colleagues
in Cambridge. So far as I know, no one has tried to measure the
heat changes during transition of soluble α-elastin or soluble
tropoelastin from the sol state to the coacervate at temperatures
in the region of 37°. I think that this might be a very useful
thing to do. Dr. Gilbert's second question can be answered in

---

[1]Sykes, B.C., and Partridge, S.M. (1972). Biochem. J.
130, 1171.

[2]Smith, D.W., Brown, D.M., and Carnes, W.H. (1972).
J. Biol. Chem. 247, 2427.

[3]Weis-Fogh, T., and Andersen, S.O. (1970). Nature 227,
718-721.

[4]Ciferri, A. (1971). J. Physical Chemistry 75, 142-150.

[5]Urry, D. (in this publication).

part from existing information. Certainly, as shown by Weis-Fogh
and Andersen, if elastin fibers are stretched and allowed to relax
when in equilibrium with solvents such as strong urea solution or
50% aqueous formamide, then the enthalpy change is reduced almost
to zero. Further, the work of Mukherjee (1969) showed that with
water as the solvent of swelling, elastin fibers showed anomalous
thermodynamic behavior when stretched at different temperatures,
and the behavior was normalized in aqueous formamide. The value
of the mean molecular weight of the kinetically free portions of
the chain between crosslinks (Mc) was calculated as 4,300 in
water, but in formamide the value for Mc was much higher at nearly
6,500. A value for Mc of this order would allow eleven crosslinks
per mole of 74,000 and could readily be accounted for on the basis
of the known crosslinkages isolated by acid or alkaline hydrolysis.
Thus in formamide, and probably in aqueous urea or guanidine salts,
the hydrophobic interactions and hydrogen bonding in elastin appear
to be abolished, and the system behaves like many synthetic elastomers as a randomly kinked network uniformly solvated.

COMPONENTS OF THE PROTEIN-LIPID COMPLEX OF ARTERIAL ELASTIN:

THEIR ROLE IN THE RETENTION OF LIPID IN ATHEROSCLEROTIC LESIONS

Dieter M. Kramsch, Carl Franzblau, and William Hollander

Boston University School of Medicine

Boston, Massachusetts

Atherosclerosis is associated with accumulations of lipids, especially ester cholesterol, in focal areas of the arterial intima and frequently in the subintimal media below plaques. The lipid accumulations commonly occur intracellularly as well as extracellularly. As many morphological studies have shown, the increased amounts of intracellular lipids are deposited mainly in proliferated and modified smooth muscle cells (Constantinides, 1965; Scott et al., 1967; Geer et al., 1968; Daoud et al., 1968). The extracellular lipids are located at the necrotic core of lesions or are associated with connective tissue which frequently has proliferated. A common finding is reduplication (or splitting) and fragmentation of the arterial elastic lamellae of the intima and subintima of lesions. These altered elastic lamellae appear to play an important role in the retention of stainable lipids in atherosclerotic lesions of all stages (Zugibe and Brown, 1960; McGill et al., 1960; Parker, 1960; Adams and Tuqan, 1961; Friedman, 1963; Lindsay and Chaikoff, 1965; Smith et al., 1967; Kramsch and Hollander, 1968).

The present studies were undertaken to achieve three goals:

(1) To correlate the structural and biochemical lipid changes occurring in arterial elastic lamellae of plaques;

(2) To determine what amount of lipids is bound by the arterial elastin and which portions of the elastin are involved in the increased lipid binding of lesion elastin; and

(3) To clarify the mechanisms involved in the binding of lipid to arterial elastin, especially to plaque elastin.

METHODS

Radioautography of arteries was performed according to the method of Kramsch et al. (1967) two to four months after intravenous injection of [^{3}H]cholesterol into moribund humans. Elastin from intimal layers of normal and atherosclerotic human aortas (containing some medial elastic lamellae) was isolated according to a modification of the method of Lansing et al. (1952), omitting delipidation of the tissues. The isolated elastin preparation was analyzed for its amino acid and lipid composition, as well as for its cholesterol radioactivity by the method described by Kramsch et al. (1971). The purity of the elastin preparation was indicated by the absence of uronic acid, neuraminic acid, and of significant amounts of hexosamine and hydroxyproline (Franzblau and Lent, 1968). Subsequent treatment of the elastin with trypsin, chymotrypsin, and hyaluronidase did not alter its amino acid or lipid composition. Portions of the non-delipidated elastin preparation were digested by elastase,which yielded in plaque elastin a soluble hydrolysate and an insoluble residue. The soluble elastase hydrolysates were separated by column chromatography on Sephadex G 200 into peptide fractions. The peptide fractions of the elastase hydrolysates of elastin and the insoluble residue after elastase were analyzed for their amino acid and lipid composition by the same methods as employed with the original elastin, and also for calcium by ashing.

The defatted elastin preparation was incubated with lipoprotein fractions of normal and hyperlipoproteinemic human plasma, as well as with lipoproteins extracted from human atherosclerotic plaques. The methods used for the incubation studies have been described previously by Kramsch and Hollander (1973). The methods for the preparation of the plasma and arterial lipoproteins were described by Hollander et al. (1967) and Hollander (1968). The lipid and protein content of the elastin was analyzed before and after incubation. In other studies the delipidated elastin was incubated with low density lipoproteins which were labeled in the lipid moiety with [^{3}H]cholesterol and labeled in the protein moiety by methods described by Hollander and Kramsch (1967). The pre-incubated elastin then was incubated again with non-labeled low density (LDL), very low density (VLDL), and high density (HDL) plasma lipoproteins (the apoproteins of these lipoproteins), and with trypsin; or it was treated again with hot alkali. The plasma HDL was delipidated by the method of Scanu (1966) and the LDL and VLDL fractions were partially delipidated by the technique of Avigan (1957).

RESULTS

Correlation of Structural and Biochemical Lipid Alterations of
Arterial Elastic Lamellae

Radioautographic Studies.   The radioautographs revealed that
dense accumulations of the intravenously injected [^{3}H]cholesterol
occurred in modified smooth muscle cells and on reduplicated (or
split) and fragmented elastic membranes of atherosclerotic lesions.
Very little cholesterol radioactivity was noted over normal smooth

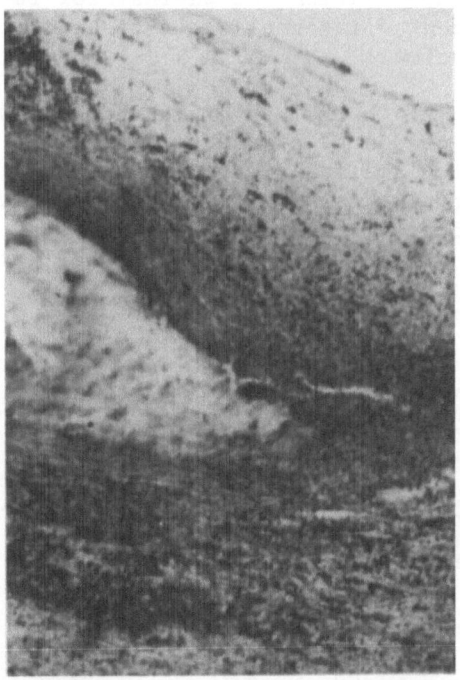

Fig. 1. Radioautograph of an advanced encapsulated plaque of
human aorta following intravenous injection of [^{3}H]cholesterol
four months prior to death. As indicated by the black granules
and bands of black granules, the radioactive cholesterol accumulated in high concentrations in cells as well as on the fragmented
and frayed elastic lamellae of the fibrous-elastic plaque capsule
around the necrotic core. In contrast,very little, if any, cholesterol radioactivity other than background artifacts was noted over
the lipid-rich gruel within the plaque capsule. Hematoxylin-Van
Gieson; exposure six weeks. (x 400). (Reduced 40% for reproduction).

muscle cells and normal elastic lamellae in uninvolved areas of
the arteries. In advanced encapsulated plaques (Figure 1) the
injected radioactive cholesterol accumulated in high concentrations in cells, as well as on the fragmented elastic lamellae of
the fibrous-elastic plaque capsule around the necrotic core. In
contrast, very little,if any,cholesterol radioactivity was observed
over the lipid-rich gruel within the plaque capsule, indicating
that the cholesterol in the plaque capsule equilibrated very slowly,
if at all,with the circulating or surrounding tissue cholesterol.
Higher magnification strikingly demonstrated the dense accumulation of the injected [^{3}H]cholesterol on the elastic membranes of
the plaque capsule (Figure 2). In fatty streaks (Figure 3) also
there were dense concentrations of cholesterol radioactivity on
the partially fragmented internal elastica as well as in the cells
of the thickened intima.

In several grossly normal arteries the only detectable microscopic abnormality consisted of reduplication (or splitting) of
the internal elastic lamella, suggesting an early elastica lesion
in an otherwise normal artery (Figure 4). Radioautography very
frequently revealed accumulations of the injected radioactive
cholesterol on the strands of the reduplicated internal elastica,

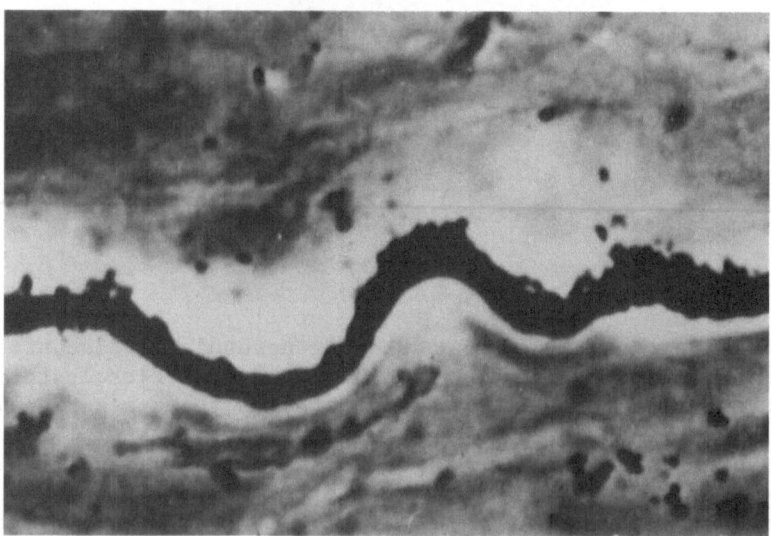

Fig. 2. Higher magnification of an elastic lamella from the
plaque capsule of the plaque shown in Fig. 1 illustrating the
dense accumulations of the intravenously injected [^{3}H]cholesterol
on the elastic lamellae. Hematoxylin-Van Gieson; exposure six
weeks. (x 2,500). (Reduced 30% for reproduction).

but not in the intima or media, suggesting that altered arterial elastica may begin very early to retain lipids.

Radiochemical Studies.   Radiochemical analysis of isolated arterial elastin revealed that the uptake of intravenously injected [3H]cholesterol by plaque elastin was five to six times higher than that by normal intimal elastin (Table I). The radiochemical findings were in agreement with the radioautographic findings, indicating a greater uptake of plasma cholesterol by plaque elastin than by normal elastin.

Elastin Protein-Lipid Complex of Normal and Plaque Elastin

Content and Composition of Elastin Protein and of Elastin Lipids. Biochemical analysis of arterial elastin revealed that elastin from normal arterial intima contained about 98% protein and one to two percent lipids (Figure 5). With increasing severity of

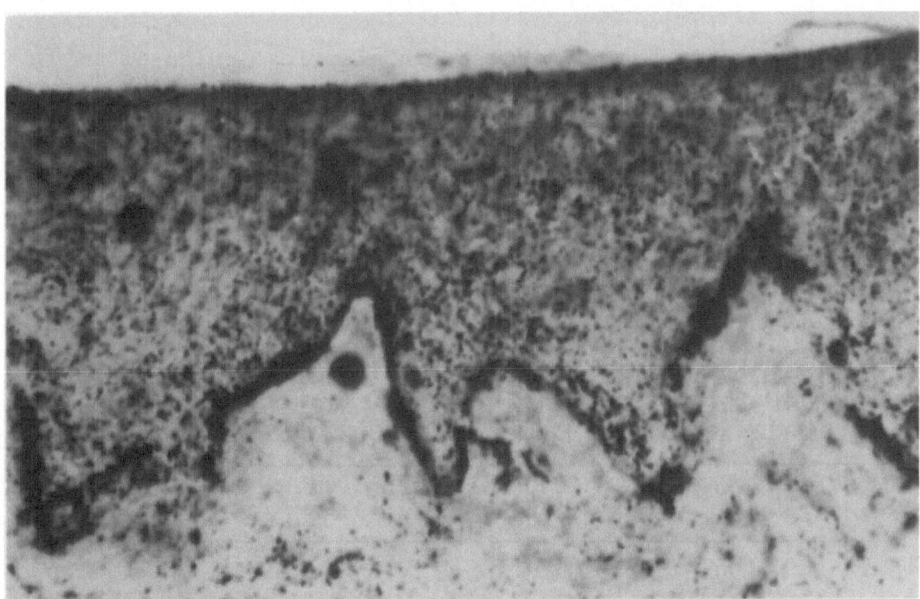

Fig. 3. Radioautograph of a fatty streak of femoral artery injected intravenously with [3H]cholesterol two months prior to death. There are dense concentrations of cholesterol radioactivity on the fragmented internal elastica as well as in cells of the thickened intima. Hematoxylin-eosin; exposure four weeks. (x 485). (Reduced 20% for reproduction).

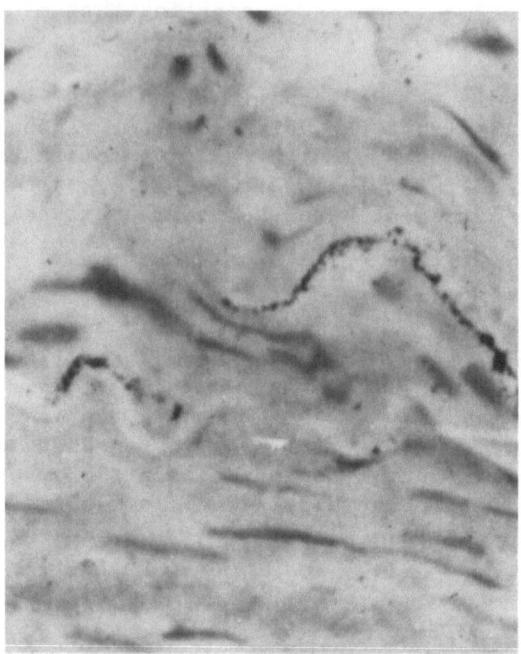

Fig. 4. Radioautograph of a microscopic elastica lesion of an otherwise normal coronary artery. Top two-thirds, intima; bottom one-third, media. The internal elastic lamella (light gray undulating bands) has reduplicated (or split). Radioactive cholesterol has accumulated on both strands of the reduplicated elastica, particularly on the upper strand. Note the absence of increased [3H]cholesterol deposition in the normal intima and media. Hematoxylin-eosin; exposure four weeks. (x 625). (Reduced 40% for reproduction).

TABLE I.   INCORPORATION OF INTRAVENOUSLY INJECTED [3H] CHOLESTEROL INTO ARTERIAL ELASTIN OF NORMAL INTIMA AND ADJACENT PLAQUE AREAS FROM HUMAN ATHEROSCLEROTIC AORTAE

	CPM/gm Elastin		Elastin Cholesterol Specific Activity	
	Free Cholesterol	Ester Cholesterol	Free Cholesterol CPM/mg	Ester Cholesterol CPM/mg
Normal	532	1072	621	530
Plaque	2760	6114	248	417

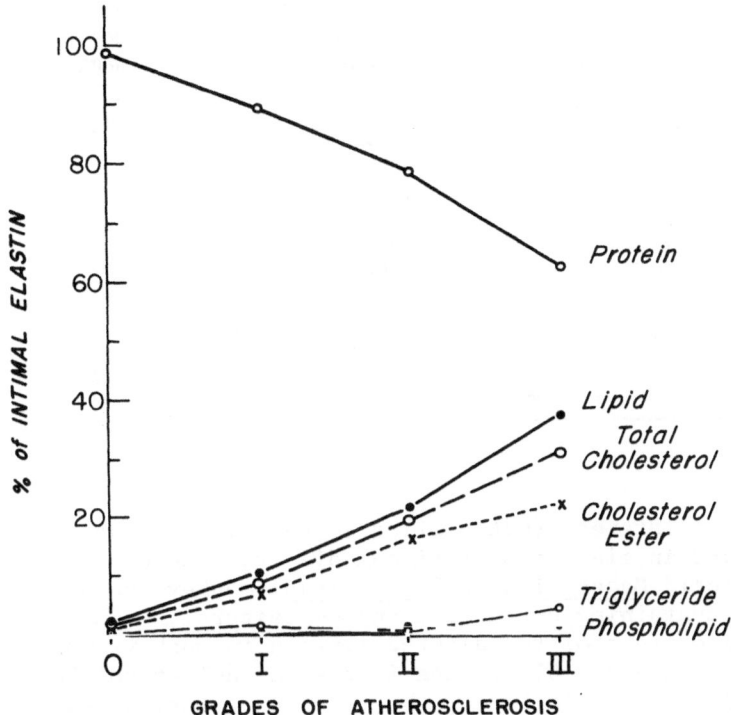

Fig. 5. Protein and lipid contents of plaque elastin with increasing severity of atherosclerosis. Grade 0 = intima with no atherosclerotic lesions; Grade I = fatty streaks and dots; Grade II = large confluent plaques; Grade III = severe calcified and ulcerated plaques.

atherosclerosis the protein moiety of plaque elastin decreased, whereas the lipid moiety increased. In severe plaques the elastin contained about 63% protein and 37% lipids. The increase in the lipid moiety was primarily due to large increases in cholesterol, mainly ester cholesterol, with minor increases in phospholipids and triglycerides. It is noteworthy that about 30% of the total intimal cholesterol of plaques was contained in plaque elastin except for very severe plaques with large amorphous centers (Figure 3). The amino acid composition of plaque elastin protein also was altered (Table II) with striking increases in polar acting amino acids (aspartic acid, threonine, serine, glutamic acid, lysine, histidine, and arginine) and decreases in the cross-linking amino acids desmosine, isodesmosine, and lysinonorleucine. However, the changes in the content of cross-linking amino acids may have been only an apparent alteration due to the large increases in polar amino acids per 1000 amino acid residues.

TABLE II.   CHANGES IN THE AMINO ACID COMPOSITION OF ELASTIN
             PROTEIN FROM PLAQUE AREAS AND ADJACENT NORMAL AREAS
             OF THE INTIMA IN HUMAN ATHEROSCLEROTIC AORTAE

Amino Acid	Normal	Plaque	% Change
	(Residues/1000 residues)		
Aspartic Acid	5.6	23.1	+ 312
Threonine	10.9	16.2	+ 48
Serine	10.6	16.6	+ 57
Glutamic Acid	20.4	40.7	+ 99
Lysine	7.9	14.8	+ 87
Histidine	2.0	5.1	+ 155
Arginine	8.9	15.2	+ 71
1/4 Isodesmosine	4.6	2.9	- 37
1/4 Desmosine	6.1	3.7	- 39
1/2 Lysinonorleucine	1.2	0.2	- 83

It is of interest that similar increases in polar amino acids
were observed in elastin of intima-media from whole aorta of
atherosclerotic Macaca fascicularis (irus) monkeys on an atherogenic diet containing butter fat and cholesterol. Likewise, the
cholesterol content of the altered elastin in monkeys was markedly
increased, with about 60% of the increased cholesterol being
cholesterol ester. Similarly, the elastin of intima-media of whole
aorta also showed marked increases in the same polar amino acids
in rabbits on an atherogenic diet of peanut oil and cholesterol,
as did elastin from human plaques (Table II) and from atherosclerotic monkey aorta. In the elastin of atherosclerotic aortae from
both animal species the content in cross-linking amino acids was
normal. The total elastin protein content of whole aorta in
atherosclerotic rabbits was about 35% higher than that of normal
rabbit aorta. As in the aortic elastin of atherosclerotic monkeys,
the elastin cholesterol content of atherosclerotic rabbit aortae
was about 10 times higher than that of aortic elastin from normal
rabbits, with 58% of the increased cholesterol being cholesterol
ester. In a few animals the elastin of normal appearing aortic
areas adjacent to plaques was analyzed. As in humans, the aortic
elastin from these normal appearing areas was normal in both
animal species, indicating that the changes in amino acid and
lipid composition were restricted to the plaques. It is noteworthy,
therefore, that the compositional changes of elastin protein and
lipids in these animals were detectable despite the fact that the
elastin alterations were diluted by large amounts of normal elastin
from the widespread aortic areas not involved by the disease.

Enzymatic Hydrolysis of Normal and Plaque Elastin. When nondeli-
pidated arterial elastin was digested with elastase (Table III),
normal elastin was completely hydrolyzed. By contrast, only 75%

TABLE III.   DEGRADATION OF NON-DELIPIDATED ARTERIAL ELASTIN BY
ELASTASE (In % of Total Dry Weight)

	Soluble Component	Insoluble Residue
Normal Elastin	100%	0%
Plaque Elastin	75.4%	24.6%

of plaque elastin became soluble,whereas 25% remained insoluble
after elastase.

Composition of Lipopeptides from Elastase Hydrolysates.   The soluble elastase hydrolysates of plaque elastin were separable into
two fractions, F_1 and F_2, by chromatography on Sephadex G 200
columns (Figure 6).   In contrast, elastase hydrolysates of normal
elastin yielded only one fraction, F_3, which showed an elution
pattern similar to that of fraction F_2 from plaque elastin.
Fraction F_1 of plaque elastin could not be separated further with
Biogel 150 or by ion exchange chromatography.   Each of the fractions (F_1, F_2, and F_3) migrated as a single band on disc electrophoresis in 3.5% polyacrylamide gel.   In duplicate gels the single
band of fraction F_1 from plaque elastin stained with Amido Schwarz
for peptides in one gel and with Oil Red O for lipids in the other
gel, indicating that fraction F_1 contained considerable amounts
of lipids which migrated with the peptides.

Protein and lipid analysis of these lipopeptide fractions
isolated from arterial elastin (Table IV) revealed that fraction
F_3 contained about 99% peptide and less than 1% lipids.   Similar
small amounts of lipids were contained in fraction F_2 from plaque
elastin.   The lipid contents of both fractions F_2 and F_3 were
comparable to those of normal elastin before digestion with
elastase (Figure 5).   In contrast, the lipopeptide fraction F_1
from plaque elastin contained about 65% peptide and 44% lipid.
The changes in the lipid composition of this lipopeptide fraction
were comparable to those seen in the original plaque elastin
before digestion with elastase (Figure 5).   The increases in the
lipid moiety of fraction F_1 was due mainly to large increases in
cholesterol, especially ester cholesterol, with smaller changes
in phospholipids and triglycerides.   From these findings it appears
that the bulk of the lipids bound to plaque elastin was incorporated in the lipopeptide fraction F_1.   It is of interest that none
of the lipopeptide fractions of normal or plaque elastin contained
measurable amounts of hexosamine, hexuronic acid, neuraminic acid,
or calcium.

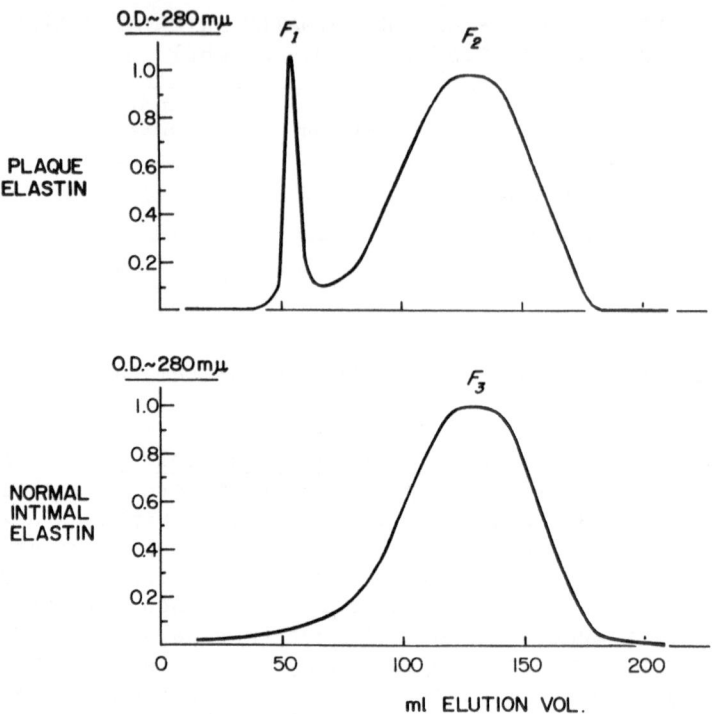

Fig. 6. Elution profiles of non-delipidated elastase hydrolysates from normal and plaque elastin chromatographed on Sephadex G200 columns.

TABLE IV. PEPTIDE AND LIPID CONTENTS OF LIPOPEPTIDE FRACTIONS ISOLATED FROM ELASTASE DIGESTS OF NON-DELIPIDATED ELASTIN FROM PLAQUES AND NORMAL AORTIC INTIMA

| mg/gm Lipopeptide | Plaque Elastin | | Normal Elastin |
	F_1	F_2	F_3
Peptide	558.8	997.9	996.8
Lipid	441.2	2.1	3.2
Free Cholesterol	100.8	0.7	1.6
Ester Cholesterol	280.0	0.5	0.3
Phospholipids	16.4	0.3	0.5
Triglycerides	44.1	0.6	0.8

As seen in Table V the amino acid composition of lipopeptide fraction F_3 from normal elastin was similar to that of fraction F_2 from plaque elastin. The amino acid compositions of both lipopeptide fractions F_2 and F_3 were comparable to that of normal

TABLE V. AMINO ACID COMPOSITION OF LIPOPEPTIDE FRACTIONS ISOLATED
          FROM ELASTIN DIGESTS OF ELASTIN FROM PLAQUES AND NORMAL
          AORTIC INTIMA

Amino Acids	Plaque Elastin		Normal Elastin
	F_1	F_2	F_3
	(Residues/1000 residues)		
Cysteic Acid	2.2	2.8	0.8
Hydroxyproline	33.4*	12.1	12.5
Aspartic Acid	51.2*	4.8	5.6
Threonine	34.1*	14.8	12.2
Serine	27.8*	11.5	9.5
Glutamic Acid	104.7*	25.1	21.2
Proline	117.8†	135.0	127.5
Glycine	200.5†	278.7	297.6
Alanine	122.2†	212.4	210.6
Valine	47.0†	135.1	130.6
Isoleucine	39.3	26.8	27.3
Leucine	65.0	62.6	64.5
Tyrosine	31.3	24.0	23.6
Phenylalanine	21.7	24.1	26.2
1/4 Isodesmosine	8.9	4.6	5.0
1/4 Desmosine	9.2	6.7	7.3
1/2 Lysinorleucine	0.6	0.8	1.3
Lysine	23.1*	6.6	6.9
Histidine	18.2*	3.1	1.9
Arginine	32.3*	9.2	7.9
Total	1,000.0	999.9	999.7

* Markedly increased from values of normal elastin.
† Markedly diminished from values of normal elastin.

elastin before elastase digestion, suggesting that these fractions
were identical and represented normal elastin. In contrast, the
amino acid composition of lipopeptide fraction F_1 of plaque
elastin revealed striking changes consisting of marked increases
in hydroxyproline, aspartic acid, threonine, serine, glutamic
acid, lysine, histidine, and arginine; whereas, proline, glycine,
alanine, and valine were markedly reduced when compared to the
composition of F_2 or fraction F_3 from normal elastin. Furthermore, it is noteworthy that the elastin cross-links were not
reduced in the abnormal lipopeptide fraction F_1.

Composition of the Elastase-Insoluble Residue of Plaque Elastin.
The insoluble residue remaining after elastase digestion of plaque
elastin consisted of about 87% inorganic matter, 10% protein, and
3% lipids (Table VI). As with the lipid moiety of the original
plaque elastin before elastase and the soluble fraction F_1 from

TABLE VI.   COMPOSITION OF THE INSOLUBLE RESIDUE REMAINING AFTER
TREATMENT OF THE HUMAN PLAQUE ELASTIN PREPARATION WITH
ELASTASE

	(mg/gm dry residue)
Inorganic Matter	868.2*
Protein	101.5
Lipid	31.3
Free Cholesterol	11.3
Ester Cholesterol	18.1
Phospholipids	0.2
Triglycerides	0.4

* 75% of the inorganic matter being calcium.

elastase hydrolysates of plaque elastin (Table IV), the lipid
moiety contained in the insoluble residue was mainly cholesterol,
especially ester cholesterol, with small amounts being triglycerides and phospholipids. The residue did not contain hexosamine,
hexuronic acid, or neuraminic acid. However, in contrast to the
soluble elastase hydrolysate, the insoluble residue did contain
calcium which accounted for 75% of the inorganic matter. The
protein, lipid, and calcium composition was not altered by a
second treatment with elastase or with collagenase, papain, trypsin,
and Nagarse. Delipidation of the residue did not render these
enzymes more effective. However, after demineralization of non-
delipidated residue with sodium EDTA the residue protein, which
still contained the lipids, was completely hydrolyzed by elastase,
papain or Nagarse, but not by collagenase or trypsin. These
findings indicate that portions of the residue calcium, perhaps
in the form of apatite, may be tightly associated with this residue
protein, protecting it from enzymatic attack.

The amino acid composition of the protein contained in the
insoluble residue revealed alterations similar to those found in
the elastase soluble fraction F_1 from the same plaque elastin
(Table V). The contents in cross-linking amino acids of residue
elastin were comparable to those of normal arterial elastin
(Table II), indicating that the residue protein was elastin, albeit
altered. The abnormal amino acid composition of the residue
elastin remained essentially unchanged after demineralization and
subsequent treatment with collagenase or trypsin. The similarities between the abnormal lipopeptide fraction F_1 (Table V) and
the abnormal residue elastin suggest that both compounds may be
essentially similar, with the difference being that the elastin-

lipid complex of the residue was protected by calcium from digestion with elastase.

Interaction of Arterial Elastin with Lipoproteins

<u>Elastin and the Lipid Moiety of Lipoproteins.</u>   <u>In vitro</u> incuba-
tions of isolated defatted aortic elastin with serum lipoproteins
revealed uptake of lipids by the elastin. After 24 hours over 75%
of the ester cholesterol from the LDL and VLDL fractions of normal
(Table VII) or hyperlipoproteinemic (Table VIII) human serum was
transferred to plaque elastin. The amounts of ester cholesterol
taken up by plaque elastin were greater from the LDL and VLDL
fractions of hyperlipemic serum than from the same fractions of
normal serum, indicating that the uptake of ester cholesterol by
plaque elastin was concentration-dependent. The findings also
indicate that plaque elastin may continue to incorporate lipids
even when the serum cholesterol levels are normal. The ester
cholesterol uptake by normal elastin was much less than that by

TABLE VII. LIPID UPTAKE BY DELIPIDATED NORMAL AND PLAQUE ELASTIN
OF HUMAN AORTIC INTIMAL INCUBATED WITH LIPOPROTEIN
FRACTIONS OF NORMAL HUMAN SERUM

		Ester Choles- terol (mg)	Free Choles- terol (mg)	Phospho- lipids (mg)	Trigly- cerides (mg)
d < 1.006	Incubation Medium (10 ml)	5.4	1.8	3.6	10.6
	Normal Elastin Plaque Elastin (50 mg)	1.6 4.1	0.1 0.4	0.2 1.1	1.7 2.4
d 1.006 to 1.063	Incubation Medium (10 ml)	8.7	4.9	5.3	3.6
	Normal Elastin Plaque Elastin (50 mg)	1.7 6.1	0.2 0.7	1.0 2.2	0.7 1.6
d 1.063 to 1.210	Incubation Medium (10 ml)	2.4	0.5	8.5	2.4
	Normal Elastin Plaque Elastin (50 mg)	0 0	0 0	0.3 0.5	0 0

TABLE VIII.   LIPID UPTAKE BY DELIPIDATED NORMAL AND PLAQUE
              ELASTIN OF HUMAN AORTIC INTIMA INCUBATED WITH SERUM
              LIPOPROTEIN FRACTION d 1.006 - 1.063 OF PATIENTS
              WITH HYPERLIPOPROTEINEMIA TYPE IIa

	Ester Cholesterol (mg)	Free Cholesterol (mg)	Phospholipids (mg)	Triglycerides (mg)
Incubation Medium (10 ml)	20.3	8.5	16.6	8.5
Normal Elastin	1.8	0.2	2.1	1.1
Plaque Elastin (50 mg)	14.8	2.1	4.2	2.7

plaque elastin and did not appear to be concentration-dependent.
Only minor amounts of free cholesterol, phospholipid, and triglycerides were transferred to both normal and plaque elastin.
Similar lipid transfers occurred with arterial lipoproteins. No
cholesterol was transferred to normal or plaque elastin from the
HDL fractions of normal or hyperlipoproteinemic serum, or from
the chylomicron fraction of patients with hyperlipoproteinemia
Type V. In some incubation studies the lipid moiety was labeled
with [^{3}H] cholesterol. Subsequent incubation of pre-incubated
plaque elastin with non-labeled serum LDL, VLDL and HDL, or the
apoproteins of these lipoproteins, did not remove the transferred
cholesterol, indicating that the affinity of cholesterol to plaque
elastin was greater than to the lipoproteins.

Elastin and the Protein Moiety of Lipoproteins.   When delipidated
elastin was incubated with LDL fractions labeled in the protein
moiety with ^{125}I, small amounts of the lipoprotein protein also
seemed to have settled with the elastin after 24 hours. However,
subsequent treatment with trypsin removed all of the lipoprotein
protein but not the transferred cholesterol, indicating that the
protein moiety of lipoproteins did not take part in the binding
of lipid by elastin. When LDL-incubated plaque elastin was
treated a second time with hot alkali, a substantial part of the
elastin protein itself was hydrolyzed. However, over 30% of the
transferred cholesterol remained associated with the elastin,
suggesting a firm binding of the lipid by plaque elastin.

CONCLUSION

    Arterial elastin is a protein-lipid complex which is altered
in atherosclerotic lesions. With increasing severity of athero-

sclerosis there is a progressive accumulation of lipid, especially ester cholesterol, in plaque elastin. The prerequisite for the lipid accumulation in plaque elastin appears to be an altered amino acid composition consisting mainly of an increase in polar amino acids. Similar alterations of arterial elastin in atherosclerosis were noted by Yu (1971). The abnormal elastin protein in atherosclerotic lesions may be newly synthetized elastin elaborated by smooth muscle cells under the atherogenic stimuli or another protein, rich in polar amino acids, may have been bound during atherogenesis to the plaque elastin rendering it also resistant to alkali extraction. The mechanism involved in the accumulation of lipid in elastin from atherosclerotic lesions appears to be an interaction of the altered elastin protein with serum or arterial LDL and VLDL. The amount of ester cholesterol incorporated into diseased elastin appears to be dependent on the concentration of these lipoproteins. The binding of lipid to diseased elastin is firm and may be irreversible. After elastase treatment a highly abnormal lipopeptide was isolated from the elastase hydrolysates of plaque elastin. This abnormal lipopeptide was responsible for the bulk of the lipids incorporated into elastin from plaques. The insoluble residue remaining after elastase treatment of plaque elastin likewise contained an abnormal elastin-lipid complex which was rich in cholesterol and calcium. The calcium minerals appeared to protect the residue elastin from enzymatic attack.

From the radioautographic and biochemical findings it appears that there may be a number of cholesterol pools in atherosclerotic lesions - one pool that equilibrates rather rapidly with the plasma cholesterol and at least two that are relatively stagnant pools. These findings are consistent with our earlier work which also indicated a greater influx of plasma cholesterol into the atherosclerotic plaque than into the normal artery (Hollander et al., 1967). One of the stagnant pools in the diseased artery appears to exist only in the necrotic core of encapsulated plaques where new cholesterol appears unable to enter and from which the encapsulated cholesterol may not be able to exit. The other stagnant pool which appears to exist in all types of atherosclerotic lesions is the cholesterol pool that is firmly bound to the elastin of plaques. This pool is a sizable one since 30% of the total intimal cholesterol of plaques appears to be contained in the protein-lipid complex of plaque elastin. The findings indicate that diseased arterial elastin plays an important role in the lipid and calcium retention of atherosclerotic lesions. Although the lipids accumulating in cells of atherosclerotic lesions may be removable (Armstrong et al., 1970), it is doubtful whether the diseased elastin can regress toward normal once the atherogenic stimuli are no longer present. This appears to be true particularly for the diseased elastin which is encrusted with calcium minerals.

ACKNOWLEDGEMENT

This work was partially supported by U.S. Public Health Service Grant HL-13262.

REFERENCES

Adams, C.W.M., and Tuqan, N.A. (1961). J. Pathol. Bacteriol. 82, 131.

Armstrong, M.L., Warner, E.D., and Connor, W. (1970). Circ. Res. 27, 59.

Avigan, J. (1957). J. Biol. Chem. 226, 957.

Constantinides, P. (1965). "Experimental Atherosclerosis." Elsevier Publishing, Amsterdam.

Daoud, A.S., Jones, R., and Scott, R.F. (1968). Exp. Mol. Pathol. 8, 3.

Franzblau, C., and Lent, R.W. (1968). In "Structure, Function and Evolution in Proteins." Brookhaven Symposia in Biology, Part 2., Vol. 21. p. 328. Brookhaven National Laboratory, Upton, New York.

Friedman, M. (1963). Arch. Pathol. 76, 318.

Geer, J.P., Catsulis, C., McGill, H.C., Jr., and Strong, P. (1968). Amer. J. Pathol. 52, 265.

Hollander, W. (1968). Exp. Mol. Pathol. 7, 248.

Hollander, W., and Kramsch, D.M. (1967). J. Atheroscler. Res. 7, 491.

Hollander, W., Kramsch, D.M., and Inoue, G. (1968). In "Recent Advances in Atherosclerosis." Progress in Biochemical Pharmacology, Vol. 4. p. 270. S. Karger, New York.

Kramsch, D.M., Franzblau, C., and Hollander, W. (1971). J. Clin. Invest. 50, 1666.

Kramsch, D.M., Gore, I., and Hollander, W.J. (1967). Atheroscler. Res. 7, 501.

Kramsch, D.M., and Hollander, W. (1973). J. Clin. Invest. 52, 236.

Kramsch, D.M., and Hollander, W. (1968). Exp. Mol. Pathol. 9, 1.

Lansing, A.I., Rosenthal, T.B., Alex, M., and Dempsey, E.W. (1952). Anat. Rec. 114, 555.

Lindsay, S., and Chaikoff, I.L. (1965). Arch. Pathol. 79, 379.

McGill, H.C., Jr., Strong, J.P., Holman, R.L., and Werthessen, N.T. (1960). Circ. Res. 8, 670.

Parker, F. (1960). Amer. J. Pathol. 36, 19.

Scanu, A. (1966). J. Lipid Res. 7, 295.

Scott, R.F., Jones, R., Daoud, A.S., Zumbo, O., Coulston, F., and Thomas, W. (1967). Exp. Mol. Pathol. 7, 34.

Smith, E.B., Evans, P.H., and Downham, M.D. (1967). J. Atheroscler. Res. 7, 171.

Yu, S.Y. (1971). Lab. Invest. 25, 121.

Zugibe, F.T., and Brown, K.D. (1960). Circ. Res. 8, 287.

DISCUSSION FOLLOWING THE PRESENTATION BY DIETER M. KRAMSCH

Unidentified Speaker: One of your earlier slides showed that the elastin which you isolated from the plaque had considerably higher content of polar amino acids and a lower content of desmosine and isodesmosine, and I think this would go along with the fact that there were considerably more of the microfibrils present. I don't know how you isolated the elastins so I can't tell whether you get rid of the microfibrillar glycoprotein while your preparations are made. If there is more, where do you think these polar amino acids are? I wouldn't like to suggest that they are in the elastin.

Dr. Kramsch: I don't really know. Either they come from another protein attached to the elastin or, I cannot exclude, that under the atherogenic stimuli the smooth muscle cell does produce indeed an elastin with more polar amino acids. This may be so with collagen, but I can't tell whether it is also true with elastin.

Unidentified Speaker: You did mention, or at least you did emphasize that there was a possibility that collagen, which is the mineralizing substrate electron, could be a part of the insoluble residue since it became digestible after you decalcified the residue.

Dr. Kramsch: I thought that too, and for that reason I incubated the elastin preparation after decalcification with collagenase several times. But the abnormal amino acid composition of the elastin preparation remained the same. I also did not mention that I subjected the demineralized elastin preparation a second time to alkali hydrolysis and that the abnormal amino acid composition of the elastin preparation did not change.

Unidentified Speaker: Did you digest it with collagenase after decalcification?

Dr. Kramsch: Yes. But collagenase had no effect on this protein.

Dr. Keeley: Dr. Partridge and I analyzed some calcified plaques from aorta, and we found similar results. Of course, the collagen was very concentrated in the areas of calcified plaques, but our findings were that after we demineralized with EDTA and then extracted for 45 minutes, the composition of the resulting elastin was identical with the composition of elastin isolated in a similar way from a 23 year old aorta.

Dr. Kramsch: I did that too, but didn't you destroy part of the elastin itself that way?

Dr. Keeley: The appearance of the elastin from calcified plaques was different from the elastin of decalcified aortas. If we just extracted the heavily calcified elastin with hot alkali, there was a considerable amount of mineral residue, sometimes up to 15% of the total residue, but if we decalcified first, we found that all of these calcified areas could be extracted in a single 45 minute period.

Dr. Kramsch: Was this delipidated elastin?

Dr. Keeley: Yes.

Dr. Sobel: Along the line suggested by Dr. Nimni, we have found that if collagen is exposed to high oxygen pressure, it becomes vastly modified so that the collagen is no longer soluble in hot water or formic acid, nor is it digested by collagenase. This material would remain behind in the "elastin" that you have isolated. Collagen and other proteins are damaged in this way to become highly insoluble. Are you suggesting this in terms of what Dr. Nimni said?

Dr. Kramsch: It is highly possible.

STUDIES ON THE CONFORMATION AND INTERACTIONS OF ELASTIN

Dan W. Urry

Laboratory of Molecular Biophysics, University of

Alabama Medical Center, Birmingham, Alabama

It is apparent at each level of microscopic examination that connective tissue components of the arterial wall are beautifully organized molecular constructs. Similarly, it is evident that transition from a healthy, elastic arterial wall to a diseased, sclerotic arterial wall involves changes in those molecular constructs - changes which can be described in terms of the forces that bind atoms, ions, and molecules together. Our interest centers on the molecular aspects of this transition, i.e., on the molecular pathogenesis of atherosclerosis.

A description of molecular pathogenesis quite naturally begins with a working model of the healthy connective tissue components. Because of the state of knowledge and because of its implication in the process of arteriosclerosis, our laboratory has focused on a study of the conformation and interactions of elastin. In the second major section of this report, we have presented a working hypothesis for the conformation of elastin and for the forces involved in maintaining a functional elastic fibrillar organization. In the first major section of the present manuscript we have demonstrated the capacity of elastin sequences to selectively bind calcium ions at peptide oxygens. The third and last major section of this report attempts to correlate these molecular descriptions with a molecular pathogenesis of atherosclerosis, and it has as its basis our 1971 paper (Urry, 1971), which can now be extended as to detail by the contents of the present report and by additional recently published accounts from other laboratories.

In the early 1970's this laboratory published a paper proposing a new mechanism for the binding of calcium ion to protein components,

e.g., elastin and collagen, of the arterial wall and discussed
possible ways in which the new mechanism could relate to pathogenic
processes associated with atherosclerosis (Urry, 1971). The paper
was based on our previous work on cation binding to ion transporting
polypeptide antibiotics. With knowledge of the amino acid composition of elastin (Petruska and Sandberg, 1968; Franzblau and Lent,
1969) and the often described affinity of elastin for calcium ion,
it was proposed that Ca^{++} bind at neutral sites, the acyl oxygen
of the peptide moiety, and that this mode of binding could be
related to other processes associated with atherosclerosis, e.g.,
lipid deposition and calcification.

More specifically, it was proposed that the presence of a
large percentage of glycine residues would, when in appropriate
sequence with bulky and hydrophobic L-amino acids, result in the
formation of conformational features called β-turns (Urry and
Ohnishi, 1970; Ohnishi and Urry, 1969) (Figure 1) which consist
of a ten atom hydrogen-bonded ring inserted into the polypeptide
backbone. The β-turn is such that the end peptide moiety has its
peptide acyl oxygen directed nearly perpendicular to the plane of
the other atoms, i.e., in an exposed position favorable for coordination of calcium ion. The glycine-containing amino acid sequences
listed as probable were:

> (a)   L - L - Gly - Gly - L - L
>
> (b)   L - Gly - L - Gly - L
>
> (c)   L - L - Gly - L - L - Gly
>
> (d)   L - Gly - L - Gly - L - L
>
> (e)   Gly - L-Pro

where L stands for an L-amino acid residue.

Subsequently, Foster et al. (in press) have determined the
amino acid sequences of some dozen peptides of soluble elastin
obtained from the aorta of copper deficient swine. Altogether,
just less than one-half of the approximately 800 amino acid residues of soluble elastin have been sequenced. In summary, all of
the sequences listed as probable (Urry, 1971) have been found.
In correspondence with the list above:

> (a)   Gly - Gly - L-Val - L-Pro - Gly - L-Ala -
>   L-Val - L-Pro - Gly - Gly - L-Val - L-Pro -
>   Gly - Gly - L-Val - L-Phe -

is the amino terminal sequence. With the exception of position 6,

a

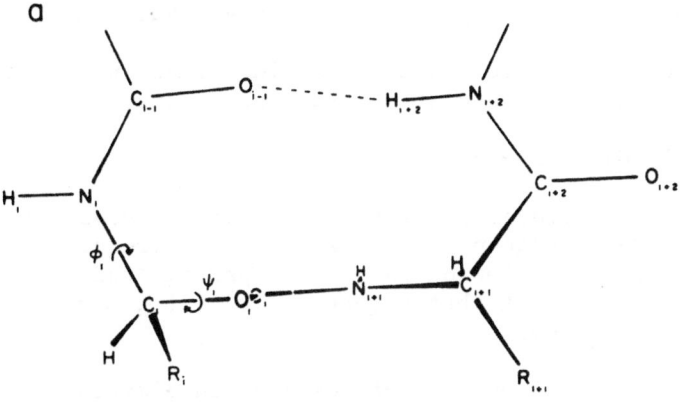

b

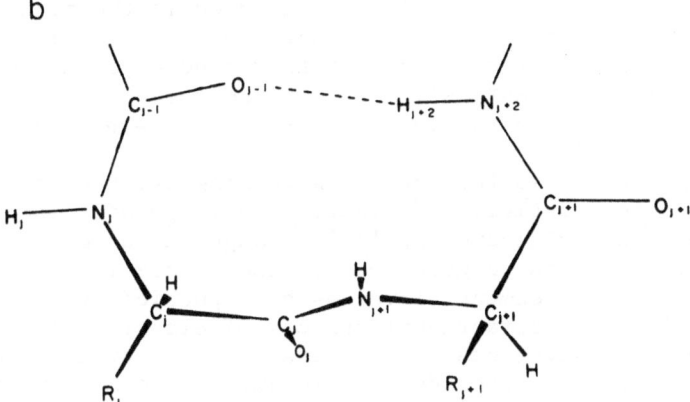

Fig. 1. β-turns.

an alanine residue, the sequence is one in which two glycine residues alternate with two hydrophobic L-amino acids, i.e., a repeating tetrapeptide.

(b)   (L-Pro - Gly - L-Val - Gly - L-Val)

This sequence is found to repeat two times in a single sequence, as well as to appear in other sequences, with alanine or isoleucine in place of valine.

(c)   L - L - Gly - L - L - Gly

This is the repeating sequence of collagen and it occurs at least twice in tropoelastin.

(d)   (L-Pro - Gly - L-Val - Gly - L-Val - L-Ala)

This sequence is found to repeat five plus times in a single sequence, as well as to appear in other sequences.

(e)   Gly - L-Pro

is found to occur several times in the sequences reported, and of course, the inverse sequence appears with high frequency. The delightful result, in view of the 1971 paper, is that not only do the sequences occur, but that sequences (a), (b), and (d) occur as regularly repeating units.

A major aspect of our recent research on elastin has been to synthesize these sequences and study their conformation and cation binding capacity. Evidence will be presented in the present manuscript that these sequences, as anticipated, form β-turns capable of binding cations, and that they bind calcium ion with a high selectivity over Na^+, K^+, Mg^{++}, making these the first characterized sequences to bind Ca^{++} over Na^+ preferentially.

In addition, gross features of a working hypothesis for the conformation and elasticity of elastin are proposed. The description is one of a serial and parallel arrangement of elastomeric segments with different degrees of stiffness, wherein the lateral association between segments involves hydrophobic forces. The conformational and interactional aspects of elastin and its repeating peptide sequences are discussed in relation to ionic and molecular associations considered relevant to the molecular pathogenesis of atherosclerosis.

STUDIES ON REPEATING SYNTHETIC SEQUENCES OF ELASTIN

Peptide Synthesis

The repeating tetra-, penta-, and hexapeptides of elastin have been synthesized for the most part by the fragment condensation method. Purity was determined by amino acid analysis, elemental analysis, thin layer chromatography, gel filtration, ion exchange resins, and nuclear magnetic resonance. A listing of the synthesized peptides is given in Table I. In addition to the simple repeating unit, linear and cyclic oligomers of the repeating unit, as well as the high polymers have been synthesized. These peptides allow conformational characterization of the repeating units, as well as a detailed study of their ion binding and other interactional capacities.

TABLE I.   SYNTHESIZED ELASTIN SEQUENCES

Tetrapeptides	Pentapeptides	Hexapeptides
$(PGGV)_1$	$(VPGVG)_1$	$(APGVGV)_1$
$(PGGV)_3$	$(VPGVG)_2$	$(APGVGV)_2$
$(PGGV)_4$	$(VPGVG)_3$	$(APGVGV)_3$
⌐$(PGGV)_3$⌐	⌐$(VPGVG)_2$⌐	⌐$(APGVGV)$⌐
⌐$(PGGV)_4$⌐		
·V-$(PGGV)_n$	$(VPGVG)_n$-V	V-$(APGVGV)_n$
$(VPGG)_1$		$(VAPGVG)_1$
$(GVPG)_1$		

G = Glycine
V = L-Valine
P = L-Proline
A = L-Alanine

Conformational Studies Using NMR

Pentapeptide Series. - Proton magnetic resonance studies have been carried out on the penta-, deca-, and pentadecapeptide of the basic sequence - L-Val$_1$ - L-Pro$_2$ - Gly$_3$ - L-Val$_4$ - Gly$_5$ -. Two methods, temperature dependence and methanol-trifluorethanol solvent mixture dependence of peptide proton chemical shift, have been used to delineate peptide protons. The pmr spectrum of the decapeptide in the peptide proton region is given in Figure 2. Assignments of all protons are indicated. The temperature dependences of peptide proton chemical shift in DMSO-d$_6$ and in methanol are given in Tables II and III, respectively. It is seen that the peptide protons of valines 4, 9, and 14 have the lowest temperature coefficient and, with the exception of the t-BOC amino terminus, that the chemical shifts are at the highest field position, i.e., at the smallest ppm for the 0° intercept. In addition, in Figure 3 the same valine residues (4 and 9) of the decapeptide show only slight upfield shifts on addition of trifluoroethanol to a methanol solution, whereas all other peptide protons shift dramatically upfield. Thus, the two methods delineate the valine 4, 9, and 14 peptide protons. In the gramicidin S model system, as well as in other systems, this delineation has been correlated with intramolecular hydrogen-bonding (Urry and Ohnishi, 1970; Ohnishi and Urry, 1969; Pitner and Urry, 1972).

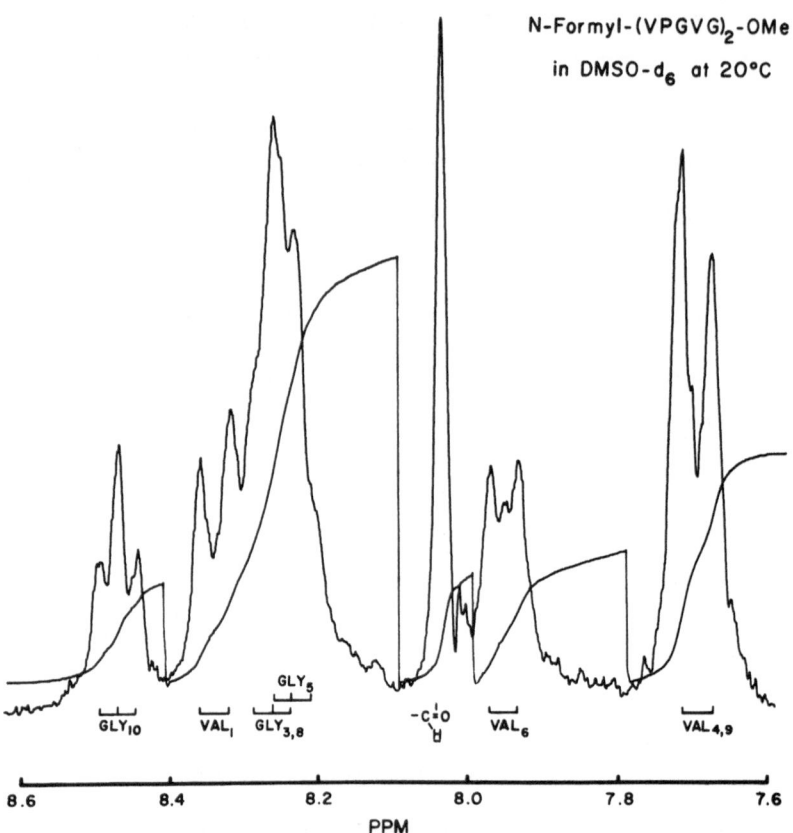

Fig. 2. Proton magnetic resonance spectrum of the peptide proton region of the decapeptide. The doublets are valine residues and the triplets are glycine residues. The formyl proton also occurs in this region. The chemical shifts are given in ppm (Hz/220 MHz) from the resonance for tetramethylsilane.

The two methods, the relatively high field position of the valine 4, 9, and 14 peptide protons (explicable by the anisotropic shielding of the end peptide of a β-turn) and the αCH-NH coupling constants for the valine residues ($^3J_{\alpha CH-NH}$ of 8 Hz or greater), are consistent with the presence of a β-turn in which L-Pro$_2$ - Gly$_3$ form the corners as indicated in Figure 4.

The Hexapeptide Series. - Proton magnetic resonance studies have been carried out on the hexa-, dodeca-, and octadecapeptides containing the repeat sequence - L-Ala$_1$ - L-Pro$_2$ - Gly$_3$ - L-Val$_4$ - Gly$_5$ - L-Val$_6$ -. As with the pentapeptide series, the assignments of the peptide proton resonances were made in dimethylsulfoxide (DMSO-d$_6$), utilizing a tracking frequency sweep decoupling accessory

TABLE II.   TEMPERATURE DEPENDENCE OF PEPTIDE PROTON CHEMICAL SHIFT OF (VPGVG) OLIGOMERS IN DMSO-d_6

PEPTIDE RESIDUE	t-BOC-(VPGVG)-OMe		N-formyl-(VPGVG)$_2$-OMe		N-formyl-(VPGVG)$_3$-OMe	
	Slope ppm/deg	0°C Intercept	Slope ppm/deg	0°C Intercept	Slope ppm/deg	0°C Intercept
Val$_1$	.0106[2]	7.03[2]	.0060[4]	8.46[4]	.0064[4]	8.49[4]
Val$_6$			.0064	8.08	.0065	} 8.13
Val$_{11}$					.0065	
Gly$_3$	.0047	8.39	.0047	8.36	.0050	
Gly$_8$			.0047	8.36	.0050	} 8.39
Gly$_{13}$					.0050	
Val$_4$	.0044	7.77	.0044	7.78	.0044	
Val$_9$			.0044	7.78	.0044	} 7.81
Val$_{14}$					.0044	
Gly$_5$	.0058[3]	8.58[3]	.0047	8.33	.0050	
Gly$_{16}$			.0057[3]	8.59[3]	.0050	} 8.39
Gly$_{15}$					.0058[3]	8.62[3]

(1) Temperature range 20°C to 70°C.
(2) This residue is displaced due to the t-BOC-derivative.
(3) This residue is the methylated carboxyl terminus.
(4) This residue is the formylated amino terminus.
(5) The slopes are all negative.

TABLE III.   TEMPERATURE DEPENDENCE OF PEPTIDE PROTON CHEMICAL SHIFT OF (VPGVG) OLIGOMERS IN METHANOL

PEPTIDE RESIDUE	t-BOC-(VPGVG)-OMe		N-formyl-(VPGVG)$_2$-OMe		N-formyl-(VPGVG)$_3$-OMe	
	Slope ppm/deg	0°C Intercept	Slope ppm/deg	0°C Intercept	Slope ppm/deg	0°C Intercept
Val$_1$	0.0103[1]	6.98[1]	0.0053	8.61	.0059	8.6
Val$_6$			0.0069	8.19	.0078	} 8.3
Val$_{11}$					.0078	
Gly$_3$	0.0071	8.71	0.0061	8.56	.0054	
Gly$_8$			0.0061	8.59	.0054	} 8.54
Gly$_{13}$					.0054	
Val$_4$	0.0045	8.03	0.0049	8.02	.0045	
Val$_9$			0.0045	8.06	.0045	} 8.06
Val$_{14}$					.0045	
Gly$_5$	0.0071[2]	8.76[2]	0.0055	8.51	.0055	
Gly$_{10}$			0.0054[2]	8.67[2]	.0055	} 8.7
Gly$_{15}$					.0055[2]	

(1) This residue is displaced due to the t-BOC derivative.
(2) This residue is the carboxyl terminus.
(3) The slopes are all negative.

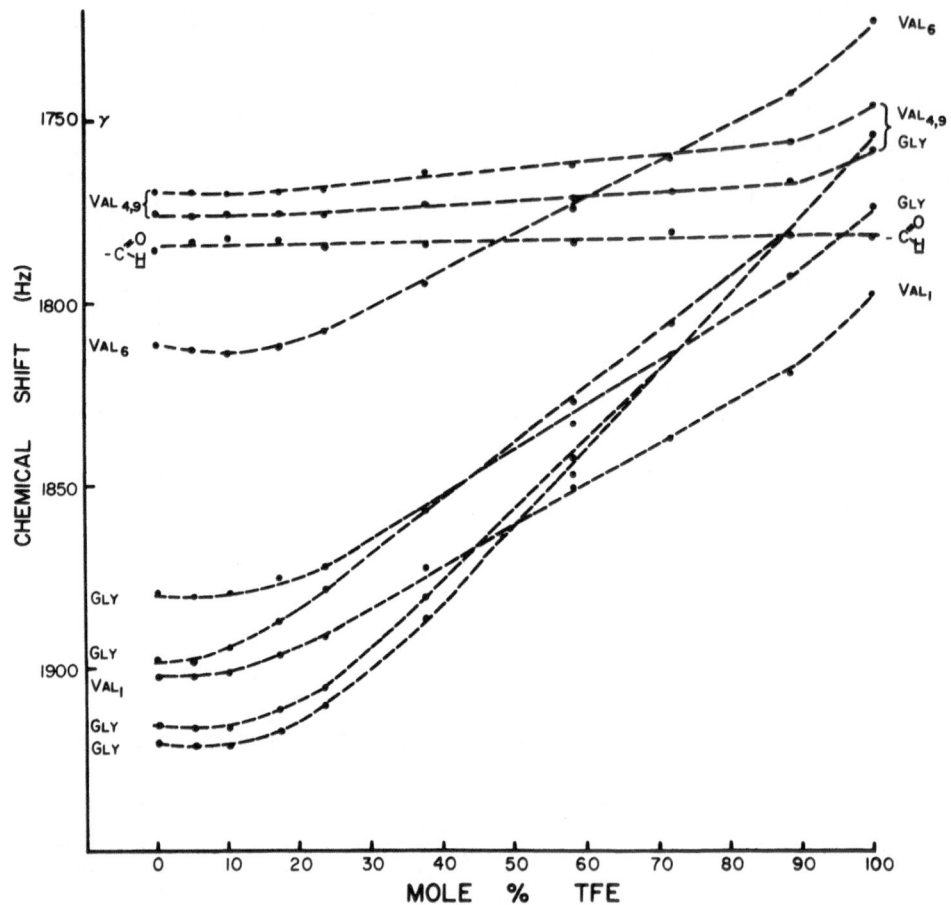

Fig. 3. Dependence of chemical shift in Hz as a function of the
mole percent of trifluoroethanol (TFE) in methanol. Solvent exposed
peptide protons shift dramatically upfield on adding TFE, whereas
solvent shielded protons, such as hydrogen-bonded peptide protons,
exhibit much less solvent dependence.

built in this laboratory for the Varian HR220 proton magnetic
resonance spectrometer. Assignments in methanol were achieved by
progressive increase in mole fraction of methanol to DMSO-d_6. The
peptide region in methanol is given in Figure 5 for the dodecapeptide at 37°C. Comparison of the hexapeptide, dodecapeptide, and
octadecapeptide allowed explicit assignment of the valines and
alanines as it was possible to distinguish the carboxyl and amino
terminal residues.

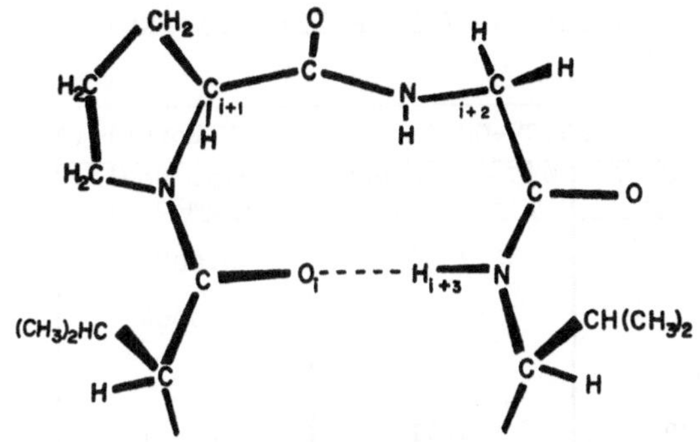

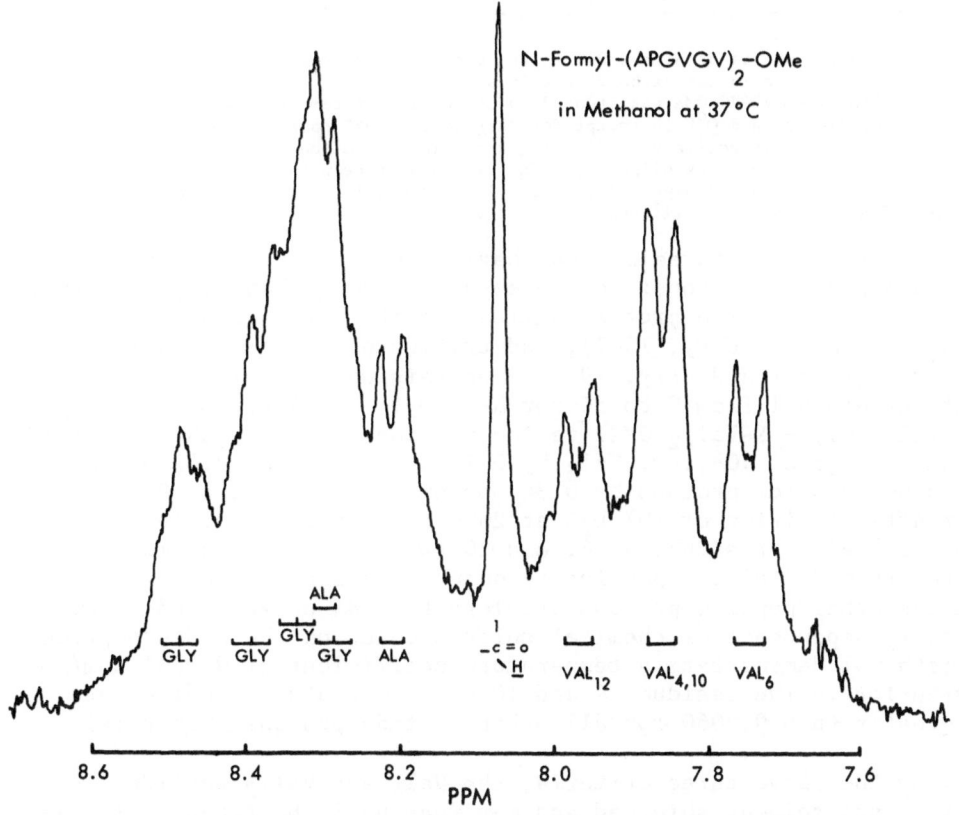

Fig. 4. Proposed β-turn of the pentapeptide, - L-Val - L-Pro - Gly - L-Val - Gly -. This conformational feature occurs in each pentapeptide of higher oligomers, i.e., in the pentapeptide, decapeptide, and pentadecapeptide.

Fig. 5. Proton magnetic resonance spectrum of the peptide proton region of the dodecapeptide. The resonance assignments for the valines and alanines are indicated.

TABLE IV.   TEMPERATURE DEPENDENCE OF PEPTIDE PROTON CHEMICAL SHIFTS
IN METHANOL

| Peptide | t-BOC-APGVGV-OMe | | N-Formyl-(APGVGV)$_2$-OMe | |
Residue	Temp. Coeff. (ppm/deg.)	0°C Intercept (ppm)	Temp. Coeff. (ppm/deg.)	0°C Intercept (ppm)
Ala$_1$	0.0085 [1]	7.08 [1]	0.0075	8.48
Ala$_7$			0.0064	8.61
Gly$_3$	0.0059	8.59		
Val$_4$	0.0040	8.01	0.0041	8.01
Val$_{10}$			0.0041	8.01
Gly$_5$	0.0067	8.68		
Val$_6$	0.0066 [2]	8.21 [2]	0.0063	7.97
Val$_{12}$			0.0062 [2]	8.20 [2]

(1) This residue is displaced due to the t-BOC derivative.
(2) This residue is the carboxyl terminus.
(3) When t-BOC-VPGVG-OMe was studied in methanol, the temperature
     coefficient and 0°C intercept for Val$_4$ were 0.0045 ppm/deg. and
     8.03 ppm, respectively, indicating a similar situation to the
     hexapeptide and its oligomers. This is consistent with a β-turn
     in which Pro$_2$ and Gly$_3$ are residues i + 1 and i + 2, respectively.
(4) The temperature coefficient is negative.

     In this case, three methods have been used to identify solvent
shielded peptide protons: hydrogen-deuterium exchange, temperature
dependence of peptide proton chemical shift (Urry and Ohnishi,
1970; Ohnishi and Urry, 1969), and trifluoroethanol-methanol solvent
mixtures (Pitner and Urry, 1972). On raising the mole percent of
trifluoroethanol from 0 to 54 for N-Formyl - (L-Ala - L-Pro - Gly -
L - Val - Gly - L-Val)$_2$-OMe, valine residues 4 and 10 shift upfield
by an average of .08 ppm, Val$_6$ by 0.25 ppm, Val$_{12}$ by 0.42 ppm and
all other peptide protons by 0.34 ppm or greater. In DMSO-d$_6$, one
hour after addition of 10% D$_2$O at 20°C to a solution of the dodecapeptide, valine residues 4, 6, and 10 (which are overlapping) have
better than 20% of the peptide resonances remaining, whereas Val$_{12}$
and the other peptide protons are less than 8% unexchanged. Temperature dependence of chemical shift studies on the dodecapeptide
in methanol demonstrate a temperature coefficient of 0.0041 ppm/
degree for valine residues 4 and 10 and temperature coefficients
of greater than 0.0060 for all other peptide protons (Table IV).

     By the above three criteria, the Val$_4$ and Val$_{10}$ peptide
protons are solvent shielded and may reasonably be taken as intra-
molecularly hydrogen-bonded. There are six hydrogen-bonded rings
possible with 13, 10, 7, 5, 8, and 11 atoms. Study of the hexapeptide t-BOC - L-Val - L-Ala - L-Pro - Gly - L-Val - Gly - OH and

TABLE V.   TEMPERATURE DEPENDENCE OF PEPTIDE PROTON CHEMICAL SHIFTS IN DMSO-d_6

Peptide Residue	t-BOC-APGVGV-OMe		N-Formyl-(APGVGV)$_2$-OMe		N-Formyl-(APGVGV)$_3$-OMe	
	Temp. Coeff.	0°C Intercept	Temp. Coeff.	0°C Intercept	Temp. Coeff.	0°C Intercept
Ala$_1$	-.0078 [1]	7.10 [1]	-.0058	8.48	-.0057	8.48
Ala$_7$			-.0062	8.37	-.0062	8.36
Ala$_{13}$					-.0062	8.36
Val$_4$	-.0042	7.58	-.0044	7.79 [3]	-.0040	7.77 [3]
Val$_{10}$			-.0044	7.79	-.0040	7.77
Val$_{16}$					-.0040	7.77
Val$_6$	-.0061 [2]	7.94 [2]	-.0053	7.86	-.0056	7.87
Val$_{12}$			-.0060 [2]	8.19 [2]	-.0056	7.87
Val$_{18}$					-.0057 [2]	8.18 [2]

[1] This residue is displaced due to the t-BOC derivative.

[2] This residue is the carboxyl terminus.

[3] When t-BOC VPGVG-OMe was studied the temperature coefficient and 0°C intercepts for Val$_4$ were .0044 ppm/degree and 7.77 ppm, respectively, indicating a similar situation for that residue. This is consistent with a β-turn in which Pro$_2$ and Gly$_3$ are residues i + 1 and i + 2, respectively.

pentapeptide t-BOC - L-Val - L-Pro - Gly - L-Val - Gly - OMe shows the same hydrogen-bond eliminating the 11 atom and making unlikely the 8 atom hydrogen-bonded rings. Consistent with this, the stereochemical criteria of Donohue (1953) allow only 13, 10, and 7 atom hydrogen-bonded rings. The 13 atom hydrogen-bonded ring is that of the α-helix with αCH-NH coupling constants for the right handed helix of about 2 or 3 Hz. Since all the Val αCH-NH coupling constants are greater than 8 Hz and those of the Ala residues are 6 Hz or greater, a regularly repeating 13 atom hydrogen-bonded ring is unlikely. Circular dichroism spectra of the 12 and 18 residue peptides demonstrate the absence of the α-helix pattern. This leaves the 10 and 7 atom hydrogen-bonded rings. The 7 atom hydrogen-bonded ring has not been observed with small linear peptides. The 10 atom hydrogen-bonded ring is known to be energetically favorable, and the high field position of the peptide protons for residues 4, 10, and 16 in DMSO-d_6 (Table V) and at low temperature in methanol has been noted as being a common diagnostic feature (Urry and Ohnishi, 1970). Also, glycine residues are known to favor β-turns (Geddes et al., 1968; Venkatachalam, 1968). The β-turn indicated for this repeating sequence is given in Figure 6. A β-turn utilizing proline as residue i + 1 was first proposed for the linear tail segment of

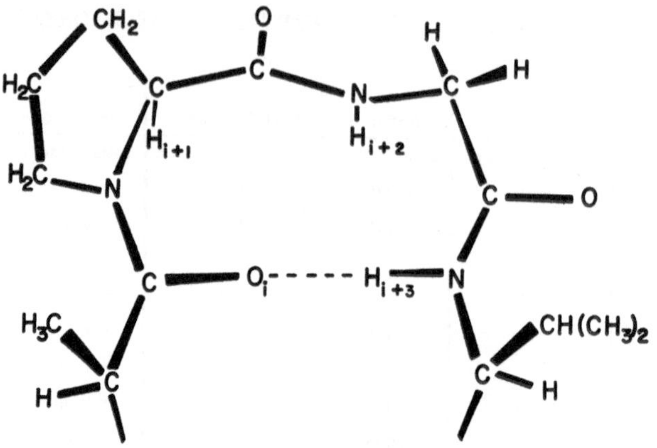

Fig. 6. Proposed β-turn of the hexapeptide, - L-Ala - L-Pro - Gly - L-Val - Gly - L-Val -. This conformational feature recurs in each repeating hexapeptide.

oxytocin (Urry and Walter, 1971) and was subsequently verified by X-ray crystallography of the tetrapeptides S-benzyl - L-Cys - L-Pro - L-Leu - Gly - NH_2 (Rudko et al., 1971). Also, Blout and co-workers (Torchia et al., 1972a; Torchia et al., 1972b; Pease et al., personal communication) have shown this to be the favored β-turn over the gramicidin S type β-turn in which the proline is residue i + 2.

As seen in Table V, this conformational feature is found to occur in the linear hexapeptide, to repeat twice in the dodeca-peptide, and to repeat three times in the octadecapeptide. The values in Table V show how regularly the conformation repeats. A regularly recurring β-turn can result in two types of non-helical conformations, the well-known cross-β-structures and the more recently proposed β-spirals (Urry, 1972). As both conformations can give rise to fibrous structures the present proposal for recur-ring β-turns provides the basis for a new description of elastin.

The Tetrapeptide Series. - The temperature dependence of peptide proton chemical shift for the high polymer of the tetrapeptide series shows one of the two glycines (the one at higher field) to have a lesser slope (Figure 7). Study of the smaller molecules, as well as the cyclododecapeptide (Urry et al., 1973), also shows a single glycine to have a low temperature coefficient. In the smaller molecules, it is possible to assign the peptide proton with a low temperature coefficient to the glycine immediately following the proline residue, i.e., Gly_1. It occurs at higher field than Gly_2 and could reasonably be in a β-turn in which - L-Val - L-Pro - form the corners. This β-turn would place proline in the same position as that found for gramacidin S.

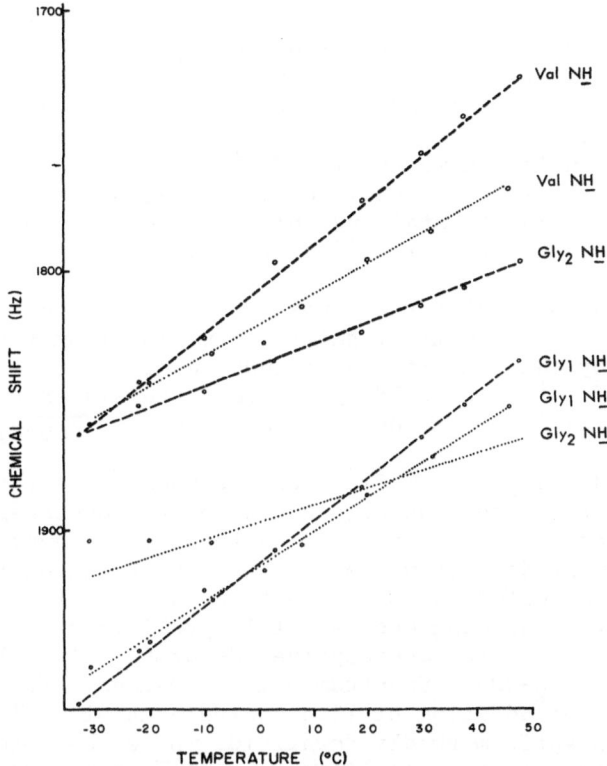

Fig. 7. Temperature dependence of peptide proton chemical shift for the high polymer N-Formyl - L-Val - (L-Pro - Gly_1 - Gly_2 - L-Val)$_n$-OMe where n is approximately nine. One glycine resonance is found at higher field and exhibits a lesser temperature coefficient. By analogy to the tetrapeptides and their oligomers it is assigned to Gly_2. Also included are the curves in the presence of Ca^{++} (dotted curves) at a mole ratio to tetrapeptide of one.

Ion Binding Studies

As will be discussed below, all of the repeating sequences of elastin bind calcium ions, each does so with differing affinities. In each case Ca^{++} is preferred over Na^+, and Mg^{++}, but the relative affinities vary. Accordingly, the set of repeating peptides of elastin preferentially bind calcium ion, but they do so with different affinities and with selectives favoring Ca^{++} over other ions.

The Tetrapeptide Series. In a recent study of the cyclododecapeptide [(GGVP)]$_3$, we have demonstrated that the repeating tetrapeptide binds Ca^{++} by the peptide oxygens (Urry et al., 1973). The cyclododecapeptide has sequence analogy to valinomycin, and as is the case with valinomycin (Ivanov et al., 1969; Pinkerton et al., 1969;

Ohnishi and Urry, 1969; Urry and Ohnishi, 1970; Mayers and Urry, 1972), it forms six intramolecular hydrogen bonds when complexed with cation (Urry et al., 1973). Further studies are required before the detailed conformation of this complex is determined. Whereas the naturally occurring cyclodecapeptide, antaminide, was the first polypeptide shown to bind Ca^{++} at the peptide oxygens (Wieland et al., 1972), synthetic cyclo $\overline{[(GGVP)}]_3$ is the first characterized peptide (containing only peptide functional groups) to exhibit a selectivity for Ca^{++} over Na^+.

Figure 7 demonstrates the binding of Ca^{++} by the tetrapeptide high polymer. By the chemical shifts resulting from interaction with Ca^{++} and by the temperature dependence of chemical shift in the presence of Ca^{++}, it would appear that the linear tetrapeptide complexes with Ca^{++} in a manner similar to cyclo $\overline{[(GGVP)}]_3$.

The Pentapeptide Series. - While there is much characterization yet to carry out on the general capacity of the pentapeptide repeating series of elastin to bind cations, it is apparent, from observing the peptide proton chemical shifts at concentrations of cations where the effect of Ca^{++} addition is essentially complete, that ion selective binding occurs. This preliminary study is given in Figure 8 for the decapeptide N-Formyl - (L-Val - L-Pro - Gly - L-Val - Gly)$_2$-OMe. Spectrum D is in methanol in the absence of any cation. On addition of 13.8 equivalents of Ca^{++}, all the peptide protons shift markedly downfield, while the formyl proton resonance shifts only a small distance. Sr^{++} at an equivalence of 14.4 causes significantly less shift (Figure 8F); while Na^+ and K^+ at equivalents of 14 and 17, respectively, cause only minor upfield shifts of selected resonances. Mg^{++} at 13.7 equivalents causes a marked broadening, particularly of the formyl proton, but no significant shifts. Magnesium ion may be catalyzing the exchange of peptide protons or there may be a paramagnetic impurity in the $MgCl_2$.

The implication of the results is a greater complexation by Ca^{++}, though the complete titrations are required for adequate comparison. Complexation has been reported with the tetrapeptide series (Urry et al., 1973), and in what follows complexation with the hexapeptide series will be considered in more detail.

The Hexapeptide Series. - As seen in Figure 9, the peptide proton chemical shifts for the dodecapeptide brought about by the presence of various cations is qualitatively similar to that observed with the decapeptide (Figure 8); Ca^{++} causes the largest downfield shifts, then Sr^{++} with Na^+ and K^+ causing only small changes in the spectra. Mg^{++} again results in a broadening.

Using circular dichroism to follow ion titrations of the hexapeptide high polymer, i.e., N-Formyl - L-Val - (L-Ala - L-Pro -

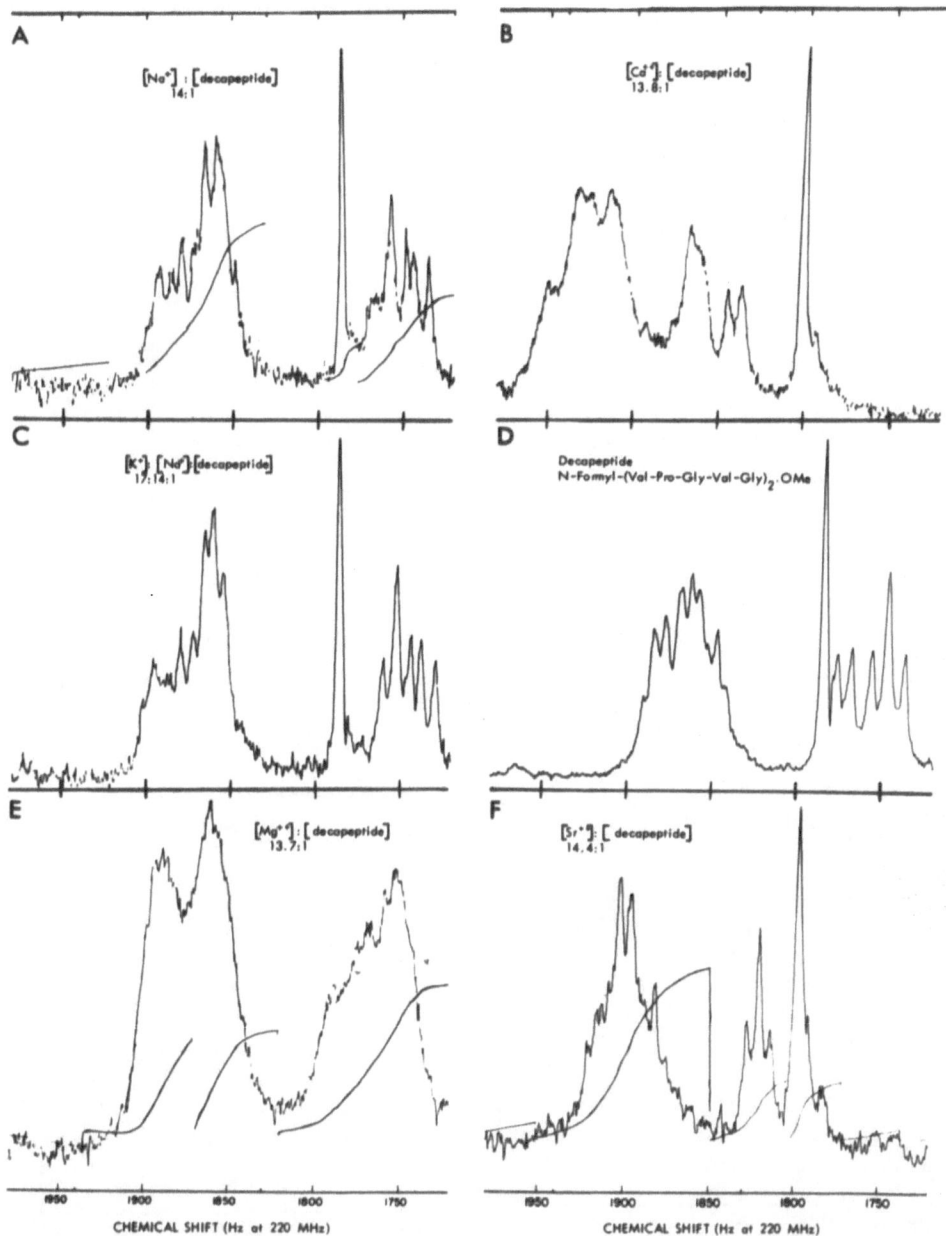

Fig. 8. Peptide magnetic resonance spectra of the decapeptide N-Formyl - (L-Val - L-Pro - Gly - L-Val - Gly)$_2$-OMe in the absence and presence of five different cations. On interacting, the cations cause a change in position of the peptide proton absorbances. These spectra indicate the highest affinity for Ca^{++}, and less affinity for Sr^{++}. Na$^+$ and K$^+$ have little effect. The effect of Mg^{++} on broadening is not necessarily one of complex formation, but could also be due to paramagnetic impurities or to catalyzing peptide proton exchange. The increased noise levels in some of the spectra are due to less time spent in multiscan averaging.

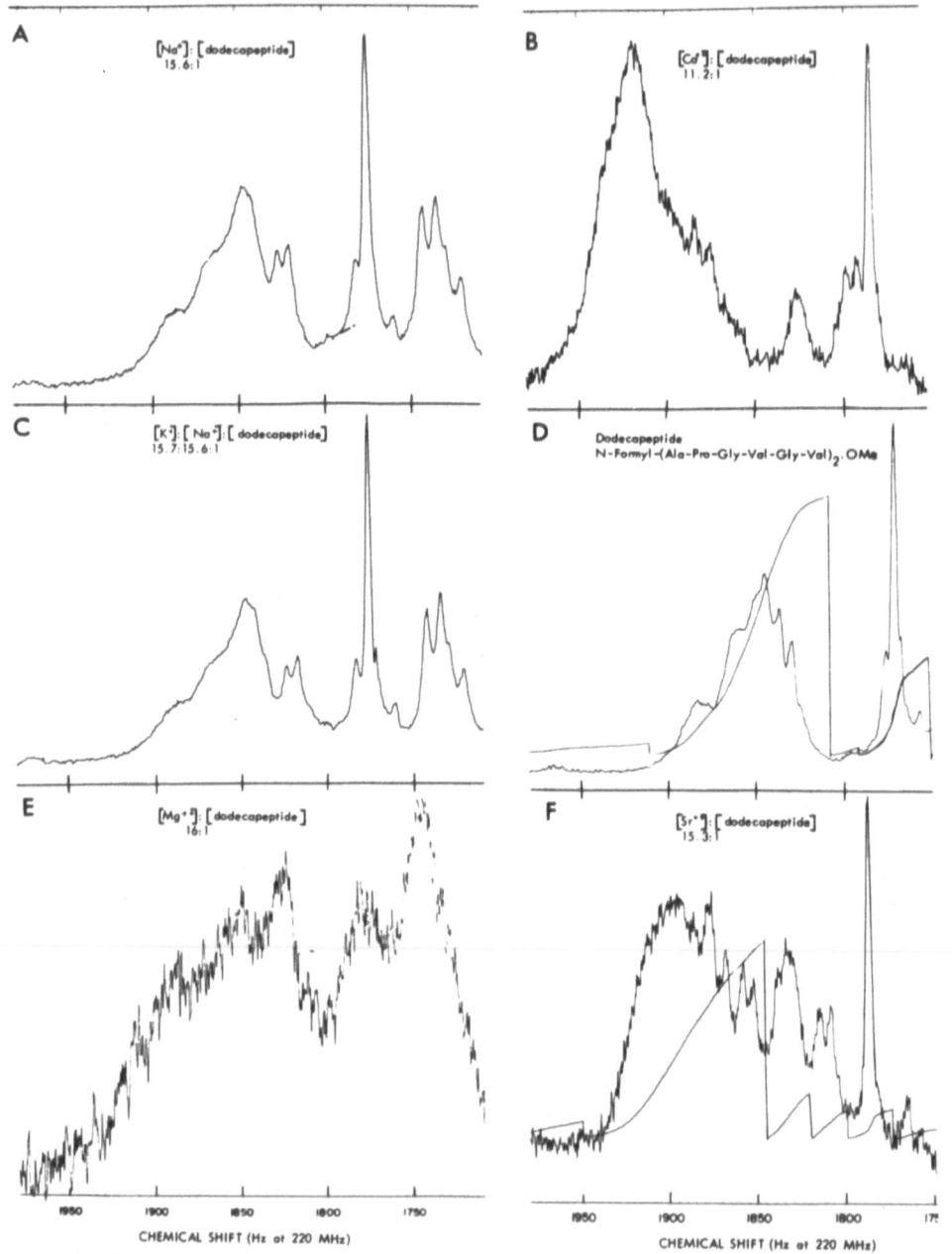

Fig. 9. Peptide proton magnetic resonance spectra of the dodecapeptide N-Formyl - (L-Ala - L-Pro - Gly - L-Val - Gly - L-Val)$_2$-OMe in the absence and presence of five different cations. These spectra indicate complexation with Ca^{++} and Sr^{++}, but only limited interaction with Na$^+$ and K$^+$. The effect of Mg^{++} on broadening is not necessarily due to complex formation, but could also be due to paramagnetic impurities or to catalyzing peptide proton exchange. The increased noise levels in some of the spectra are due to the averaging of a fewer number of scans.

Gly - L-Val - Gly - L-Val)$_n$-OMe, Figure 10 dramatically demonstrates
the relative binding of Ca^{++}, Sr^{++}, Mg^{++}, Na$^+$, and K$^+$. The ions Mg^{++},
Na$^+$, and K$^+$ cause no detectable change in the CD spectrum. Ca^{++}
causes large changes in the CD spectrum; the curve in Figure 10 follows the ellipticity changes at 222 nm. The formation constant for
the calcium ion complex is greater than 10^3; this is two orders of
magnitude greater than that observed for the cyclododecapeptide

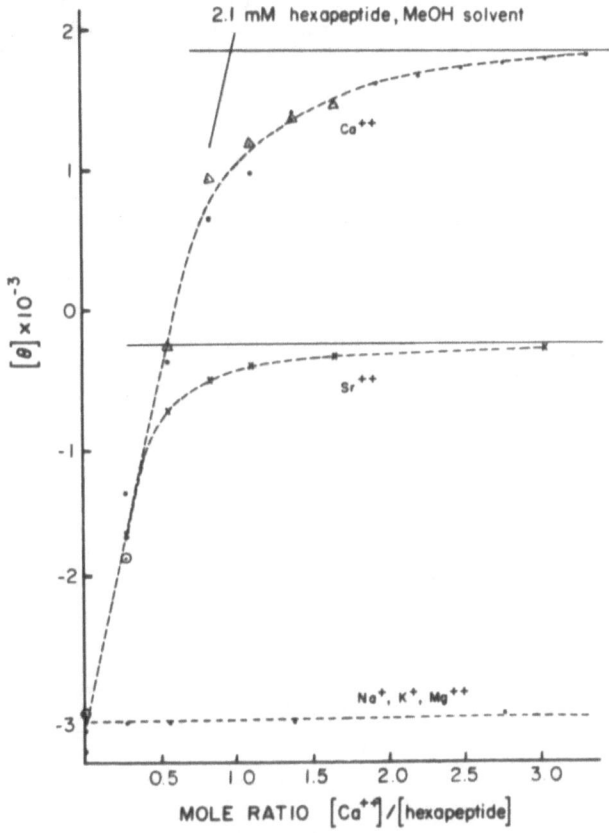

Fig. 10. Changes in the ellipticity at 222 nm of the higher polymer
of the hexapeptide, i.e., N-Formyl - (L-Ala - L-Pro - Gly - L-Val -
Gly - L-Val)$_n$-OMe and the addition of cations. This molecule exhibits a high affinity for calcium ion with a formation constant of a-
bout 10^3. The intercept of the initial slope and the asymptote of
the values at high Ca^{++} concentration indicate the binding of one
Ca^{++} per hexapeptide unit. This implies that each hexapeptide unit
represents a calcium ion binding site. With this method, there is
no detectable interaction with Na$^+$, K$^+$, and Mg^{++}.

containing the tetrapeptide repeat sequence (Urry et al., 1973). The curve indicates the binding of one Ca^{++} per hexapeptide and of approximately one Sr^{++} per dodecapeptide. Thus, the high polymer of the hexapeptide demonstrates the highest absolute affinity for Ca^{++} and the greater degree of selectivity for Ca^{++} over Mg^{++}, Na^{+}, and K^{+}.

Having noted the high affinity for the high polymer and the stoichiometry of one Ca^{++} per hexapeptide unit, it becomes of interest to examine individual hexapeptides. Figure 11 contains a titration of t-BOC - L-Ala - L-Pro - Gly - L-Val - Gly - L-Val - OMe, followed by plotting the peptide proton chemical shifts on

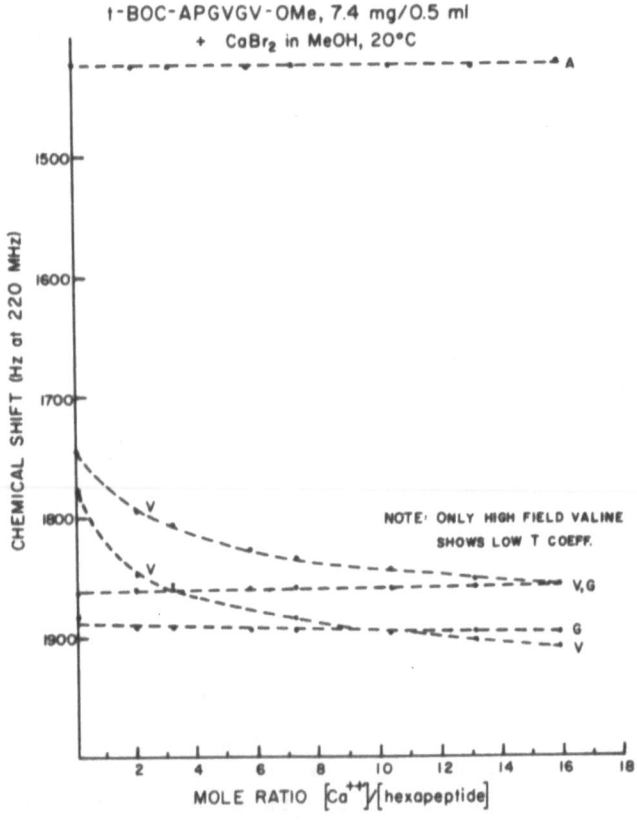

Fig. 11. Changes in the peptide proton chemical shift on the hexa-peptide t-BOC - L-Ala - L-Pro - Gly - L-Val - Gly - L-Val - OMe on titration with Ca^{++}. Two protons indicate interaction, whereas with the dimer and trimers of the above sequence all protons titrated.

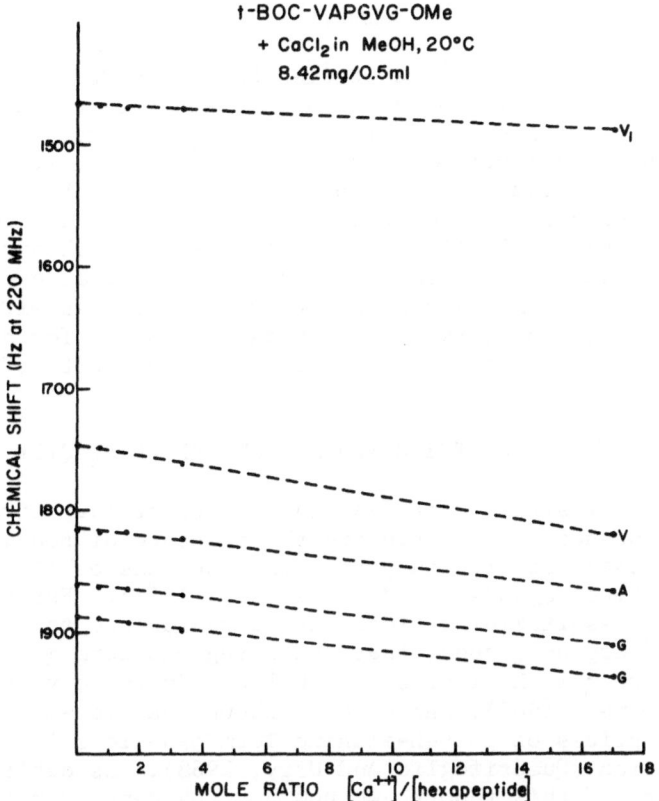

Fig. 12. Titration of the hexapeptide t-BOC - L-Val - L-Ala-L-Pro - Gly - L-Val - Gly - OMe with Ca⁺⁺. The straight line curves give no evidence of complex formation. The result indicates that this sequence of six residues is not the hexapeptide binding site, i.e., the site does not include the three L-amino acid sequence.

addition of Ca⁺⁺. In this case, only the two peptide protons of the valyl residues indicate a selective binding, whereas in the dodeca and octadecapeptides all the peptide protons shift, i.e., reflect complexation. The situation is even more striking with the hexapeptide permutation t-BOC - L-Val - L-Ala - L-Pro - Gly - L-Val - Gly - OMe. As seen in Figure 12, there is no titration curve indicative of complex formation - only a general downfield shift. Thus, the binding sequence is not L L L Gly L Gly, but could be L L Gly L Gly L, or L Gly L Gly L L with end effects considered. The fundamental point of a hexapeptide binding site with high Ca⁺⁺ affinity has been established.

Summary

Proton magnetic resonance studies have provided an argument
for the presence of β-turns in repeating sequences of elastin; and
proton magnetic resonance and circular dichroism studies have been
carried out which demonstrate binding of Ca^{++} to the neutral polypeptides at the peptide oxygen. Binding of Ca^{++} can be of high
affinity with high ion selectivity. This work provides an explicit basis for the previously proposed neutral site theory for the
binding of calcium ion to elastin wherein the peptide oxygens
directly coordinate the calcium ion (Urry, 1971). As will be
discussed further, the work also provides the basis for a new
fibrous description of the conformation and elasticity of elastin.

A WORKING HYPOTHESIS FOR THE CONFORMATION AND ELASTICITY OF ELASTIN

The two most significant features of the primary structure, or
amino acid sequence, of elastin are the presence of repeating oligopeptides (Foster et al., in press) and the runs of alanine in
the cross-linking regions (Sandberg et al., 1971). For the alanine
runs in the cross-linking regions, it is reasonable to deduce, as
Gray and Sandberg have done, that these regions form α-helices;
this is because poly-L-alanine is α-helical in the dry state
(Arnott and Dover, 1967), and we have shown that low-molecular-
weight polypeptides of poly-L-alanine form α-helices in trifluoroethanol solution (Quadrifoglio and Urry, 1968). As outlined in
the first part of this report, we now have evidence for the
presence of β-turns in the repeating oligopeptides of elastin.
Two types of conformations can occur which contain regularly
repeating β-turns. These are the recently proposed β-spirals
(Urry, 1972) and the well-known anti-parallel-β-pleated sheets,
or cross-β-conformations, of Pauling and Corey (1953). Figure 13
contains a schematic representation of cross-β-conformations which
differ in the number of residues per β-turn. The β-turn is the
conformational feature which folds a chain back on itself. The
backbone structure is schematically represented as straight lines
connecting positions of the α-carbons, and the hydrogen-bonding
is indicated by the sets of parallel lines connecting between
chain segments. The significant point to be made by Figure 13
is that the cross-β-conformations require an even number of residues
in the repeating units, i.e., per β-turn.

The second class of conformations containing regularly
repeating β-turns, the β-spirals, is shown schematically in cyclic
representations in Figure 14. Instead of actually being cyclic
as a complete turn of the spiral is completed, one β-turn stacks
above another in a manner making it possible for the end peptides
to hydrogen-bond between β-turns. Depending on the actual spiral

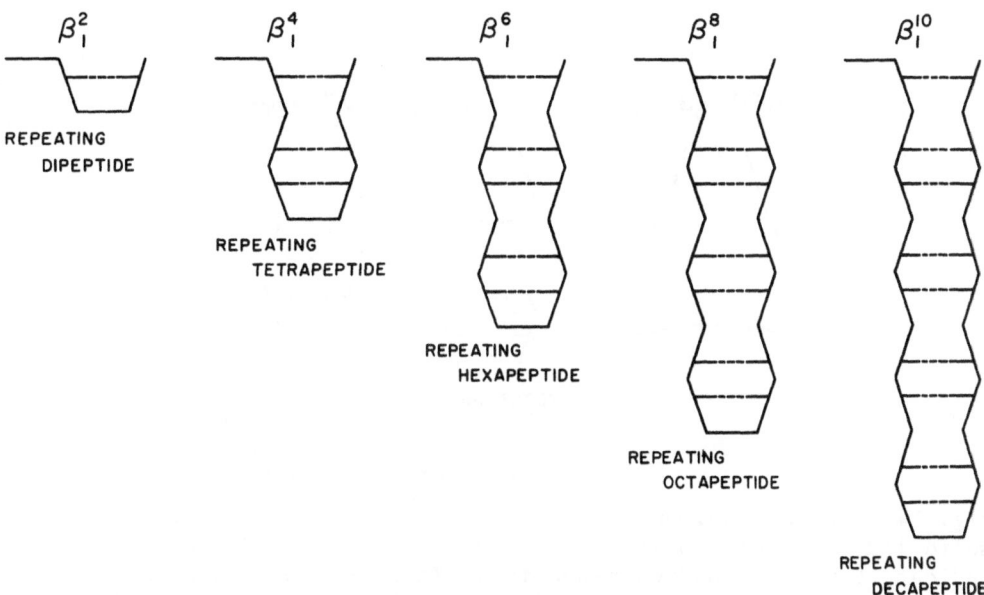

β_I^2 β_I^4 β_I^6 β_I^8 β_I^{10}

REPEATING
DIPEPTIDE

REPEATING
TETRAPEPTIDE

REPEATING
HEXAPEPTIDE

REPEATING
OCTAPEPTIDE

REPEATING
DECAPEPTIDE

Fig. 13. Cross-β-conformations. In this representation of polypeptide structure, the peptide residue is represented simply by
straight lines connecting the positions of the α-carbons; the
horizontal lines containing dashes indicate hydrogen-bonding
between chain segments. The structural feature formed when one
chain segment folds and runs anti-parallel to the preceding chain
segment is a β-turn (for details of a β-turn see Figures 1, 4,
and 6). This polypeptide structure is also called the anti-parallel-
β-pleated sheet because of the sheet-like result when long chains
align in an anti-parallel manner. When a single chain regularly
turns or folds back on itself making a ribbon-like structure and
the chain length between turns is not large, the structure is
commonly termed a cross-β-conformation. For regularly repeating
sequences this structure requires an even number of residues in
the repeating unit.

conformation, the stacking of one β-turn may not be exactly above
the other as in the left-handed β_2^6-spiral indicated in Figure 15.
In this conformation, there are about 6.3 residues per turn, such
that one β-turn does not sit directly above the other. The cross-
hydrogen-bonding is not indicated in Figure 15.

The significant feature of β-spirals in relation to the
repeating peptides of elastin is that these conformations can

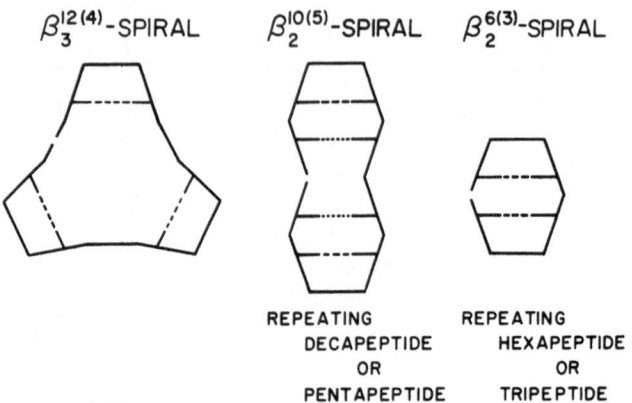

$\beta_3^{12(4)}$-SPIRAL $\beta_2^{10(5)}$-SPIRAL $\beta_2^{6(3)}$-SPIRAL

REPEATING
DECAPEPTIDE
OR
PENTAPEPTIDE

REPEATING
HEXAPEPTIDE
OR
TRIPEPTIDE

Fig. 14. Spiral Conformations. As in Figure 13, the straight
solid lines connect positions of α-carbons and the dashed lines
indicate C-O...H-N-hydrogen-bonding. It should be visualized for
linear peptides that, at the position of the break in the cyclic
representation, the continuing polypeptide chain may spiral
around above or below the indicated structure to form a left-handed
or right-handed β-spiral respectively. Also, depending on the
actual structure formed, there may be a fractional number of
residues per complete turn of the spiral (see Fig. 15).

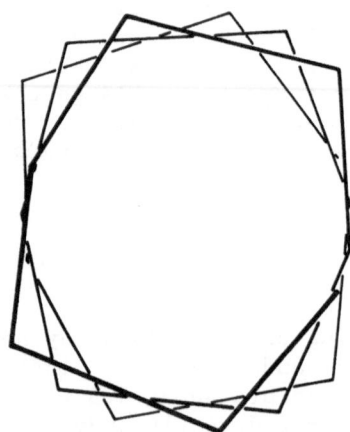

Fig. 15. Axis view of a left-handed β_2^6-spiral in which there are
approximately 6.3 residues per complete turn.

exist with an odd or an even number of residues in the repeating unit. Therefore, the repeating pentapeptide of elastin cannot have the regular repeating β-turns (Tables II and III) and occur in the cross-β-conformation. The repeating pentapeptide can form β-spirals, e.g., β_2^{10}, β_3^{15}, etc., and in these conformations have identically repeating units. In regard to conformational analysis, it is the regularly repeating pentapeptide containing a β-turn that allows discrimination between the cross-β and β-spiral classes of conformation. The presence of a proline residue also disfavors the cross-β-conformation, as it prevents one of the interchain hydrogen bonds holding the pleated sheet together, but the β-spiral does not require this hydrogen bond when the proline is in the β-turns, as indicated for the penta- and hexapeptide (Figures 4 and 6).

On the basis of the above conformational analysis, we are proceeding with the following hypothesis for the conformation of elastin. As it turns out, it is a conformation which has interesting elastic properties and is consistent with many of the other physical properties of elastin. As indicated in Figure 16, the conformation, in its ordered regions, is one of a sequential arrangement of β-spiral and α-helical segments along a single chain. The segments are determined by the amino acid sequence. The β-spirals occur in the repeating pentapeptide and hexapeptide sequences and the α-helix occurs in the runs of alanine associated with cross-linking regions. The single chains can associate by cross-linking and by hydrophobic interactions to form an alignment of chains. This gives rise to serial and parallel arrangements of elastic segments, such that as a softer segment is extended; a stiffer segment can begin extending before the softer segment passes out of its dynamic range.

It is well-known that dry elastic fibers are not elastic, but become so on hydration. In terms of the β-spirals, hydrogen-bonding between stacked β-turns would prevent extension; hydration would allow disruption of these hydrogen bonds and allow the bellows-like structure to extend.

When coacervate forms, for example, at elevated (body) temperature, an inverse transition indicative of hydrophobic interactions is represented (Urry et al., 1969). Also, we have observed that a small amount of dimethyl sulfoxide, which disrupts hydrophobic interactions, dissolves the coacervate. In the β-spiral conformations, the hydrophobic side chains are in a position largely tucked between the turns of the spiral, but with a hydrophobic side exposed, such that association of chains would involve

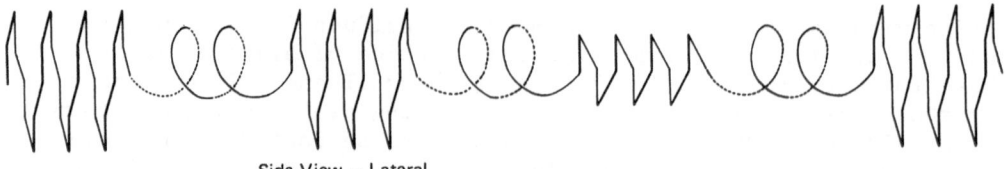

Side View — Lateral

Side View — β-Turn End

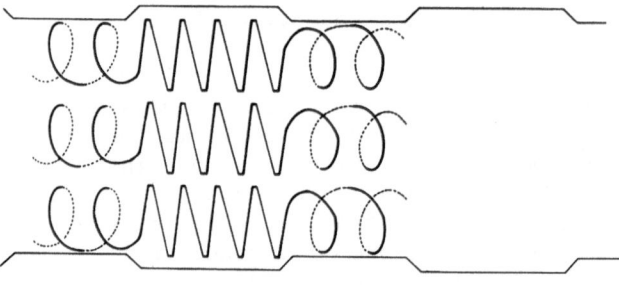

Associating Chains and Cross Linking

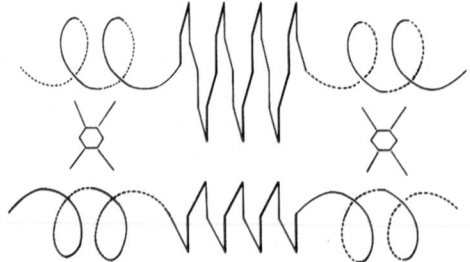

Fig. 16. This working model for the conformation of elastin is
one of a sequential arrangement of β-spiral and α-helical segments
along a single chain. The segments are determined by the amino
acid sequence. The β-spirals occur in the repeating pentapeptide
and hexapeptide sequences and the α-helix occurs in the runs of
alanine associated with cross-linking regions. The single chains
can associate by cross-linking and by hydrophobic interactions to
form an alignment of chains. This gives rise to serial and parallel
arrangement of elastic segments so that as a softer segment is
extended, a stiffer segment can begin extending before the softer
segment passes out of its dynamic range. The association between
chains would in large measure involve interaction of the hydrophobic
side chains of valines and prolines, which, though tucked to some
extent between turns of the spirals, constitute hydrophobic sides of
the spiral.

hydrophobic interactions. Accordingly, DMSO would be expected to dissolve the coacervate. On extension of the β-spiral, the hydrophobic side chains would become more exposed to an aqueous medium. The exposing of hydrophobic groups by stretching is a conclusion of the Weis-Fogh and Anderson analysis of the thermodynamic properties of elastin (Weis-Fogh and Anderson, 1970).

Gotte et al. (1968) have observed 30 $\overset{o}{A}$ wide fibrils in electron microscope studies of sonicated and alkali-treated elastin. They also reported diffuse X-ray diffraction rings at 8.9 $\overset{o}{A}$ and 4.4 $\overset{o}{A}$. In terms of the proposed conformation, lateral association of three β-spirals, each about 9 $\overset{o}{A}$ in width, would be consistent with a 30 $\overset{o}{A}$ filament and the 8.9 $\overset{o}{A}$ repeat in the diffraction pattern. The 4.4 $\overset{o}{A}$ repeat in dry elastin is explicable by the stacking of β-turns along the spiral. Gotte et al. (1968) also report that addition of water results in loss of the 4.4 $\overset{o}{A}$ ring, but not the 8.9 $\overset{o}{A}$ ring. This corresponds with the breaking of the hydrogen bond between turns of the spiral and the onset of elasticity. The same authors report that addition of DMSO results in loss of the 8.9 $\overset{o}{A}$ ring, but retention of the 4.4 $\overset{o}{A}$ ring. This is consistent with DMSO disrupting the hydrophobic interactions between associating spirals, but not the hydrogen-bonding between turns of a given spiral.

The above correlation of the conformations depicted in Figure 16 and the known physical data are sufficient to warrant consideration of this conformation as a working hypothesis. Further detailed physical studies on the synthetic and natural products should allow full development of the detailed elastin conformation.

It should also be appreciated that elastin could just as well be comprised of globular units containing many β-turns perhaps with short runs of β-spiral with their axes being other than parallel to the fiber axis. The fundamental points are the recurring of β-turns and hydrophobic association.

It has been suggested above that the association of single chains involves hydrophobic forces. It follows then that these forces for condensation could contribute to the fibrillar organization of elastin, first described by Gotte et al. (1968). Accordingly, one would like to examine at high resolution the coacervate which forms from the association of α-elastin, the 70,000 molecular weight solubilized protein comprised of approximately 16 cross-linked chains (Partridge and Davis, 1955). A finding of fibrous structures in the coacervate would demonstrate the significance of hydrophobic interactions in maintenance of the integrity of the elastin fiber. Such a result would bring us one step closer to relating the conformation of elastin to the pathogenesis of atherosclerosis.

ON THE RELATIONSHIP OF CONFORMATION TO THE MOLECULAR PATHOGENESIS
OF ATHEROSCLEROSIS

Lipid Infiltration

In a recent publication Kramsch and Hollander (1973) have
reported cholesterol esters and other lipids bound to elastin
isolated from atherosclerotic plaques. In view of the proposed
hydrophobic association between single polypeptide chains comprising an elastic fiber, it is reasonable to expect that under
appropriate circumstances cholesterol esters and other lipids
could become interposed between chains, and that once this dispersing
of the fiber begins, lipid deposits could result. Once lipid deposition is initiated, then the rate of accumulation would depend on
the serum lipid levels and lipid types and on the rate of transport
of the lipids from the serum to the initiating site.

Calcium Ion Binding

Yu and Blumenthal (1963a,b,c; 1965) have long argued the
significance of calcium salt accumulation in the arterial wall and
have pointed to the internal elastic membrane and the elastic
fibers as foci. With the proposal and demonstration of Ca^{++} binding
at the oxygen of the peptide moiety (Urry et al., 1971), insight is
obtained into an initiating mechanism. The affinity of calcium
ion for an uncharged binding site can result in a positively charged
elastin matrix which would attract negatively charged ions. These
counter ions could then relax charge repulsion between bound calcium ions and allow more Ca^{++} to bind the elastin matrix in a
propagating step. Particularly if the geometry of the sites were
regular and favorable, an initiating site for calcification (hydroxyapatite growth) is obtained. Quite conceivably, the repeating
hexapeptide sequence discussed previously, where one ion binds
each hexameric unit (Figure 10), could provide favorable geometry.

The Valinomycin Paradox

In general it has been appreciated by both chemist and biolo-
gist that the charging of a molecular species will increase its
affinity for, or partition in, an aqueous phase. The ion transporting antibiotic, valinomycin, belies this general consideration
and it does so by virtue of the detailed conformation of the charged
complex. The valinomycin molecule is a cyclododecadepsipeptide
containing alternating ester and peptide groups and hydrophobic
side chains with no charge on the uncomplexed molecule. It resides
at the aqueous-hydrophobic interface of biomembranes. Valinomycin

has a substantial affinity for K^+ not unlike the affinity of the repeating elastin hexapeptide for Ca^{++}. On binding of K^+ while at the interface, one might expect the molecule to increase its solubility in the aqueous phase. This is not the case. If anything, the valinomycin-K^+ complex is more soluble in the lipid phase. This is due to the conformation of the complex (Urry and Ohnishi, 1970). On complexation, C-O moieties which were directed into the aqueous medium in the uncomplexed molecule turn inward and form a polar core for the cation, and at the same time, the hydrophobic side chains turn outward providing an enveloping hydrophobic coat for the complex. The hydrophobic coat, which is a result of the specific conformation of the complex, provides solubility in the lipid interior of the biomembrane.

In direct analogy to the valinomycin-K^+ complex, complexation of Ca^{++} by elastin sequences can result in the turning outward of hydrophobic side chains and in the formation of a lipid region. Accordingly, within a localized area, there can be a synergism between Ca^{++} binding and lipid deposition. Overall charge neutrality is, of course, a requirement but it need not be achieved by direct charge-charge interaction. Indeed, the charged species may be separated by many Angstroms, with each charge being locally satisfied by appropriate dipolar interactions not dissimilar to those which result in dissolution of salts in aqueous media. In the case of cation dissolution in, or complexing to, polypeptide the dipolar interactions are provided by the oxygen end of the peptide dipole. It is also reasonable that a polypeptide conformation may exist wherein the positive end of the peptide dipole, i.e., the peptide proton, would interact with an anion (e.g., phosphate). While there is as yet no model system demonstrating this possibility, it need also be investigated as an initiating mechanism for calcification. What has recently been demonstrated (Starcher and Urry, 1973) is that the elastin coacervate, formed from α-elastin in which the free amino and carboxyl functions have been blocked, serves well as an initiator of in vitro calcification.

Susceptibility of Elastic Fibers to Molecular Pathogenesis

Meyer (1971) has called attention to locations in the arterial tree where hemodynamic stress results in rupture of the internal elastic membrane and has noted that in newborn infants and stillborns such ruptures in the internal iliac and common iliac arteries result in calcification of the exposed fibers. The observation is one of paired, calcific ridges bordering gaps in the internal elastic membrane with calcification progressing from the ruptured edge into the defined internal elastic membrane. Accordingly, rupture due to hemodynamic stress is one means whereby a fiber becomes susceptible to molecular pathogenesis.

It is conceivable, in view of the working model for the conformation of elastin (Figure 16), that an extended fiber may be more susceptible to calcium ion penetration into the folds of the bellows-like regions. It is not unlikely that chronic extension of the fibers could provide greater opportunity for calcium ion penetration and initiation of pathogenesis. Accordingly, exposure of sites during stretching is a second mechanism whereby pathogenesis may be initiated.

Furthermore, it seems quite natural that a molecular construct such as the elastic fiber would have a chemically protective coating. For reasons previously discussed (Urry, 1971) mucopolysaccharides would seem to provide the properties for a protective coating. In an entirely similar manner so also could glycoproteins and proteoglycans provide a protective sheath. Within the context of the molecular mechanisms discussed here it would be of great interest to know whether connective tissue components, which are known to tightly adhere to the elastin fibers, may have genetic determinants and species variations that could be correlated with the susceptibility to atherosclerosis. In view of the perspective developed above, the efficacy of a protective sheath for the elastic fiber could be of fundamental significance in the pathogenesis of atherosclerosis.

ACKNOWLEDGEMENTS

The author gratefully acknowledges research assistants T. Ohnishi and W.D. Cunningham for synthesizing the elastin peptide sequences and obtaining nmr spectra respectively, and C. Yarborough and D. Hopper for technical assistance in both the nmr and circular dichroism studies.

The author is particularly indebted to W.R. Gray and L.B. Sandberg for communicating their results on tropoelastin sequences prior to publication.

Special thanks are due William T. Kirby, Jr. for his contributions to the continuity of this research program.

This work was supported in part by National Institutes of Health Grants HL-14510 and HL-11310 and by the Mental Health Board of Alabama.

REFERENCES

Arnott, S., and Dover, S.D. (1967). J. Mol. Biol. 30, 209.

Donohue, J. (1953). Proc. Nat. Acad. Sci., U.S.A. 39, 470.

Foster, J.A., Bruenger, E., Gray, W.R., and Sandberg, L.B.
     (In press). J. Biol. Chem.

Franzblau, C., and Lent, R.W. (1969). Brookhaven Symp. Biol. 21,
     358.

Geddes, A.J., Parker, K.D., Atkins, E.D.T., and Beighton, E.J.
     (1968). J. Mol. Biol. 32, 343.

Gotte, L., Mammi, M., and Pezzin, G. (1968). In "Symposium on
     Fibrous Proteins, 3rd, 1967" (W.G. Crewther, ed.). pp. 236-
     245. Plenum Press, New York.

Ivanov, V.T., Laine, I.A., Abdulaev, N.D., Senyavina, L.B.,
     Popov, E.M., Ovchinnikov, Y.A., and Shemyakin, M.M.
     (1969). Biochem. Biophys. Res. Commun. 34, 803.

Kramsch, D.M., and Hollander, W. (1973). J. Clin. Invest. 52,
     236.

Mayers, D.M., and Urry, D.W. (1972). J. Amer. Chem. Soc. 94, 77.

Meyer, W.W. (1971). In "The Artery and the Process of Arterio-
     sclerosis, Pathogenesis." Advances in Experimental Medicine
     and Biology, 16-A. (S. Wolf, ed.), p. 15. Plenum Press,
     New York.

Ohnishi, M., and Urry, D.W. (1970). Science 168, 1091.

Ohnishi, M., and Urry, D.W. (1969). Biochem. Biophys. Res.
     Commun. 36, 194.

Partridge, S.M., and Davis, H.F. (1955). Biochem. J. 61, 21.

Pauling, L., and Corey, R.B. (1953). Proc. Nat. Acad. Sci.,
     U.S.A. 39, 253.

Pease, L.G., Deber, C.M., and Blout, E.R. (Personal communication).

Petruska, J.A., and Sandberg, L.B. (1968). Biochem. Biophys.
     Res. Commun. 33, 222.

Pinkerton, M., Steinrauf, L.K., and Dawkins, P. (1969). Biochem.
     Biophys. Res. Commun. 35, 512.

Pitner, T.P., and Urry, D.W. (1972). J. Amer. Chem. Soc. 94, 1399.

Quadrifoglio, F., and Urry, D.W. (1968). J. Amer. Chem. Soc.
    90, 2755.

Rudko, A.D., Lovell, F.M., and Low, B.W. (1971). Nature,
    [New Biol.] 232, 18.

Sandberg, L.B., Weissman, N., and Gray, W.R. (1971). Biochemistry
    10, 52.

Starcher, B.C., and Urry, D.W. (1973). Fed. Proc. 32, 315.

Torchia, D.A., di Corato, A., Wong, S.C.K., Deber, C.M., and
    Blout, E.R. (1972a). J. Amer. Chem. Soc. 94, 609.

Torchia, D.A., Wong, S.C.K., Deber, C.M., and Blout, E.R. (1972b).
    J. Amer. Chem. Soc. 94, 616.

Urry, D.W. (1972). Proc. Nat. Acad. Sci., U.S.A. 69, 1610.

Urry, D.W. (1971). Proc. Nat. Acad. Sci., U.S.A. 68, 810.

Urry, D.W., Cunningham, W.D., and Ohnishi, T. (1973). Biochim.
    Biophys. Acta 295, 853.

Urry, D.W., Krivacic, J.R., and Haider, J. (1971). Biochem.
    Biophys. Res. Commun. 43, 6.

Urry, D.W., and Ohnishi, M. (1970). In "Spectroscopic Approaches
    to Biomolecular Conformation" (D.W. Urry, ed.), pp. 263-300.
    American Medical Association Press, Chicago.

Urry, D.W., Starcher, B., and Partridge, S.M. (1969). Nature 222,
    795.

Urry, D.W., and Walter, R. (1971). Proc. Nat. Acad. Sci., U.S.A.
    68, 956.

Venkatachalam, C.M. (1968). Biopolymers 6, 1425.

Weis-Fogh, T., and Anderson, S.O. (1970). Nature 227, 718.

Wieland, Th., Faulstich, H., and Burgermeister, W. (1972).
    Biochem. Biophys. Res. Commun. 47, 984.

Yu, S.Y., and Blumenthal, H.T. (1963a). J. Gerontol. 18, 119.

Yu, S.Y., and Blumenthal, H.T. (1963b). J. Gerontol. 18, 127.

Yu, S.Y., and Blumenthal, H.T. (1963c). Lab. Invest. 12, 1154.

Yu, S.Y., and Blumenthal, H.T. (1965). J. Atheroscler. Res. 5, 159.

DISCUSSION FOLLOWING THE PRESENTATION BY DAN W. URRY

Dr. Robert: Dr. Urry, I enjoyed your presentation very much, and I think your suggestion that calcium can aid lipid binding is very interesting. Would you make any prediction of lipid binding first and how that would affect calcium binding?

Dr. Urry: Well, calcium ion binding to carbonyl oxygens is going to turn the carbonyl oxygens inward and the hydrophobic R groups of the amino acids outward into the surrounding milieu. Such a process would be facilitated by having hydrophobicity available in the milieu. At this stage the detailed environment of the elastic fiber is unknown, but the hydrophobicity could come from the elastin fiber itself, or it could come from bound lipid molecules. By virtue of the conformation, lipid binding and calcium binding can be cooperative or synergistic. They could occur simultaneously, or one may precede the other. Only a knowledge of the detailed molecular environment would allow determination of a probable sequence of events. Hopefully it will be possible to experimentally approach the question with carefully controlled in vitro systems.

Dr. Robert: Would there be a change of conformation or calcium or lipid binding in fibrous elastin?

Dr. Urry: The thing about molecular interactions and associations is that one really needs to know the details of conformation before such questions can be adequately answered. In this case of the interactions and associations of elastin we have generalized, but just as we can be surprised by a molecule increasing its lipophilicity after becoming charged, as with the valinomycin-potassium ion complex, we can be surprised by virtue of a specific conformation imparting previously unexpected properties. A change in conformation, however, is surely associated with Ca^{++} binding and could readily occur on lipid binding.

Dr. Yu: How does Ca^{++} binding in calcified tissue compare with your proposed mechanism in which all the Ca^{++} in the tissue is bound to protein.

Dr. Urry: When we discuss Ca^{++} binding to neutral sites in relation to calcification, the emphasis is on an initiation process. An area of a protein which would be favorable for initiating calcification would be one in which the relative orientation of calcium binding sites would be of a geometry just right for initiating crystal growth. The Ca[++] deposition during crystal growth obviously would be within the crystal and not bound to the protein.

Dr. Yu: If the temperature increases in your experimental model, what kind of affinity constant for metalic ions are you going to get on this type of model?

Dr. Urry: Oh goodness, there are so many interactions with different temperature dependencies that it would be hard to predict the effect of increasing temperature on lipid and calcium ion affinity. We have shown that the conformation of elastin changes on coacervation and that there is an implied increase in order with increase in temperature. This is an inverse temperature effect.[1] This is relevant since we have also shown that the elastin coacervate can initiate calcification.[2] In addition, there is the competition between water and peptide oxygens as ligands for the calcium ion. Each has its own complicated temperature dependence. We can show, for specific repeat elastin sequences, that as long as the concentration of water is less than 5%, the carbonyl oxygens can compete well at one-hundredth the concentration of the water. First of all, there is the competition of carbonyl oxygen and water as ligands; second, there is the energy required for the peptide sequence to attain a favorable conformation, and with a given conformation, there is the energy required to turn hydrophobic groups outward. If the environment is highly aqueous all three effects are not as favorable.

Dr. Muir: May I ask a rather naive question, and that is presumably if you have lipid binding elastin, would it be less elastic?

Dr. Urry: I would suspect that.

Dr. Muir: I wondered whether you have considered testing your hypothesis perhaps on a different protein.

Dr. Urry: No, we haven't studied other proteins in detail, but preliminary studies on albumin, poly-L-alanine, and other

---

[1]Cox, B.A., Starcher, B.C., and Urry, D.W. (1973). Biochim. Biophys. Acta 317, 209.

[2]Starcher, B.C., and Urry, D.W. (1973). Biochim. Biophys. Res. Commun. 53, 210.

proteins and polypeptides do show calcium ion binding under
appropriate conditions. For example, at the peptide level the
capacity of the repeat hexapeptide of elastin to bind Ca^{++} does
appear to be quite exceptional.

SECTION III

TISSUE CULTURE APPLICATION IN

CONNECTIVE TISSUE RESEARCH

TISSUE CULTURE TECHNOLOGY APPLICABLE TO ARTERIAL MESENCHYME

Sergey Fedoroff

Department of Anatomy

University of Saskatchewan, Saskatoon, Canada

Tissue culture, since its inception at the turn of this century, has undergone several stages in its evolution. During the first 40 or 50 years the main emphasis was on observation of cell growth and an overall fascination with the technique. During the second phase of 15 to 20 years the emphasis was on growing large numbers of cells, producing cell populations for quantitative work,and studying neoplastic transformation. Methods were developed which produced cells by the pound. In the third and present phase emphasis is placed on the analysis of cellular interaction, cell differentiation, cell function and, in general, on finding answers to specific questions related to in vivo phenomena.

Tissue culture technology has advanced to the point at which it is flexible and adaptable to various problems. Difficulties which seemed insurmountable not so long ago, such as frequent accidental contaminations, toxicity of the media, etc., have been partially overcome, although contamination of the cells with mycoplasma is still a major threat (Fedoroff et al., 1972; Fogh et al., 1971). With the introduction of laminar flow hoods which provide an organism-free environment, tissue culture laboratories can be set up with ease,and expensively constructed culture rooms have become unnecessary (Coriell et al., 1967; Coriell and McGarrity, 1968; McGarrity and Coriell, 1971). A number of excellent courses in tissue culture technology are now available, varying from two to four weeks, and the Tissue Culture Association is putting considerable effort into improvement and standardization of the quality of tissue culture media available from commercial sources (Morton, 1970). A large variety of well-defined cell lines is available through the American Type Culture Collection (Stulberg et al., 1970).

In spite of advances the size of the piece of tissue which can be successfully cultured in vitro still is limited to 1 to 2 mm. Larger fragments are nourished with difficulty and as a result extensive necrosis develops within a short time. The problem is the same as that encountered in vivo with tissues which do not have a blood supply and are nourished through diffusion. Therefore, the choice is either small fragments of tissue or tissues separated into individual cells by various enzymes. By using fragments one can study cell reactions within the framework of histological organization (organ culture), or by encouraging cell outgrowth from the fragments one can study reactions in a framework of unorganized populations similar to the situation when cells are separated by means of enzymes.

Probably most work in tissue culture has been done on cells in unorganized cell populations. This is also true of the work related to the arteries. In unorganized cell populations it is very difficult to identify specific cell types. Therefore, in the earlier days of tissue culture it was said that all cells in vitro revert to either epithelial-like, fibroblast-like, or ameboid cells. Now we know that methods of classical cell morphology are not always adequate to identify cells. For example, T and B lymphocytes appear to be the same morphologically but can be distinguished by their function or special markers, such as cell surface antigens (Reif and Allen, 1964; Boyse and Old, 1969; Schlesinger, 1970) or sensitivity to various agents (Sultzer and Nilsson, 1972; Stockman et al., 1973; Nordling et al., 1972).

Because of the difficulties in recognizing cells in vitro Lazzarini-Robertson (1961) classified cells which grew out of fragments of the arterial wall as Type I and Type II cells. He believed Type I cells to be endothelial cells because of their morphology, growth behaviour and histochemistry, and Type II cells to be connective tissue fibroblasts. Later these were renamed "atherophils" and "fibrophils" (Robertson, 1965). Atherophils apparently can rapidly incorporate extracellular lipids under unfavorable environmental conditions resulting in lipid-laden "foam cells" or "atherocytes"; whereas "fibrophils" are characterized by their reluctance to incorporate extracellular lipids and their tendency to synthesize acid mucopolysaccharides and collagen in vitro (Robertson, 1967). Similarly, Kokubu and Pollak (1961), who studied cells from various regions of rabbit aorta, classified the cells, based on morphology and growth behaviour, as Type I, the "intermediate" cells; Type II, the "fibrocytic" cells; and Type III, the "endothelial" cells. Type III cells were further subdivided into Type IIIa and Type IIIb, depending on the number of granules they had in their cytoplasm. The population of these three types of cells apparently varied depending on the part of the aorta from which the explants were taken and on whether it was a normal or a diseased aorta.

The need to devise new terminology in order to describe cells
in vitro only emphasizes the difficulty in relating any particular
cell type observed in vitro to a specific histotype as we know it
in organized tissues. In order to overcome these difficulties
three basic approaches are being used: first, to isolate cells
from specific anatomical sites which would ensure an overwhelming
population of one specific cell type; second, to isolate specific
cells, because of their inherent properties, from a mixed population of cells; and third, to limit the studies to organized tissues
in which individual cells can be identified, based on histological
criteria.

An example of the first approach is the method developed to
isolate endothelium from the umbilical vein. The endothelium of
the vein is in direct contact with the internal elastic lamina
and there are no other cells in between. Therefore, it is an
easy procedure to trypsinize the endothelial cells inside the
umbilical vein which has no tributaries. The effect of trypsin
on the wall of the vein can be verified in histological sections.
Maruyama (1963), who developed this method, found that the trypsin
solution usually frees only the endothelial cells and does not
damage the underlying elastic lamina. On the other hand, the
umbilical artery has no distinct elastic lamina and, therefore,
depending on the extent of trypsinization, cells from the subendothelial layer as well as endothelial cells are released. Mixed
cell cultures result from such cell suspensions, and it is interesting that the cells from the subendothelial layer always overgrow
the endothelial cells (Pollak and Kasai, 1964; Fryer et al., 1966).

I think that if one combined the cell cloning technique with
this method, or propagated the cells for several passages, one
could isolate pure populations of subendothelial cells free of
endothelial cells, since, unless they behave differently in the
presence of fibroblasts, smooth muscle cells, and macrophages,
endothelial cells apparently begin to degenerate in cultures after
14 to 21 days (Maruyama, 1963). Given methods to separate pure
populations of endothelial cells, it would be only a matter of
time before antisera will become available for precise identification of endothelial cells in mixed cultures, similar to the anti-
Θ-serum for identification of T type lymphocytes (Reif and Allen,
1964; Schlesinger, 1970).

A pure population of smooth muscle cells can be isolated from
the tunica media of the aorta or large blood vessels. The tunica
media of blood vessels which do not have vasa vasorum are composed
only of smooth muscle cells and intercellular connective tissue

components which the smooth muscle cell synthesizes (Pease and Paule, 1960; Buck, 1963; Wissler, 1968). Therefore, if the adventitia and intima are stripped off such vessels, the remaining tunica media is an excellent source for pure cultures of smooth muscle cells.

In cultures, smooth muscle cells first acquire a fibroblast-like appearance. During this stage many cells degenerate but others proliferate (Jarmolych et al., 1968). After a few weeks in culture the cells again acquire the appearance of smooth muscle cells (Jarmolych et al., 1968; Fritz et al., 1970; Ross, 1971; Ross, 1972; May and Paule, 1972). Their identity can be easily established by electron microscopy because, by then, they again contain considerable amounts of myofilaments in their cytoplasm, and because other smooth muscle characteristics become visible (Fritz et al., 1970; Ross, 1971; Ross, 1972). The actomyosin in the cells can be demonstrated by immunohistochemical methods (Knieriem et al., 1968; Dzoga et al., 1971a). There is little doubt that the cells in culture are indeed smooth muscle cells even if they came from tunica media of vessels which had vasa vasorum. It seems that the cells of vasa vasorum do not contribute greatly, if at all, to the final cell population (Fritz et al., 1970).

In cultures, the smooth muscle cells grow in "hills and valleys" and may form, in some parts of the culture, as many as 10 to 13 layers of cells (Ross, 1972). It is significant that smooth muscle cells in culture continue to synthesize collagen fibers, elastic fibers, and mucopolysaccharides (Jarmolych et al., 1968; Ross, 1972; May and Paule, 1972). It is not known whether one and the same cell can synthesize all these connective tissue intercellular components or whether the jobs are divided among the cells.

The growth of smooth muscle cells can be estimated by the addition of homologous hyperlipemic blood serum to the culture (Florentin et al., 1969; Daoud et al., 1970; Dzoga et al., 1971a). It seems that it is the low density lipoproteins in the hyperlipemic serum which are responsible for the growth stimulating effect (Dzoga et al., 1971b), although the situation may be much more complex because normal sera, at least in some animal species, may contain natural components which may regulate the rates of proliferation of smooth muscle cells (Fritz et al., 1972).

At present we do not know whether the observations made on smooth muscle cells derived from aortae or large blood vessels are generally applicable to all smooth muscle cells from different anatomical regions such as the uterus, the gastrointestinal tract, and even to small arteries and veins. It would not be surprising if, for example, it were found that smooth muscle cells from the

uterus behave in cultures quite differently from smooth muscle
cells from the tunica media of large blood vessels.

Instead of taking advantage of specific anatomical sites for
obtaining cultures of the desired cell types, occasionally advantage can be taken of specific cell properties. One such property
is the affinity of cells to attach to glass or other surfaces.
For example, macrophages have a very great affinity for glass
surfaces; they attach very rapidly and cannot be removed from the
glass by treatment with 0.02 percent trypsin solution. Evans
(1972), using this technique, was able to separate macrophages
from various tumors and to determine the number of macrophages
present in the various types of tumors. I see no reason why this
technique could not be applied to the isolation of macrophages
from subendothelial tissues or atherosclerotic lesions.

Kasten (1972), using this principle, succeeded in isolating a
pure population of endothelial cells from the hearts of three to
four day old rats. The isolation procedure was based on the
observation that endothelial cells attach to the glass more rapidly
than myocardial cells. The optimum time for the separation of the
two cell types was found to be 90 minutes. Endothelial cells
separated by trypsinization from human umbilical veins (Maruyama,
1963) did not proliferate in culture, but endothelium separated
by Kasten (1972) from the hearts of rats proliferated rapidly.
This interesting discrepancy could be due to regional differences
in endothelial cells, differences in species, or differences in
culturing conditions.

Methods to isolate fat cells from adipose tissue (Rodbell,
1964) have been adapted to the isolation of foam cells from
atherosclerotic lesions in rabbits (Day et al., 1966). The
method consists of treating stripped intima with collagenase and
elastase in a solution of bovine albumin in Krebs Ringer phosphate
to which glucose has been added. Apparently such preparations, in
addition to foam cells, contain approximately five percent fibroblasts (Tume et al., 1969). The foam cells rapidly attach to the
glass; however, they apparently do not divide in vitro (Tume et al.,
1969). By careful timing, it might be possible to separate macrophages loaded with fat granules from real foam cells by the
rapidity with which the macrophages attach to the glass surfaces.
It is also possible that foam cells may be stimulated to divide by
using methods which have been quite successful in stimulating the
division of macrophages in vitro. I refer to procedures such as
the addition of media collected from cultures of syngeneic or allo-
geneic fibroblasts. Such media contain macrophage growth factor
(MGF),which induces dormant (G_0 state) macrophages to divide
(Virolainen and Defendi, 1967).

By experimenting with various types of surfaces it might be possible to differentiate between various cell types,because not all cells have the same degree of affinity to different surfaces. For example, recently it has been demonstrated that fibroblasts do not attach well to acrylamide gel, whereas the epithelial cells, especially those from tumors, readily do so (Haskill, 1973).

Up to now I have considered approaches to the isolation of specific cell types which would grow in cultures as unorganized, single-cell populations. It is possible to use such cell populations for reconstruction of tissues in vitro and for the study of specific cell interactions. For this purpose collagen-coated cellulose sponges provide a three-dimensional matrix (Leighton et al., 1967).

Leighton et al. (1970) were able to use unorganized,single-cell populations of mouse fibroblasts (line 3T6) in the reconstruction of an excellent three-dimensional connective tissue by using collagen-coated cellulose sponges and increasing the ascorbic acid content of the medium to 250 µg/ml. It was found previously that most tissue culture media are deficient in ascorbic acid,which is conducive to collagen synthesis (Goldberg and Green, 1964; Schafer et al., 1967).

Such three-dimensional connective tissue can be effectively tested for its interactions with other types of cells under various experimental conditions. For example, Leighton (1969) studied extensively the interactions between tumor cells and connective tissue. Among his experiments he demonstrated beautifully the effect of embryonic connective tissue on the polarity of kidney epithelial cells. Collagen-coated sponges might be very useful in studying the interactions between the cell types found in the walls of blood vessels. The effects of factors which normally stimulate the growth of blood vessels in vivo probably could be tested by this means. Instead of using isolated cells from formed blood vessels, one could use embryonic tissue which is destined to form blood vessels. A good source of such tissue is the primordia of the retinal vessels in rabbits (Ashton, 1966). In rabbits under two weeks of age the developing vascular plexus lies on the surface of the retina and can be lifted from the retina and transferred into tissue cultures. This material should be excellent for the study of the formation of capillaries and differentiation of mesenchymal cells, either in a sponge matrix or in other tissue culture systems in which cells can be easily observed throughout the culturing period.

The principle of reconstruction of tissues by single-cell populations is also being used to reconstruct the lining of blood vessels on microfabric-lined artificial vascular prostheses. This approach is of very practical importance because it will make possible the lining of such prostheses with autologous cells, making the prostheses more compatible to the recipients (Kahn et al., 1972; Burkel and Kahn, 1973).

In contrast to the unorganized monolayer cultures, in organized cultures in which the in vivo histological organization of the tissue is preserved, recognition of the cells is based on the usual histological criteria. The main disadvantage of such cultures over the unorganized monolayer cultures is that the cells cannot be observed continuously under the microscope during culturing. At the end of the culturing period the fragments must be fixed, and thin sections must be cut and stained before the cells can be examined.

For example, thin cross-sections of rabbit aorta were cultured in Millipore chambers, i.e., chambers which are tightly covered on both sides by Millipore filters, and were incubated either subcutaneously or in the abdominal cavity of another rabbit. In such in vivo cultures the cells in the subendothelium proliferate, resulting in a thickened intima. However, the endothelium remained intact (Wada and Pollak, 1967; Iwanaga et al., 1969). Wada and Pollak (1967), after culturing such sections of aorta in vivo for two weeks, transferred the sections into culture vessels which were then incubated in vitro. While in vitro, the endothelium proliferated. If they started to grow sections of aorta first in vitro, then the endothelium proliferated, and on culturing in vivo the cells in the subendothelial layer proliferated. It seems that different conditions are required to stimulate proliferation of the endothelium than for stimulation of cells in the subendothelial layer.

However, when Wada and Pollak (1967) everted the sections of aorta in such a way that the adventitia was lining the lumen and the endothelium formed the outer surface, the endothelium proliferated instead of the cells in the subendothelial layer, in the in vivo cultures. During two weeks of culturing, two to five layers of endothelial cells formed. Because Wada and Pollak (1967) fed a high cholesterol diet to the rabbits which were used as "incubators," the proliferated endothelial cells in the incubated sections, on prolonged cultivation, were replaced by foam cells. When such everted sections with proliferating endothelium were transferred into in vitro conditions, the subendothelial layer began to proliferate. It seems that such experiments could be expanded fruitfully by determining more precisely the physical and biochemical conditions required in vitro to stimulate proliferation of endothelial cells or cells in the subendothelial layer. In such studies the interrelationships between the endothelium and cells in the subendothelial layer could not be disregarded.

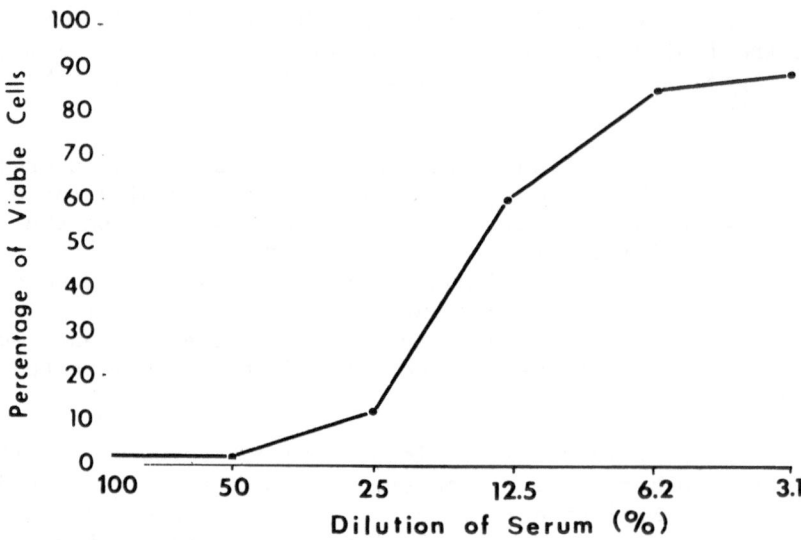

Fig. 1. Trypsinized cells from rabbit kidney cortex were suspended for one hour at 37°C in various dilutions of serum taken
from the same animal. Serum was diluted with Hanks' BSS. After
incubation, cell viability was determined in haemocytometer by
dye exclusion test.

     The primary goal in tissue culture work is to reproduce in
vitro phenomena which occur in vivo, in order to study these
phenomena in a simplified, defined environment in which observation is more feasible. Originally, it was a logical choice to use
blood serum as a major component of culture media since, after all,
cells are nourished by blood in vivo. However, only a few cell
types in the body are exposed directly to the blood. Most cells
are nourished by components of the serum which have filtered
through the capillary endothelium to varying extents in different
parts of the body, through the ground substance and the meshwork
of various extracellular fibers. Therefore, it is not surprising
that in vitro 100 percent serum is not necessarily conducive to
the survival of autologous cells. Figure 1 indicates the effect
of serum in various concentrations on the cells of the renal
cortex of the rabbit. The serum and the cells came from the same
animal, but the cells could survive only in very dilute serum.

     With the help of the Bellco Company, we devised "twin cultures"
(Figure 2) consisting of two spinner cultures linked with an additional vessel which is separated from the spinner cultures by
cellophane membranes. The spinner culture vessels were filled
with chemically-defined medium (medium 199) and the vessel in the

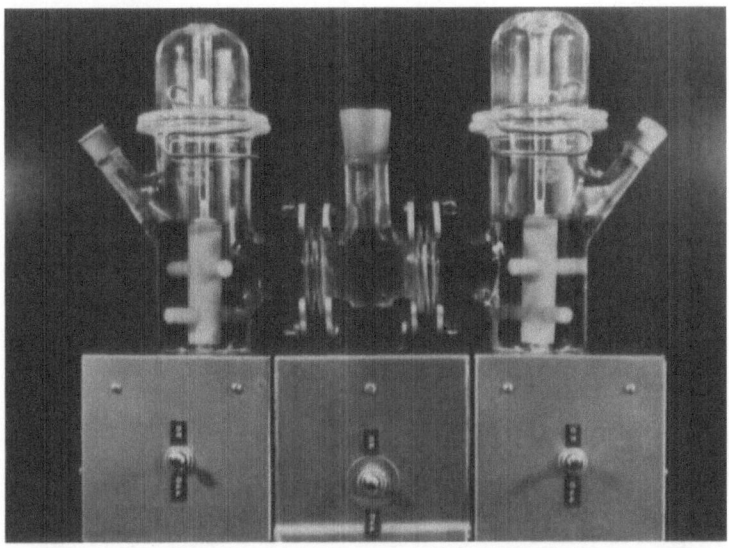

Fig. 2. "Twin culture" apparatus, consisting of two Bellco
spinner-flasks joined by a middle vessel. Various membranes can
be inserted to separate the middle vessel from the spinner-flasks.
Serum in middle vessel can be agitated by a small, magnetic bar.

middle with 100 percent horse blood serum. We allowed the system
to equilibrate and then added line L cells to the spinner culture
vessels. Figure 3 shows that cells in chemically-defined medium
only were unable to survive, but when serum components were allowed
to dialyze through a cellophane membrane into the chemically-
defined medium, the cells thrived. Similar findings were made by
Eagle (1960) and Metzgar and Moskowitz (1960).

It is well known that human serum contains naturally
occurring antibodies which, in the presence of human complement,
lyse mouse cells (Fedoroff and Doerr, 1962). If, however, human
serum is added to the central vessel in the "twin cultures", it
can sustain growth of mouse line L cells in the spinner cultures,
provided it is separated from the cells by a cellophane membrane.

These experiments demonstrated that the components of the
serum necessary for cell growth can be partitioned from deleterious
components by a cellophane membrane. Rose (1957), and Rose et al.
(1958) who originally introduced the use of cellophane strips in
tissue culture for other reasons, realized its importance and in
his later papers he writes about the microenvironment which surrounds the cells underneath the cellophane and the macroenvironment which is above the cellophane. The microenvironment is

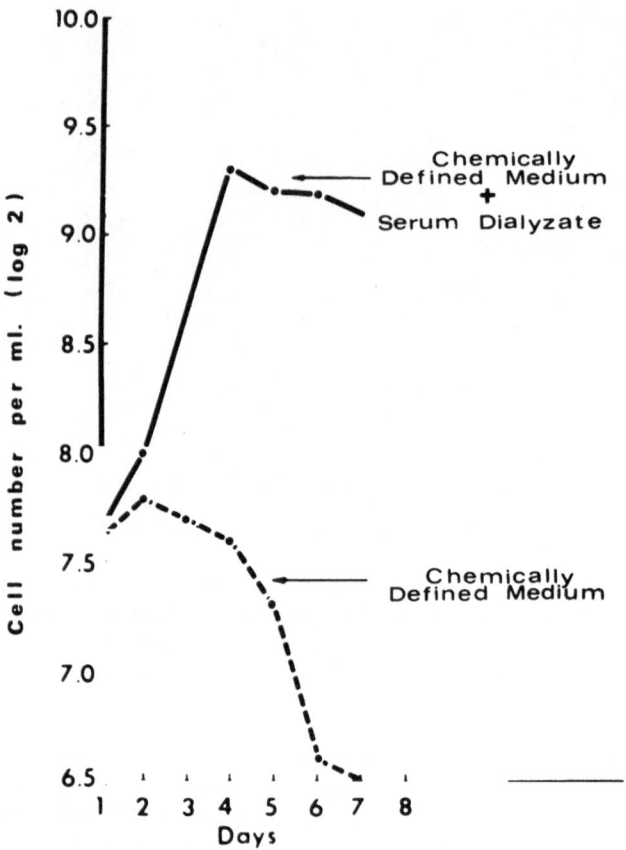

Fig. 3. Growth curves of line L cells in "twin cultures."
Middle vessel was filled with 100 percent horse serum. On one
side the middle vessel and spinner-flask were separated by a
cellophane membrane. On the other side they were separated by
an impermeable membrane. The cell population declined in the
flask into which serum could not dialyze. In the flask into
which serum could dialyze through the cellophane membrane the
cell population increased.

serum-free; the macroenvironment contains the serum, and both
environments are in equilibrium through the cellophane membrane
(Rose, 1967; Rose et al., 1970).

For years tissue culture workers were concerned with what
to feed cells in order to make them divide. However, since the
removal of metabolic by-products from the cells is just as
important as introducing various substrates into the cell, the
cells must be in proper osmotic relationship to their environment.

Only in the last few years has more attention been paid to what
is isotonic to various cell types. In our laboratory we have
observed that epithelium from the renal medulla requires considerably higher osmolality of the medium than epithelial cells from
the cortex (Fedoroff and Munkacsi, unpublished). There is also
some indication that embryonic cells equilibrate with lower osmolalities than adult cells. An excellent review on this subject has
been published recently (Waymouth, 1970).

    One of the major differences between _in vivo_ and _in vitro_ situ-
ations is that the former is an open system; the body fluids continuously flow by the cells and the by-products are removed. Tissue
cultures, on the other hand, represent closed systems, in which the
cells draw the required components from a pool which is gradually
depleted. As the cells metabolize there is an accumulation of
metabolic by-products. Periodic changing of the medium results
in stress to the cells and requires the cells to readjust to the
new environmental conditions. In order to overcome these defects
and to approach more closely an open system and a steady state,
numerous attempts have been made to devise a continuously perfusing
tissue culture system in which nutrients would be perfused through
the cultures at predetermined rates. Although the first attempts
in this direction were made by Burrows in 1912 more attention has
been given to perfusion systems only recently.

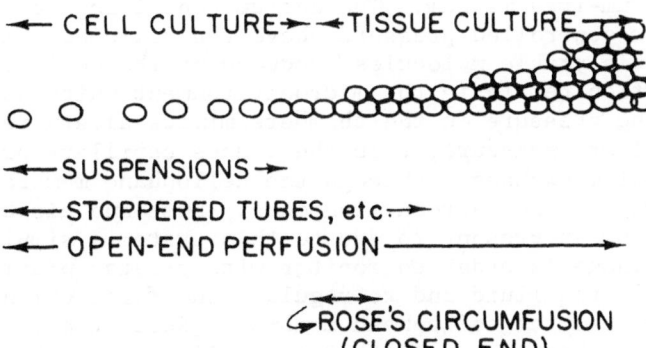

<— CELL CULTURE— —TISSUE CULTURE—

<—SUSPENSIONS—>

<—STOPPERED TUBES, etc.—>

<— OPEN-END PERFUSION————————>

ROSE'S CIRCUMFUSION
(CLOSED END)

(P.F. Kruse et al.

In Vitro 6: 75-88, 1970)

Fig. 4. Comparison of layering of cells by various culture
methods. (Reproduced with permission from the Tissue Culture
Association, Incorporated).

Interest in the perfusion system was stimulated after Kruse
et al. (1963, 1969, and 1970) and Kruse and Miedema (1965)
demonstrated that by perfusing monolayer cultures of diploid or
heteroploid cell lines in T-flasks the cell populations could be
raised to much higher numbers than by any other culturing method.
With continuous perfusion the cells pile up in multiple layers,
resembling a tissue. Kruse et al. (1970) in Figure 4 summarize
the relative relationship between various techniques and possible
cell densities. The system developed in Kruse's laboratory and
other similar systems are based on continuous perfusion of the
medium through the culture; therefore, any substance which the
cells may produce will be carried away. There is no evidence so
far of cell differentiation in such cultures in spite of multi-
layering of the cells, which may reach as many as 16 to 20 layers.
In perfusion systems conditions can be set up so that the cells
proliferate until they reach a state in which most of the cells
do not divide. Such populations may contain only 0.5 percent
dividing cells. The cells can be maintained in this state without
deterioration for at least several weeks. Such cultures should be
ideal for biochemical studies because they resemble the cell populations in vivo much more closely than do exponentially growing
cell populations (Kruse et al., 1969).

However, the work started by Rose in Pomerat's laboratory in
Galveston twenty years ago and continued in Rose's laboratory in
Houston has taken a different approach. They developed systems
which approximate in vivo conditions more and more closely (Rose,
1957, 1967; Rose et al., 1958, 1970). In the Dual-Rotary Circumfusion System the tissue fragments are covered by a cellophane membrane in a serum-free medium. The medium containing serum is
perfused under controlled pressure above the cellophane membrane.
Thus any non-dialyzable molecules produced by the cells and vital
to their function remain in the microenvironment which surrounds
the cells. The pressure in the chambers mimics alternately the
arterial capillary pressure, then the venous capillary pressures,
thus facilitating exchanges through the cellophane membrane
between the micro- and macroenvironments. Rose and his collabora-
tors are working at present to add to this system a simulation of
lymphatic drainage in order to monitor with greater precision the
osmolalities of the fluid and to regulate the force which moves
the solutes across the cellophane membrane (Rose et al., 1970).
An advantage of this system is that the cells can be observed
under the phase microscope, and cinematographic records can be made
all through the culturing period.

In circumfusion systems the tissues develop a higher degree
of differentiation than they do in any other system devised so far
(Rose et al., 1969). It is obvious that many future developments
in the study of cell reactions will depend on circumfusion or like

systems. A review of the developments in this area has been written recently by Kruse (1972).

The more closely the in vivo conditions are being mimicked and the more closely the cells begin to perform in vitro as they do in vivo, the more carefully the interacting factors will have to be considered, e.g., interactions between similar (homotypic) and different (heterotypic) cell types, interactions with the media, the substrate on which the cells are grown, the genetic make-up, and the immediate environment from which the cells came. The environment from which the cells came depends on the anatomical site, age, diet, and the physiological state of the animal.

My assignment in this workshop was to consider the technology which can be applied to the growing of arterial mesenchyme in tissue cultures. However, I have not dealt with mesenchyme as such because practically any tissue culture method can be used to grow it. In general, the important point is not just to grow the mesenchyme, but to grow it for a specific purpose; the problem should dictate the technology to use.

REFERENCES

Ashton, N. (1966). Oxygen and the growth and development of retinal vessels. In vivo and in vitro studies. Amer. J. Opthalmol. 62, 412.

Boyse, E.A., and Old, L.J. (1969). Some aspects of normal and abnormal cell surface genetics. Annu. Rev. Genet. 3, 269.

Buck, R.C. (1963). Histogenesis and morphogenesis of arterial tissue. In "Atherosclerosis and its Origin." (M. Sandler and G.H. Bourne, eds.), pp. 1-38. Academic Press, New York.

Burkel, W.E., and Kahn, R.H. (1973). An ultrastructural study of human pseudoendothelium propagated in vitro. Anat. Rec. 175, 281.

Burrows, M.T. (1912). A method of furnishing a continuous supply of new medium to a tissue culture in vitro. Anat. Rec. 6, 141.

Coriell, L.L., and McGarrity, G.J. (1968). Biohazard hood to prevent infection during microbiological procedures. Appl. Microbiol. 16, 1895.

Coriell, L.L., McGarrity, G.J., and Horneff, J. (1967). Medical application of dust-free rooms. I. Elimination of airborne bacteria in a research laboratory. Amer. J. Pub. Health 57, 1824.

Daoud, A.S., Fritz, K.E., and Jarmolych, J. (1970). Increased DNA synthesis in aortic explants from swine fed a high cholesterol diet. Exp. Mol. Pathol. 13, 377.

Day, A.J., Newman, H.A., and Zilversmit, D.B. (1966). Synthesis of phospholipid by foam cells isolated from rabbit atherosclerotic lesions. Circ. Res. 19, 122.

Dzoga, K., Vasselinovitch, D., Fraser, R., and Wissler, R.W. (1971a). The effect of lipoproteins on the growth of aortic smooth muscle cells. Amer. J. Pathol. 62, 32a.

Dzoga, K., Wissler, R.W., and Vasselinovitch, D. (1971b). The effect of normal and hyperlipemic low density lipoprotein fractions on aortic tissue culture cell. Circulation 44, 4.

Eagle, H. (1960). The sustained growth of human and animal cells in a protein-free environment. Proc. Nat. Acad. Sci. U.S.A. 46, 427.

Evans, R. (1972). Macrophages in syngeneic animal tumors. Transplantation 14, 468.

Fedoroff, S., and Doerr, J. (1962). Effect of human blood serum on tissue culture. III. A natural cytotoxic system in human blood serum. J. Nat. Cancer Inst. 29, 331.

Fedoroff, S., Evans, V.J., Hopps, H.E., Sanford, K.K., and Boone, C.W. (1972). Summary of proceedings of a workshop on serum for tissue culture purposes. In Vitro 7, 161.

Fedoroff, S., and Munkacsi, I. (1970). (Unpublished).

Florentin, R.A., Choi, B.H., Lee, K.T., and Thomas, W.A. (1969). Stimulation of DNA synthesis and cell division in vitro by serum from cholesterol-fed swine. J. Cell Biol. 41, 641.

Fogh, J., Holmgren, N., and Ludovici, P.P. (1971). A review of cell culture contaminations. In Vitro 7, 26.

Fritz, K.E., Jarmolych, J., and Daoud, A.S. (1970). Association of DNA synthesis and apparent dedifferentiation of aortic smooth muscle cells in vitro. Exp. Mol. Pathol. 12, 354.

Fritz, K.E., Jarmolych, J., Daoud, A.S., and Peters, T. (1972). Factors influencing DNA synthesis and degradation present in swine serum and aortic tissue. Exp. Mol. Pathol. 16, 54.

Fryer, D.G., Birnbaum, G., and Luttrell, C.N. (1966). Human endothelium in cell culture. J. Atheroscler. Res. 6, 151.

Goldberg, B., and Green, H. (1964). An analysis of collagen
    secretion by established mouse fibroblast lines. J. Cell
    Biol. 22, 227.

Haskill, J.S. (1973). (Personal communications).

Iwanaga, Y., Takimura, A., Kitsukawa, H., Tanigawa, J., Aihara,
    M., Kawashima, T., Mae, A., and Nakashima, T. (1969). The
    role of endothelial cells in the pathogenesis of
    atherosclerosis. Acta Pathol. Jap. 19, 161.

Jarmolych, J., Daoud, A.S., Landau, J., Fritz, K.E., and McElvene,
    E. (1968). Aortic media explants. Cell proliferation and
    production of mucopolysaccharides, collagen, and elastic
    tissue. Exp. Mol. Pathol. 9, 171.

Kahn, R.H., Burnel, W., and Rabin, S. (1972). Development of
    intimal linings for artificial vascular prostheses. In
    Vitro 7, 267.

Kasten, F.H. (1972). Rat myocardial cells in vitro: mitosis and
    differentiated properties. In Vitro 8, 128.

Knieriem, H.J., Kao, V.C.Y., and Wissler, R.W. (1968).
    Demonstration of smooth muscle cells in bovine arteriosclerosis.
    J. Atheroscler. Res. 8, 125.

Kokubu, T., and Polla,, O.J. (1961). In vitro cultures of aortic
    cells of untreated and of cholesterol-fed rabbits. J.
    Atheroscler. Res. 1, 229.

Kruse, P.F., Jr. (1972). Use of perfusion system for growth of
    cell and tissue culture. In "Growth, Nutrition, and Metabolism
    of Cells in Culture." (G.H. Rothblat and V.J. Cristofalo,
    eds.), pp. 11-66. Academic Press, New York.

Kruse, P.F., Jr., Keen, L.N., and Whittle, W.L. (1970). Some
    distinctive characteristics of high density perfusion cultures
    of diverse cell types. In Vitro 6, 75.

Kruse, P.F., Jr., and Miedema, E. (1965). Production and
    characterization of multiple-layered populations of animal
    cells. J. Cell Biol. 27, 273.

Kruse, P.F., Jr., Myhr, B.C., Johnson, J.E., and White, P.B.
    (1963). Perfusion system for replicate mammalian cell
    cultures in T-60 flasks. J. Nat. Cancer Inst. 31, 109.

Kruse, P.F., Jr., Whittle, W., and Miedema, E. (1969). Mitotic and nonmitotic multiple-layered perfusion cultures. J. Cell Biol. 42, 113.

Lazzarini-Robertson, A., Jr. (1961). Effects of heparin on the uptake of lipids by isolated human and animal arterial endothelial type cells. Angiology 12, 525.

Leighton, J. (1969). Propagation of cancer: Targets for future chemotherapy. Cancer Res. 29, 2457.

Leighton, J., Estes, L.W., Goldblatt, P.J., and Brada, Z. (1970). The formation of histotypic fibrous collagen in matrix tissue culture by 3T6 mouse fibroblasts: a response to ascorbic acid. In Vitro 6, 153.

Leighton, J., Justh, G., and Esper, M. (1967). Collagen-coated cellulose sponge: three dimensional matrix for tissue culture of Walker Tumor 256. Science 155, 1259.

Maruyama, Y. (1963). The human endothelial cell in tissue culture. Z. Zellforsch Mikrosk. Anat. 60, 69.

May, J.F., and Paule, W.J. (1972). Light and electron microscopic observations of cultured pig aortic smooth muscle cells. J. Cell Biol. 55, 335.

McGarrity, G.J., and Coriell, L.L. (1971). Procedures to reduce contamination of cell cultures . In Vitro 6, 257.

Metzgar, D.P., Jr., and Moskowitz, M. (1960). Separation of growth promoting activity from horse serum dialysis. Proc. Soc. Exp. Biol. Med. 104, 363.

Morton, H.C. (1970). A survey of commercially available tissue culture media. In Vitro 6, 89.

Nordling, S., Andersson, L.C., and Hayry, P. (1972). Thymus-dependent and thymus-independent lymphocyte separation: Relation to exposed sialic acid on cell surface. Science 178, 1001.

Pease, D.C., and Paule, W.J. (1960). Electron microscopy of elastic arteries; the thoracic aortae of the rat. J. Ultrastruct. Res. 3, 469.

Pollak, O.J., and Kasai, T. (1964). Appearance and behavior of aortic cells in vitro. Amer. J. Med. Sci. 248, 105.

Reif, A.E., and Allen, J.M.V. (1964). The AKR thymic antigen and
    its distribution in leukemias and nervous tissue. J. Exp.
    Med. 120, 413.

Robertson, A.L., Jr. (1965). Metabolism and ultrastructure of the
    arterial wall in atherosclerosis. Cleveland Clin. Quart. 32,
    99.

Robertson, A.L., Jr. (1967). Transport of plasma lipoproteins and
    ultrastructure of human arterial intimacytes in culture.
    (G.H. Rothblat and D. Kritchevsky, eds.). In "Lipid Metabolism
    in Tissue Culture Cells." Wistar Institute Press, Philadelphia.

Rodbell, M. (1964). Metabolism of isolated fat cells. I. Effects
    of hormones of glucose metabolism and lipolysis. J. Biol.
    Chem. 239, 375.

Rose, G.G. (1967). The circumfusion system for multipurpose
    culture chambers. I. Introduction to the mechanics,
    techniques, and basic results of a 12-chamber (in vitro)
    closed circulatory system. J. Cell Biol. 32, 89.

Rose, G.G. (1957). Special uses of the multipurpose tissue
    culture chamber. Tex. Rep. Biol. Med. 15, 310.

Rose, G.G., Kumegawa, M., Nikai, H., Bracho, M., and Cattoni, M.
    (1970). The dual-rotary circumfusion system for Mark II
    culture chambers. I. Design, control, and monitoring of
    the system and the cultures. Microvasc. Res. 2, 24.

Rose, G.G., Kumegawa, M., Nikai, H.,Cattoni, M., and Hu, F. (1969).
    The HFH-18 mouse melanoma in roller tube, chamber, and
    circumfusion system cultures. Cancer Res. 29, 2010.

Rose, G.G., Pomerat, C.M., Shindler, T.O., and Trunnel, J.B.
    (1958). A cellophane-strip technique for culturing tissue
    in multipurpose culture chambers. J. Biophys. Biochem.
    Cytol. 4, 761.

Ross, R. (1972). The arterial smooth muscle cells. (R.W. Wissler,
    J.C. Geer, and N. Kaufman, eds.). In "The Pathogenesis of
    Atherosclerosis, 1971." Williams and Wilkins, Baltimore,
    Maryland.

Ross, R. (1971). The smooth muscle cell. II. Growth of smooth
    muscle in culture and formation of elastic fibers. J. Cell
    Biol. 50, 172.

Schafer, I.A., Silverman, L., Sullivan, J.C., and Robertson, W.V.B. (1967). Ascorbic acid deficiency in cultured human fibroblasts. J. Cell Biol. 34, 83.

Schlesinger, M. (1970). Anti-Θ antibodies for detecting thymus-dependent lymphocytes in the immune response of mice to SRBC. Nature 226, 1254.

Stockman, G.D., Heim, L.R., South, M.A., and Trentin, J.J. (1973). Differential effects of cyclophosphamide on the B and T cell compartments of adult mice. J. Immunol. 110, 277.

Stulberg, C.S., Coriell, L.L., Knaizeff, A.J., and Shannon, J.E. (1970). The animal cell culture collection. In Vitro 5, 1.

Sultzer, B.M., and Nilsson, B.S. (1972). PPD-Tuberculin-a B-Cell mitogen. Nature [New Biol.] 240, 198.

Tume, R.K., Bradley, T.R., and Day, A.J. (1969). An investigation by tissue culture techniques on the growth of foam cells isolated from rabbit atherosclerotic lesions. J. Atheroscler. Res. 9, 151.

Virolainen, M., and Defendi, V. (1967). Dependence of macrophage growth in vitro upon interaction with other cell types. (V. Defendi and M. Stoker, eds.). In "Growth Regulating Substances for Animal Cells in Culture." pp. 67-83. Wistar Press, Philadelphia.

Wada, A., and Pollak, O.J. (1967). Extracirculatory cholesterol. Atherosclerosis in rabbits. Arch. Pathol. 84, 460.

Waymouth, C. (1970). Osmolality of mammalian blood and of media for culture of mammalian cells. In Vitro 6, 109.

Wissler, R.W. (1968). The arterial medial cell, smooth muscle or multifunctional mesenchyme? J. Atheroscler. Res. 8, 201.

STUDIES OF PRIMATE ARTERIAL SMOOTH MUSCLE CELLS IN RELATION TO

ATHEROSCLEROSIS

Russell Ross and John Glomset

Departments of Pathology and Medicine, and The Regional
Primate Research Center, University of Washington,
Seattle, Washington

Arterial smooth muscle cells play a major role in the genesis
of the lesions of atherosclerosis (French, 1966; Haust and More,
1963; Jones et al., 1967; McGill and Geer, 1963; Wissler, 1967).
Other cells, such as hematogenously derived macrophages, have been
found within the lesions, but there is little evidence that they
play a principal part in lesion development. Numerous observations
of human lesions and of lesions produced in experimental animals
have provided clear evidence that the lesions of atherosclerosis
are fundamentally proliferative, and have suggested that they
result from the migration of arterial smooth muscle cells from the
media into the intima followed by their subsequent proliferation.
Concomitant with or subsequent to this cell migration and proliferation, intracellular and extracellular lipids are deposited in
association with formation of new extracellular connective tissue
matrix constituents, including collagen, elastic fibers, and glycosaminoglycans.

We have been investigating the possibility that the proliferation
and subsequent metabolism of smooth muscle cells that characterize
atherosclerosis occur in response to "injury" to the arterial
endothelium. Our hypothesis, a modification and extension of the
hypotheses of earlier investigators (Duncan, 1963; French, 1966;
Haust, 1970; Virchow, 1856), can be summarized as follows: Continuous or intermittent, subtle injury to the endothelium by
factors such as local hydrodynamic stress and antigen-antibody
complexes (Minick et al., 1966) alters endothelial permeability
and increases diffusion of plasma proteins from the arterial lumen
into the intima. Under these conditions medial smooth muscle cells
immediately subjacent to the internal elastic lamina become exposed

to increased concentrations of certain plasma factors which
stimulate the cells to migrate into the intima, proliferate, and
form extracellular connective tissue matrix components. This type
of injury could occur continuously or intermittently. In the
absence of elevated plasma lipoprotein concentrations and other
complicating factors, lesions of this type may be reversible and
thus may be continually forming and regressing in man. However,

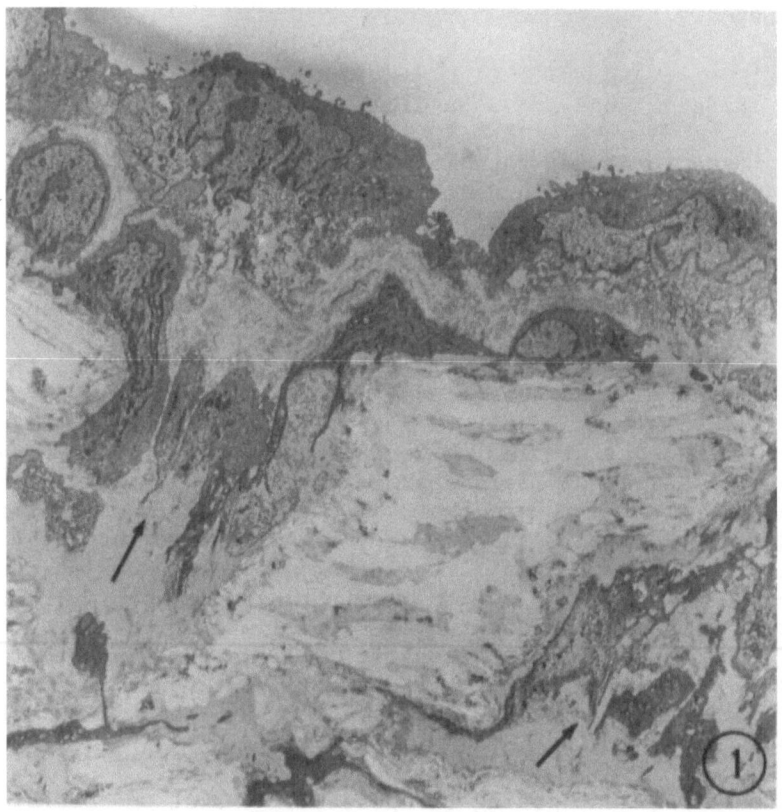

Fig. 1. This is a low power electron micrograph of an arterial
lesion that has formed two weeks after de-endothelialization with
an intravascular balloon catheter. The endothelium has regenerated
and beneath it is seen a segment of the internal elastic lamina
with two fenestrae. In these fenestrae, smooth muscle cells can
be seen in the process of migrating from the media into the intima
(arrows). Several of these cells are partially extended into the
intima, whereas others are completely within the intima. Observations such as these are common between seven days and two weeks
after injury. (x 3,000). (Reproduced with permission from
Stemerman, M., and Ross, R., 1972, J. Exp. Med. 136, 769).

when the initial lesion occurs in the presence of complicating
factors, or when repeated injury occurs to the same locus, progressive and irreversible development of the lesion may occur.   To
test this hypothesis, we have been studying the in vivo and in
vitro responses of arterial smooth muscle cells from subhuman
primates, specifically Macaca nemestrina, the pig-tail macaque
(Ross and Glomset, 1973).

PRODUCTION OF EXPERIMENTAL ATHEROSCLEROSIS IN VIVO

We have produced lesions in vivo in monkey iliac arteries that
appear strikingly similar to the "fibromusculoelastic lesion"
(Stemerman and Ross, 1972) considered by many (DHEW Publication
No. NIH 72-219) to antecede the fatty streaks and fibrous plaques
of human atherosclerosis. The arterial intima is removed with an
intravascular, Fogarty type, balloon catheter, and this causes a
proliferative response of the arterial smooth muscle cells
(Björkerud, 1969; Helin et al., 1971; Stemerman and Ross, 1972).
One week after de-endothelialization, smooth muscle cells can be
seen protruding from the media into the intima through fenestrae
in the internal elastic lamina (Figure 1); after two weeks, endothelial cells again line the intimal surface; and within one to
three months marked intimal thickening is produced by a proliferative lesion consisting of five to fifteen layers of smooth muscle
cells surrounded by glycosaminoglycan, collagen, and small elastic
fibers (Figure 2). In normo-lipemic animals the lesions appear
to be reversible since six months after injury only two to three
layers of smooth muscle cells remain. Thus, these results support
our hypothesis if it is assumed that an endothelial "barrier" to
the diffusion of plasma constituents is disrupted by the balloon
catheter; that the barrier requires many weeks to be re-established;
and that upon being reformed, the barrier limits further cell
proliferation and permits or promotes cell removal.

We are currently investigating the "complicating" effects of
hyperlipemia on the development, character and reversibility of
these lesions. Figures 3 and 4 demonstrate the characteristic
appearance of a lesion three months after injury in a monkey which
was fed a continuous high fat diet. This monkey was hypercholesterolemic six weeks prior to injury and remained so during the
entire period of the experiment (plasma cholesterols 300 - 400 mg%).
In the presence of hyperlipidemia, the appearance of the lesions
strikingly resembles that of human atherosclerotic plaques and
differs from the lesions seen in the normo-lipemic animals in that
smooth muscle cells in the deeper portion of the intima are laden
with large lipid droplets, and extracellular lipid aggregates are
present in the spaces between the collagen and elastic fibers
(Figure 4). A detailed report presenting other aspects of these
experiments will be published elsewhere.

PROLIFERATION OF ARTERIAL SMOOTH MUSCLE CELLS IN VITRO

To identify possible plasma constituents that might act to
promote migration and proliferation of medial smooth muscle cells
in vivo, we are examining the effects of serum protein fractions
on the behavior of arterial smooth muscle cells in vitro. To
facilitate comparison with the in vivo experiments we obtain the
cells from primates of the same genus (Macaca nemestrina) and age
(approximately one year), acquired from the breeding colony of the
Regional Primate Research Center at the University of Washington.
Explants are prepared from the inner one-third of the media of the
thoracic aorta, and the cells are subsequently trypsinized into

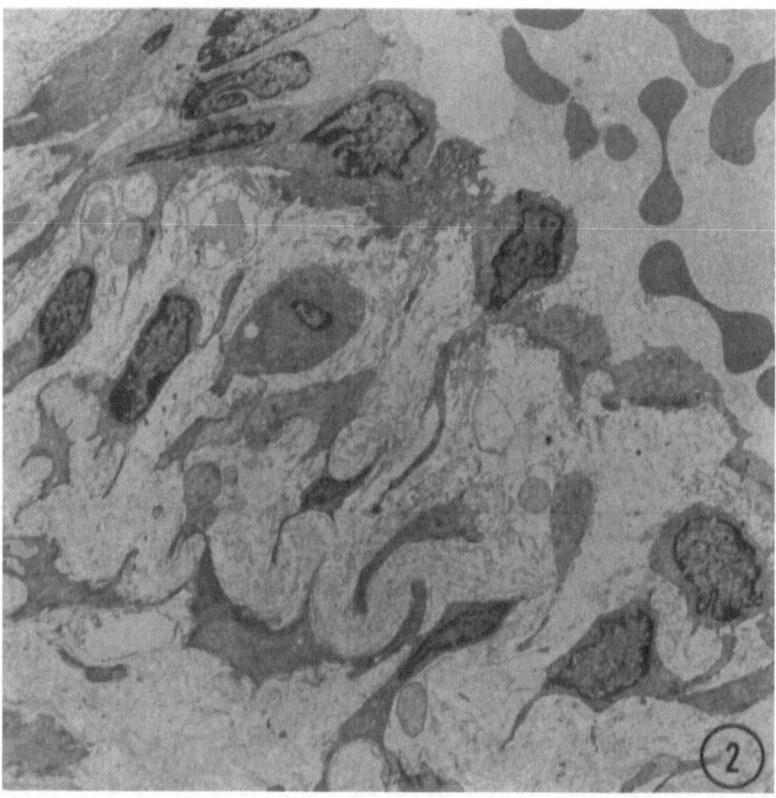

Fig. 2. This is an electron micrograph of a small portion of an
arterial lesion that has formed three months after de-endothelialization. The endothelium covers a lesion consisting entirely
of numerous smooth muscle cells surrounded by small collagen fibers,
large amounts of glycosaminoglycan (which cannot be clearly seen in
this micrograph), and numerous small elastic fibers. (x 3,000).

subcultures by methods described previously (Ross, 1971; Ross, in press; Ross and Glomset, 1973) except that 6 oz. Falcon plastic culture flasks rather than Leighton tubes are employed for the outgrowth of the explants (Ross, 1971). Thirty to fifty explants are placed in these flasks together with a small amount of modified Dulbecco-Vogt medium containing 5% pooled monkey (<u>Macaca</u> <u>nemestrina</u>)

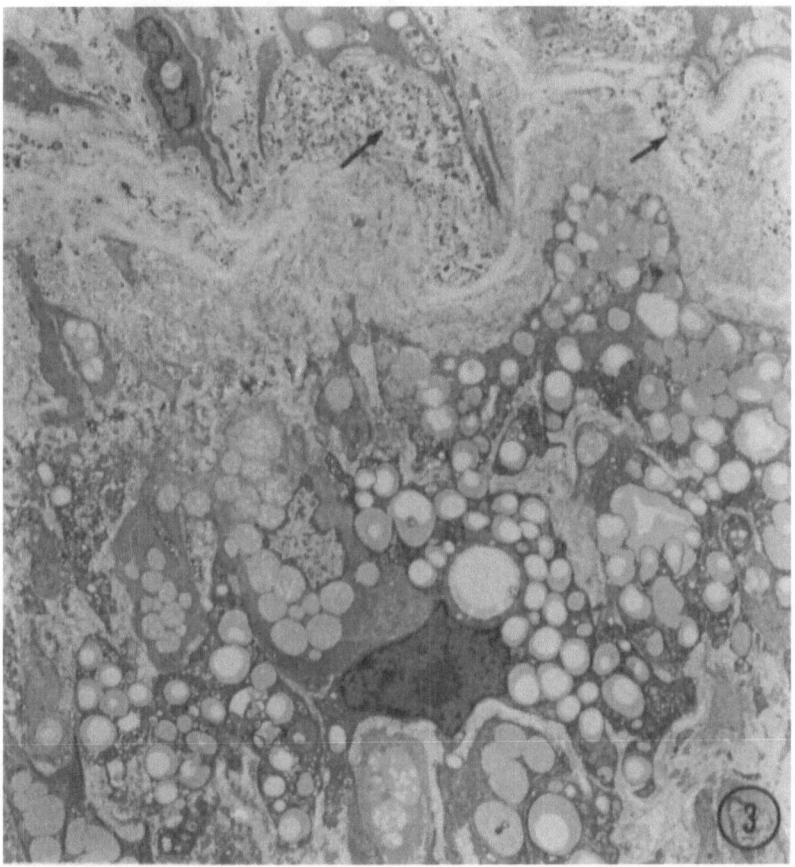

Fig. 3. This electron micrograph represents a small segment of a three month lesion in a pig-tail monkey that was continuously hyperlipemic for the entire duration of the experiment. In this low power electron micrograph, the deeper portion of the lesion contains numerous fat-filled smooth muscle cells. The extensive lipid deposits fill the cells and severely extend them. Many of these lipid deposits have been partially extracted and appear as central clear areas. In the more superficial portion of the lesion, numerous small deposits of extracellular lipid can be seen in the connective tissue matrix (arrows). (x 2,700).

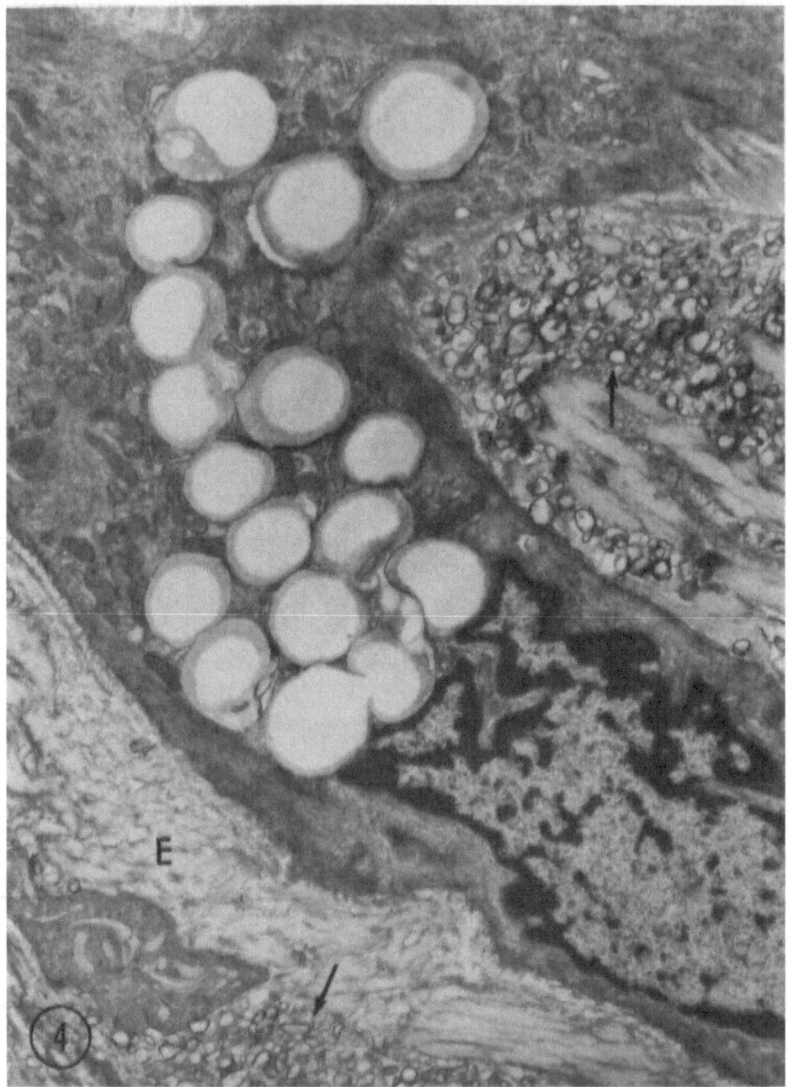

Fig. 4. This electron micrograph is a higher magnification of one
of the lipid filled smooth muscle cells from a lesion similar to
that seen in Fig. 3. The numerous, partially extracted lipid
droplets can be seen to fill the cytoplasm which is also abundant
in myofilaments and other cell organelles. This cell is surrounded
by young elastic fibers (E), and the spaces occupied by glycosaminoglycan contain numerous aggregates of small lipid deposits (arrows)
(x 13,000).

serum (Ross, 1972) and left relatively undisturbed for minimally
one week until outgrowth of cells has begun. After the cells in
the outgrowth have become confluent, which generally requires
approximately four weeks, the cells are trypsinized and subcultured
in large quantities using similar plastic flasks and the same
medium. Finally, cells for the various experiments are passed to
60 mm Falcon plastic petri dishes containing 4 ml of medium.

In experiments such as the one described below, equal numbers
of cells (approximately 10^5) are added to each dish with a
Cornwall syringe in aliquots of medium containing 1% pooled monkey
serum. The cells are grown in this medium for seven days, by which
time they reach a stationary phase of growth, and the dishes are
then randomly subdivided into appropriate categories. Enough
dishes are included in each category not only to permit examination
of the cells by phase microscopy and replicate cell counting at
each time period in the experiment, but also to permit fixation
and examination of the cells by light and electron microscopy.

Arterial smooth muscle cells from Macaca nemestrina divide
minimally, if at all, when incubated in serum-free medium. However,
in the presence of 5% serum from the same genus of monkey they
proliferate logarithmically for 10 - 14 days before entering
stationary growth (Ross, 1972). Therefore, we study the effects
of serum fractions on cell proliferation by adding the fractions
to serum-free medium in concentrations comparable to those present
in 5% monkey serum. Since the rate and extent of cell proliferation
vary from donor to donor and from batch to batch of serum, we
include controls in which the cells are grown in medium containing
0% and 5% monkey serum. The same batch of serum is used to prepare
the controls and the serum fractions to be tested.

Figure 5 shows the results of an experiment comparing the effect
of combinations of three serum fractions on cell proliferation.
The serum fractions, prepared by differential flotation (Havel
et al., 1955) in the preparative ultracentrifuge, were: the low
density lipoprotein (LDL) of d 1.006 - 1.063 g/ml, the high density
lipoprotein (HDL) of d 1.063 - 1.25 g/ml, and the remaining plasma
proteins of d >1.25 g/ml ("1.25 bottom"). Each of the dishes in
the three test categories contained the proteins of d >1.25 g/ml in
a concentration similar to that in the 5% whole serum controls.
In addition, the dishes of one of the test categories contained
sufficient LDL to provide the same amount of cholesterol (154
nmoles/ml medium) provided by the 5% serum, and the dishes in the
third test category contained a comparable amount of HDL. The
experiment shows that the serum proteins of d >1.25 g/ml stimulate
cell proliferation, and that the rate and extent of cell proliferation essentially double when LDL is added. Note that HDL also
increases the rate and extent of cell proliferation, but to a

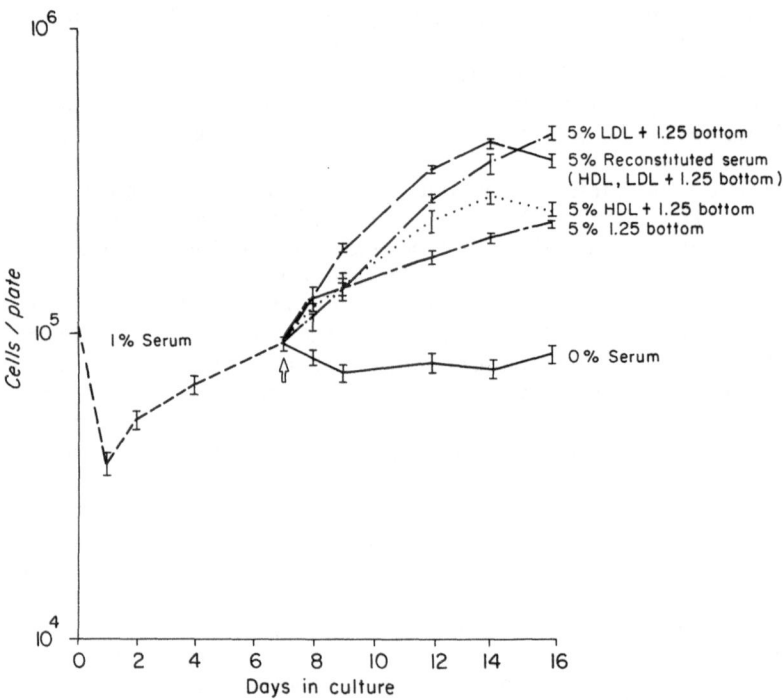

Fig. 5. Response of arterial smooth muscle to serum fractions.
Equal numbers (10^5) of smooth muscle cells were added to a large
series of petri dishes and incubated in a modified Dulbecco-
Vogt modification of Eagle's medium (Ross, 1971) containing 1%
serum pooled from several Macaca nemestrina. After seven days
(arrow) the dishes were separated into five groups and were
incubated further. One group was incubated in serum-free medium.
The remaining groups were incubated in media containing proteins
of d > 1.25 g/ml from the equivalent of 5% serum; this protein
fraction contained very little high density lipoprotein (HDL) or
low density lipoprotein (LDL); proteins of d > 1.25 g/ml plus HDL
(154 nmoles cholesterol per ml medium); proteins of d > 1.25 g/m
plus LDL (154 nmoles per ml medium); and reconstituted serum
containing proteins of d > 1.25 g/ml plus HDL (77 nmoles HDL
cholesterol per ml medium) plus LDL (77 nmoles LDL cholesterol
per ml medium). The pooled primate serum used as a source of
lipoprotein in these experiments contained 154 nmoles lipoprotein
in 5% whole serum. Vertical bars represent standard error of the
mean. (Reproduced with permission from Ross, R., and Glomset, J.,
1973, Science 180: 4039, 1332-1339. Copyright 1973 by the
American Association for the Advancement of Science).

lesser extent than that produced by LDL which was equivalent to the effect of whole serum. The foregoing observations support the notion that in vivo exposure of arterial smooth muscle to serum constituents could result in proliferation of these cells in a fashion similar to that induced by increased concentrations of serum proteins and lipoproteins in vitro. We are pursuing studies to examine the role of in vitro subfractions of the serum

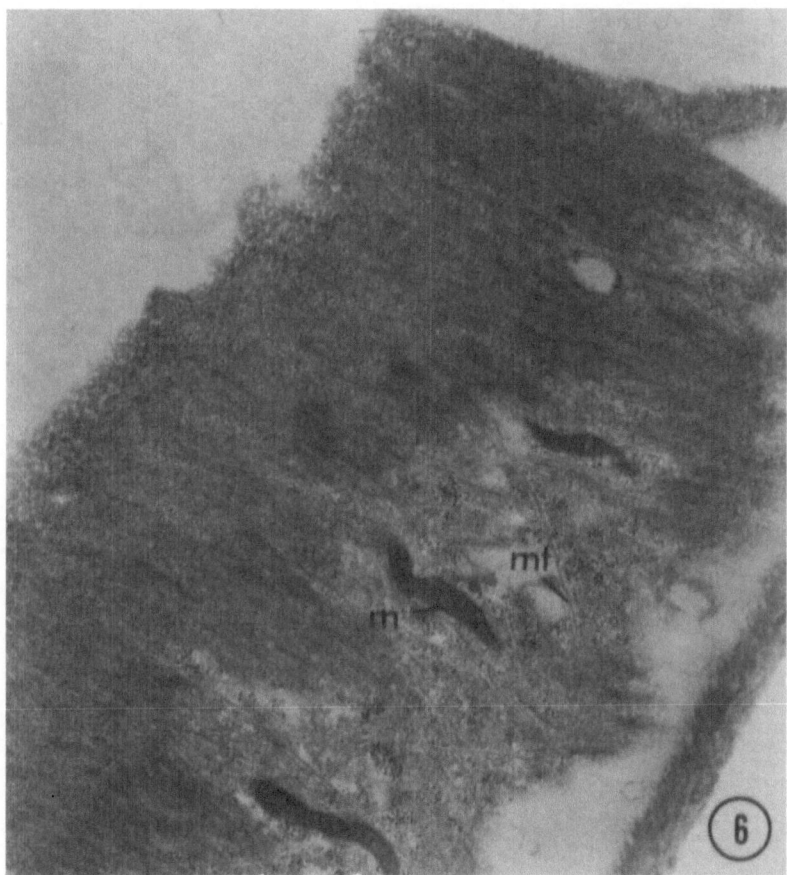

Fig. 6. This electron micrograph demonstrates a portion of an arterial smooth muscle cell grown in culture for seven days in medium containing no serum. The numerous parallel myofilaments can be seen together with microtubules (mt) and a few mitochondria (m). In other regions of the cell there are some cisternae of rough endoplasmic reticulum. This micrograph represents an en face view of the cell due to tangential sectioning in the plane of the surface of the cell. (x 18,000).

proteins of d > 1.25 g/ml and to clarify the mechanisms of the
effects of LDL and HDL.

Electron micrographs of the arterial smooth muscle in these in
vitro experiments demonstrate that as they are grown in 0% serum
(Figure 6) versus serum containing 5% LDL plus 1.25 bottom (Figures

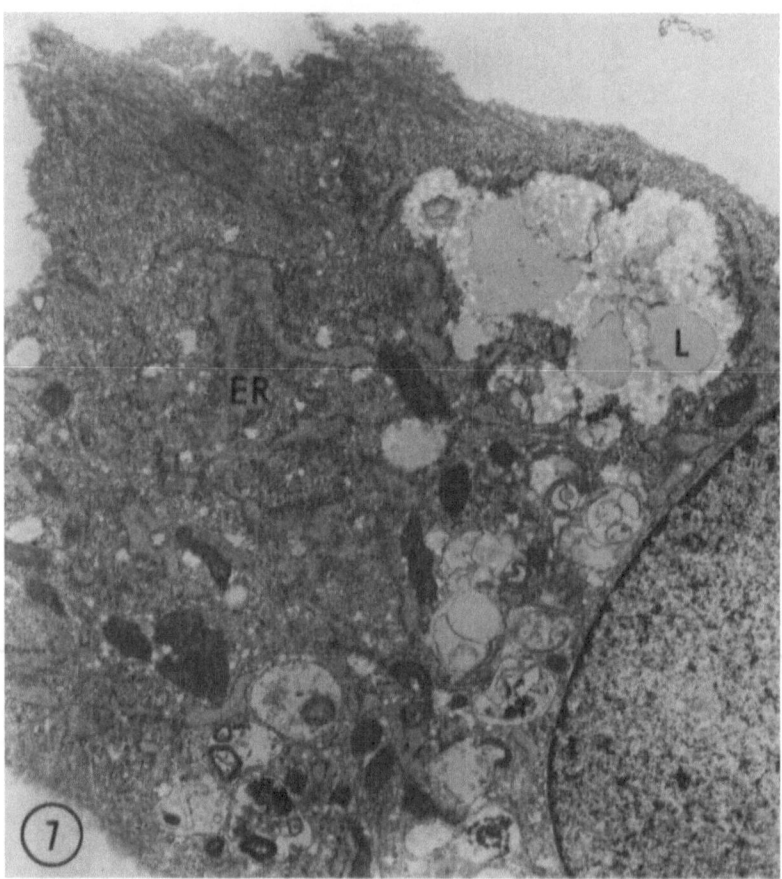

Fig. 7. This is a low power electron micrograph of a portion of
a pig-tail macaque arterial smooth muscle cell that has been in
culture for seven days in the presence of LDL, 1.25 bottom, and
cholesterol in amounts equivalent to that of 5% whole serum. The
cell can be seen to contain numerous lipid deposits (L), some of
which are morphologically associated with glycogen deposits. Many
membrane bounded structures are present in the cell, together with
mitochondria and reasonably well developed rough endoplasmic reticulum (ER). (x 10,000).

7 and 8) in the presence of LDL the cells not only proliferate but begin to accumulate numerous lipid deposits, many membrane bound bodies containing intramembranous whorls, and autophagic vacuoles. The cells also contain well developed rough endoplasmic reticulum after exposure to low density lipoprotein. In medium containing no serum (Figure 6) the cells remain relatively differentiated in their appearance in terms of their content of myofilaments, and the other organelles usually associated with smooth muscle. It is noteworthy that the proliferative effect of

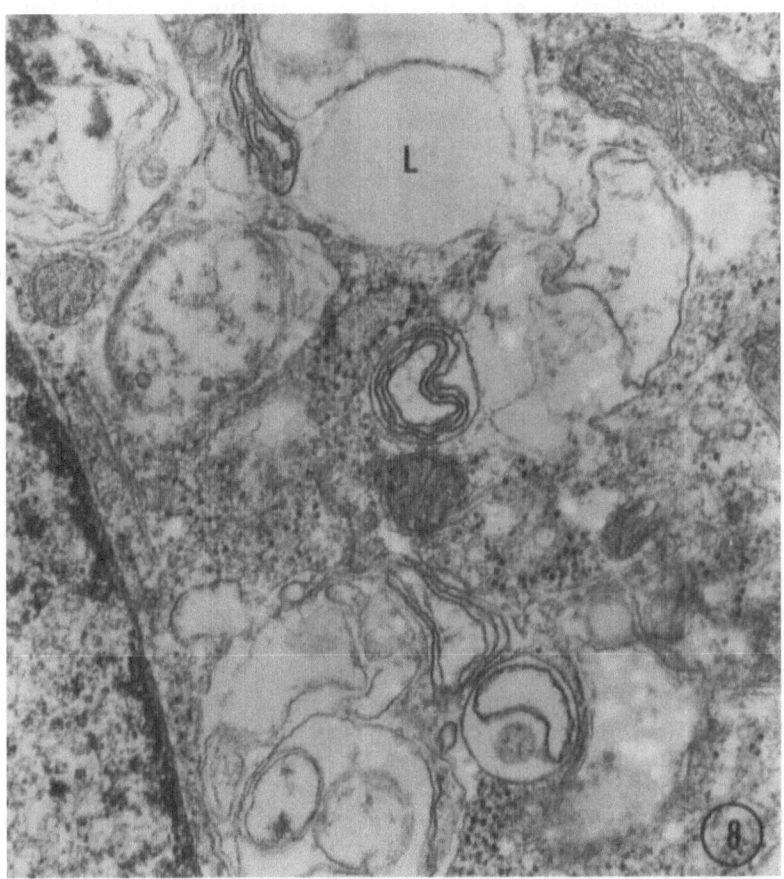

Fig. 8. This is a higher magnification of a small segment of the arterial smooth muscle cell seen in Fig. 7. The lipid deposits (L) do not appear to be membrane bounded. Several membrane bounded structures containing membranous whorls within them are seen within the cell. An autophagic vacuole can be seen in the upper left hand corner of the micrograph. (x 40,000).

the low density lipoproteins in culture is associated with both a
marked uptake of lipid in the form of intracellular lipid droplets,
and the development of their protein synthetic apparatus associated
with formation of secretory proteins, the rough endoplasmic reticulum.

Our observations on the behavior of smooth muscle cells in vitro
are somewhat different from those of Fisher-Dzoga et al. (this
volume), in that the latter did not detect a response from HDL
in their system. Their studies differ from ours in several regards:
1. They were measuring the size of the outgrowth of cells from
explants, rather than counting cells in cultures; 2. The lipoproteins were added to a base medium containing 5% whole fetal calf
serum, and 3. The lipoproteins were obtained from serum from
hyperlipoproteinemic monkeys.

Thus, comparisons between these two studies become difficult.
The lack of response to HDL in their studies may be due to the
greater effect of whole serum, thus masking any effect of HDL. In
addition, and of particular interest, is the suggestion in their
studies that the effect of LDL obtained from hyperlipoproteinemic
serum is different from that of LDL from normal serum. If these
differences are real, it will be important to explore them further.

CONNECTIVE TISSUE FORMATION BY SMOOTH MUSCLE CELLS IN VITRO

In previous studies, we demonstrated that arterial smooth muscle
cells synthesize the extracellular connective tissue matrix components of the artery wall (Ross, 1972; Ross and Klebanoff, 1971).
In this sense these cells are analogous to fibroblasts, chondro-
blasts, osteoblasts, and odontoblasts. It will be of interest to
determine whether the formation and secretion of extracellular
matrix components are affected by plasma factors in vitro and in
vivo. We have already observed that arterial smooth muscle cells,
under appropriate circumstances in vitro, form elastic fiber microfibrils and collagen, and we are pursuing studies of the synthesis
of elastin and glycosaminoglycans in vitro. The nature of all the
connective tissue constituents that are formed in vitro and the
factors that control and alter their formation will be of principal
interest. These studies will provide further insight into how the
cells elaborate connective tissue matrix and they should lead to a
better design of in vivo studies of the role played by smooth muscle
cells in the development of atherosclerotic lesions.

ACKNOWLEDGEMENTS

The authors wish to express their gratitude to Ms. Beverly
Kariya, Jocelyn Phillips, and Mary Stewart for their assistance in

these studies. This work was supported in part by grants from NIH No. HL 14823, RR 00166, and GM 13543.

REFERENCES

Björkerud, S. (1969). Virchows Arch. Abt. A. Pathol. Anat. 347, 197.

DHEW Publication No. (NIH) 72-219. A Report by the National Heart and Lung Institute Task Force on Arteriosclerosis. National Institutes of Health. Vol. 2, 1971.

Duncan, L.E. (1963). In "Evolution of the Atherosclerotic Plaque" (R.J. Jones, ed.). pp. 171-182. Chicago University Press, Chicago.

French, J.E. (1966). In "International Review of Experimental Pathology" (G.W. Richter and M.A. Epstein, eds.), pp. 253-342. Academic Press, New York.

Haust, M.D., and More, R.H. (1963). In "Evolution of the Atherosclerotic Plaque" (R.J. Jones, ed.), pp. 51-63. Chicago University Press, Chicago.

Haust, M.D. (1970). In "Atherosclerosis: Proceedings of the Second International Symposium" (R.J. Jones, ed.), pp. 12-20. Springer-Verlag, New York.

Havel, R.J., Eder, H.A., and Bragdon, J.H. (1955). J. Clin. Invest. 34, 1345.

Helin, P., Lorenzen, I., Garbarsch, C., and Matthiessen, M.E. (1971). Atherosclerosis 13, 319.

Jones, R., Daoud, A.S., Zumbo, O., Coulston, F., and Thomas, W.A. (1967). Exp. Mol. Pathol. 7, 34.

McGill, H.C., Jr., and Geer, J.C. (1963). In "Evolution of the Atherosclerotic Plaque" (R.J. Jones, ed.), pp. 65-81. Chicago University Press, Chicago.

Minick, C.R., Murphy, G.E., and Campbell, W.G., Jr. (1966). J. Exp. Med. 124, 635.

Ross, R. (1971). J. Cell Biol. 50, 172.

Ross, R., and Klebanoff, S. (1971). J. Cell Biol. 50, 159.

Ross, R. (1972). Proceedings of the Sigrid Juselius Foundation Symposium, Finland. (In Press).

Ross, R., and Glomset, J. (1973). Science. 180, 1332.

Stemerman, M., and Ross, R. (1972). J. Exp. Med. 136, 769.

Virchow, R. (1856). In "Gesammelte Abhandlungen zur
    Wissenschaftlichen Medicin" Meidinger Sohn u. Comp.,
    Frankfurt-am-Main.

Wissler, R.W. (1967). Circulation 36, 1.

DISCUSSION FOLLOWING THE PRESENTATION BY RUSSELL ROSS

Dr. Haust: Dr. Ross, since you have made no reference to the original work in this field carried out by the Russian investigators by light microscopy, I wonder whether you are familiar with their work and if so, how do your results differ from theirs? Secondly, you did refer to the criteria indicating intracellular lipid accumulation in cultures "fed" various lipids, i.e., biochemical analysis or morphologically demonstrable "myelin" figures and other lipid-like intracytoplasmic structures. Whereas the former criterion is tenable (whether all lipid is intracellular, extracellular, or both is another question), the morphological criteria alone are not, for even in my short experience with tissue culture work with arterial smooth muscle cells, I do find "myelin" figures and lipid-like inclusions in explants from normal animal arterial wall and under normal feeding conditions.

Dr. Ross: You are referring to the work of Myasnikov, and I am very familiar with the studies. They were very early studies, and I think they represent an early stage of what we did, but I also think we carried the studies to a much further degree. Yes, I am very familiar with them. I don't know the relationship of the question.

Dr. Wissler: I believe that they used hyperlipemic serum.

Dr. Ross: Well, we haven't used hyperlipemic serum and so the studies are not analogous. We used lipids but not the same ones. My answer to your second question apparently wasn't clear. The only criteria for cell proliferation we have used are cell numbers and nothing else. What was of interest to us was that in vivo one sees all kinds of dense bodies as well as lipid accumulation and that in vitro LDL did not produce many myelin figures or autophagic vacuoles as HDL did. There were clearly different effects from LDL vs HDL. LDL had a much greater stimulatory effect in terms of smooth muscle proliferation than did HDL, so that we begin to see some separate effects from the two different lipoproteins.

Dr. Fisher-Dzoga: Dr. Myasnikov, whose work was mentioned by Dr. Haust, found that rabbit cultures were stimulated if he used hyperlipemic serum instead of normal serum; that is, he got much faster growth. However, he also observed more degenerative changes in the rabbit cultures; this he didn't find in cultures of normal human aortic cells with human serum from hyperlipemic patients.

Dr. Ross: Maybe I ought to say just one more thing briefly. I think it is important to point out in relation to Katti's studies, and in contrast to the things she is doing at present, that the lipoproteins we have been looking at have all been from monkeys which are normocholesterolemic. We have not taken lipoproteins from hyperlipemic serum, and I think that is important.

PRODUCTION OF MUCOPOLYSACCHARIDES, COLLAGEN AND ELASTIC TISSUE BY AORTIC MEDIAL EXPLANTS

A.S. Daoud, K.E. Fritz, J. Singh, J.M. Augustyn, and
J. Jarmolych

Departments of Pathology, Veterans Administration
Hospital and Albany Medical College, Albany, New York

Early atherosclerotic lesions consist mainly of smooth muscle cells and extracellular substances, the principal constituents of which are mucopolysaccharides, collagen, and elastic tissue. Varying amounts of intracellular and extracellular lipids are present. In the late phase of the disease the lesion is complicated by necrosis, hemorrhage, and calcification (Daoud et al., 1964; Haust et al., 1960; Geer et al., 1961). The role of the extracellular substances in the progression of the lesion and the occurrence of complications is not clear. One can postulate that the presence of large amounts of these substances in the lesion leads to an increase in its size and encroachment upon the lumen. It is also possible that these substances may influence the accumulation of lipids in the atheroma, thus aggravating the atherosclerotic process. On the other hand, the presence of collagen and elastic tissue may be beneficial in preventing extensive necrosis or in causing healing of necrotic lesions.

Of interest to us is the role of some extrinsic factors involved in atherogenesis in the production of these substances. For instance, what is the effect of lipoprotein fraction of serum or of various types of injury? Since a study of the effect of any single factor such as a lipoprotein fraction of serum or some type of injury in the production of connective tissue in the whole organism is virtually impossible, we have developed a swine aortic medial explant system which develops a peripheral growth having many of the characteristics of the early atherosclerotic plaque. In this communication we report on two experiments. The first was designed to characterize the explant system and was carried for 21 days, in the course of which explants were terminated at 1, 2, 4, 7, 9, 14, and 21 days. The second experiment was designed primarily

to study collagen synthesis quantitatively in the presence of
either swine or human serum, and was carried for 18 days.

METERIALS AND METHODS

Blood is collected, allowed to clot, and the serum removed
with sterile conditions maintained throughout the entire procedure.
Serum is stored at 4°C for no longer than one month. It is
neither frozen nor subjected to sterilization by filtration.
Maintenance of sterility is checked by culture in Eugon broth.

Swine aortic explants are prepared as previously described
(Jarmolych et al., 1968, and Daoud et al., 1970). Briefly, the
swine thoracic aorta is stripped of both adventitia with subjacent
outer media and intima with subjacent inner media. The remaining
middle media is cut with a multibladed instrument into equidimen-
sional (1.2 mm^2) segments, and four randomly selected segments are
transferred to each plastic culture flask. Cultures are incubated
at 37°C in 4.0 ml growth medium which is changed three times per
week, at each of which times the air atmosphere is replaced with
5% CO_2 in air, with a resultant pH of 7.2.

Growth medium consists either of chemically defined medium
alone (M199 Hanks' base including antibiotics) or with serum added
at 20% concentration. Sterility is monitored by culturing samples
in Eugon broth culture.

In Experiment I, [^{3}H] thymidine was added at 4 µc/ml during
the last two hours of the culture. In Experiment II, 10 µc [^{3}H]
proline were added to each flask at the time of the last change
of medium, 48 hours before termination, and again at 24 hours prior
to termination. Details of the termination procedure, processing
for light microscopy including autoradiography, and for electron
microscopy have been previously described (Jarmolych et al., 1968,
and Daoud et al., 1970).

Cultures for chemical determinations, after brief exposure to
non-isotopic precursors, three brief saline washes, and 5% trichloroacetic acid (TCA) are freeze-dried, homogenized in 5% TCA, lipid
extracted, and the nucleic acids extracted with hot TCA. The TCA-
insoluble residue after nucleic acid extraction is solubilized in
1N NaOH and autoclaved 20 hours at 15 psi in 6N HCl. The resultant
hydrolysate is neutralized by repetitive drying under vacuum after
reconstitution with distilled H_2O. One fraction is transferred
directly to scintillation vials and dried; Soluene and toluene
cocktail are added. Another fraction is applied to an AA15 column
of a Beckman Model 120B Amino Acid Analyzer, and chromatographed
with pH 2.8 citrate buffer at 50°C. The hydroxyproline and

proline fractions are diverted; collected; de-salted on 0.5 cm x
5.5 cm Dowex 50W-X8 columns; and the amino acids are eluted with
2N NH₄OH into scintillation vials, dried, and Soluene and toluene
cocktail are added. Radioactivity is counted in a Packard 3320
Liquid Scintillation Spectrometer, with counting efficiency determined by automatic external standardization.

RESULTS

Experiment I

    The sequential changes in the medial explants, with respect
to the development of peripheral growth, have been previously
reported (Jarmolych et al., 1968) and are schematically represented in Figure 1. Briefly, cell proliferation, as demonstrated
autoradiographically by [3H] thymidine incorporation into nuclei
of smooth muscle cells (SMC) and by an apparent increase in the
number of cells in the explant proper, occurred by the second
day. A growth at the periphery of the explant developed by the
fourth day and increased in amount until the 21st day, when the
experiments were terminated (Figure 2). In the early states of
formation (four days), most cells in the peripheral growth showed
few, if any, myofilaments (Figure 3). They were rich in organelles
and generally had a partial or no basement membrane at the plane
of section. As the explant aged, the cells began to modify toward
SMC, and by the 21st day most cells were modified SMC. Not only
was there an increase in the proportion of modified SMC, but also
the number of filaments per cell was greater. A few of these cells
appeared morphologically very similar to the mature medial SMC of
the original explants (Figure 4). However, the relative volume of
cells occupied by organelles varied from cell to cell, and even at
21 days many cells had few or no myofilaments. The bulk of the
cytoplasm was occupied by dilated granular endoplasmic reticulum
which contained electron-dense material.

    Histochemical staining for mucopolysaccharides, collagen, and
elastic tissue showed that mucopolysaccharides were present at the
end of the first week, while collagen and elastic tissue were
demonstrated only at 14 days but in some instances were abundant
by 21 days.

    Electron microscopy of the peripheral growth showed the typi-
cal electron opaque granules and thin fibrils characteristic of
mucopolysaccharides (Matukas et al., 1967) as early as seven days

CHANGES IN MEDIAL EXPLANT

(1 - 21 Days)

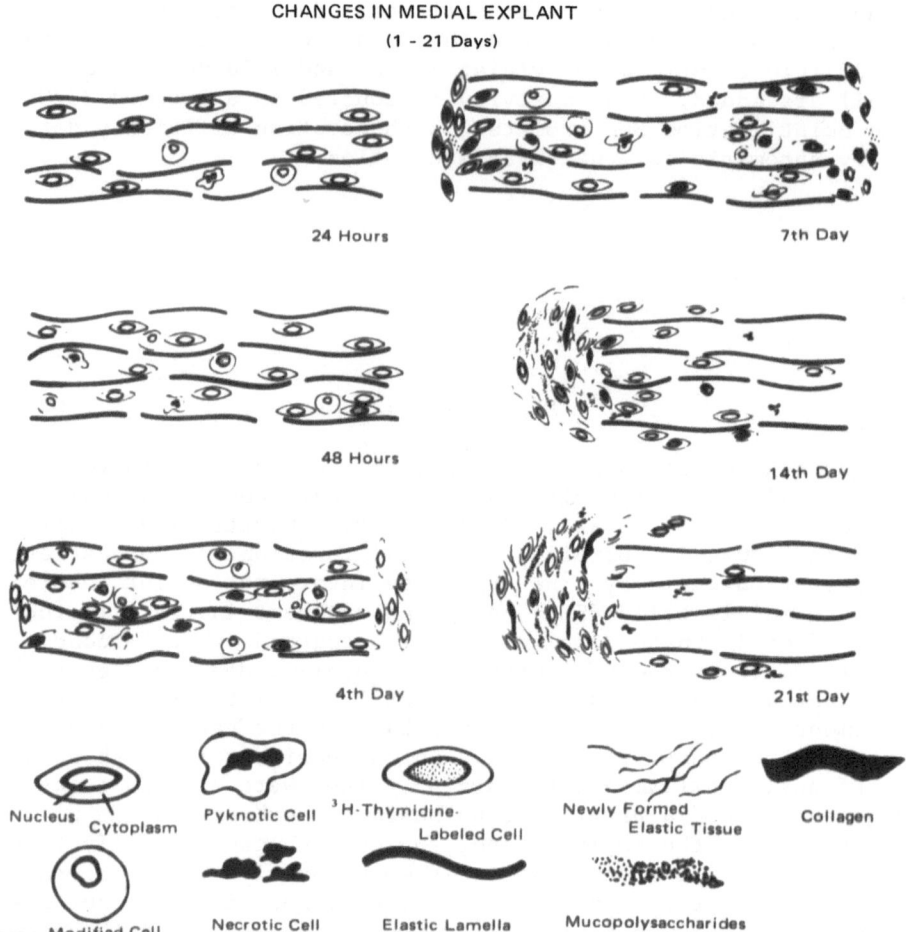

Fig. 1. Schematic diagram representing sequential changes in the explant proper and development of the peripheral growth. In the explant proper, from 24 hours through seven days there was an increase in the number of modified smooth muscle cells and in the number of nuclei showing [^{3}H] thymidine incorporation by autoradiography. Degeneration, minimal at early stages, became more pronounced by seven days and increased variably through the 21st day.

The earliest appearance of a peripheral growth was detected at four days, and it increased in amount variably through 21 days. Labeled nuclei increased in number until day 14, after which they were less numerous, although still demonstrable at day 21. Some degeneration of nuclei of the peripheral growth became noticeable by day 14.

Mucopolysaccharides first appeared in the peripheral growth at seven days, collagen and elastic tissue at 14 days, each persisting through 21 days. (Reproduced with permission from Jarmolych et al., 1968 and Academic Press).

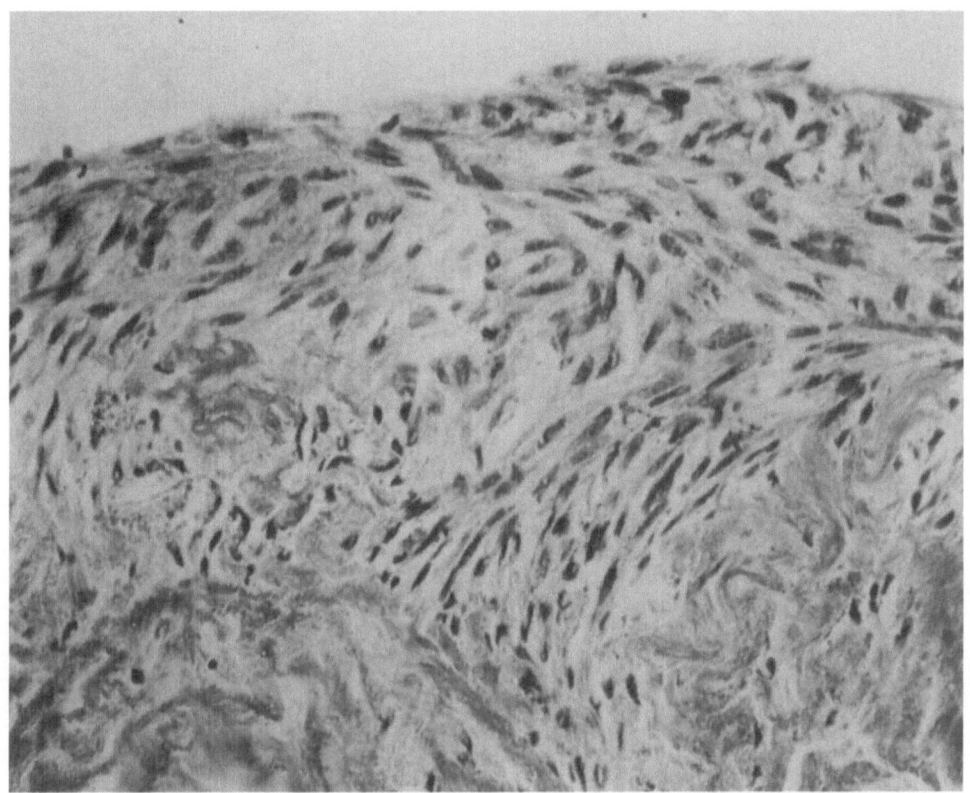

Fig. 2. Photomicrograph of peripheral growth from an explant at
21 days. The peripheral growth is several cell layers thick with
varying amounts of extracellular substance. In the deeper layers,
cells undergoing necrosis are present. H & E (x 360). (Reproduced
with permission from Jarmolych et al., 1968 and Academic Press).

and continuing thereafter (Figure 4). From this early stage on,
the extracellular space also contained amorphous osmiophilic
material and microfilaments varying in size from 5 to 15 mμ. The
amorphous material had an appearance similar to that of basement
membrane and sometimes was mixed with a few microfilaments. The
microfibrils were similar in appearance to those described by Ross
(1971) and by Haust et al. (1965) as elastic microfibrils and by
Goldberg and Green (1964) as collagen fibrils. In addition to the
microfibrils, fibers showing the periodicity typical of collagen
fibers (Figure 5), singly or in groups, were demonstrated at 14
days and were most abundant at 21 days. Electron microscopy at 14

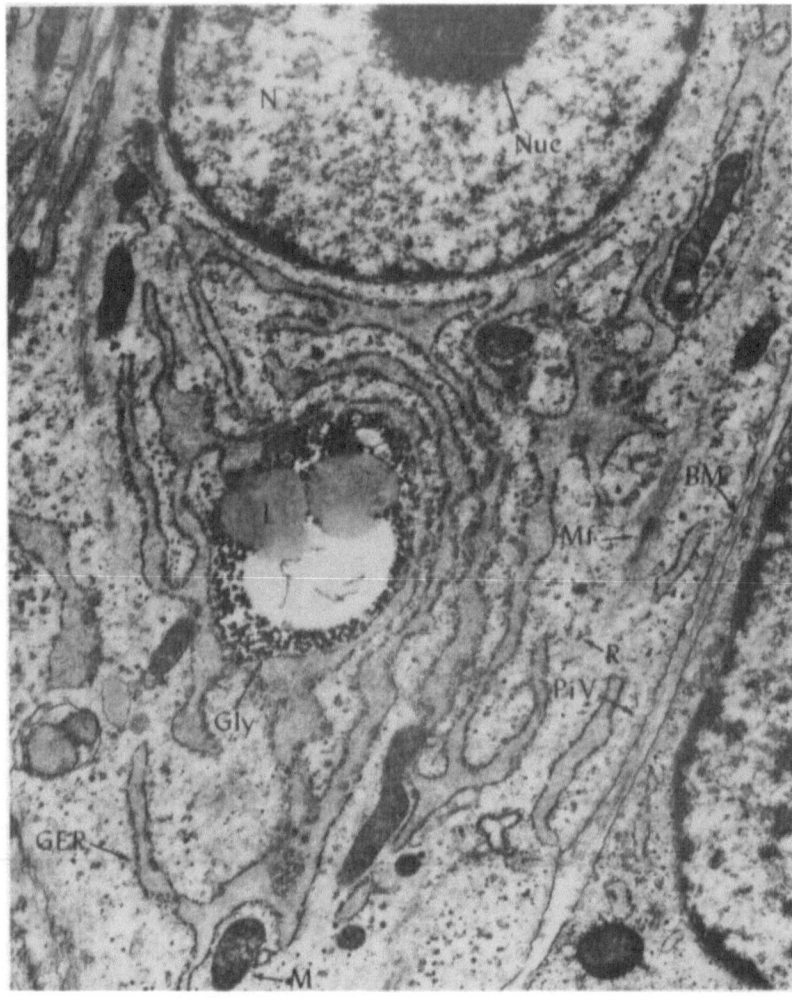

Fig. 3. Electron micrograph of fibroblast-like cells in the
peripheral growth of a seven day culture. There are abundant
granular endoplasmic reticulum (GER) filled with an electron
opaque substance and numerous scattered free ribosomes. A cluster
of glycogen granules (Gly) and two lipid droplets are present. A
nucleus (N) having the dispersed chromatin and large nucleolus
(Nuc) characteristic of an immature cell is in one cell which
also contains myofilaments (Mf), pinocytotic vesicles (PiV), and a
partial basement membrane (BM) (x 15,000). (Reproduced with permission from Jarmolych et al., 1968 and Academic Press).

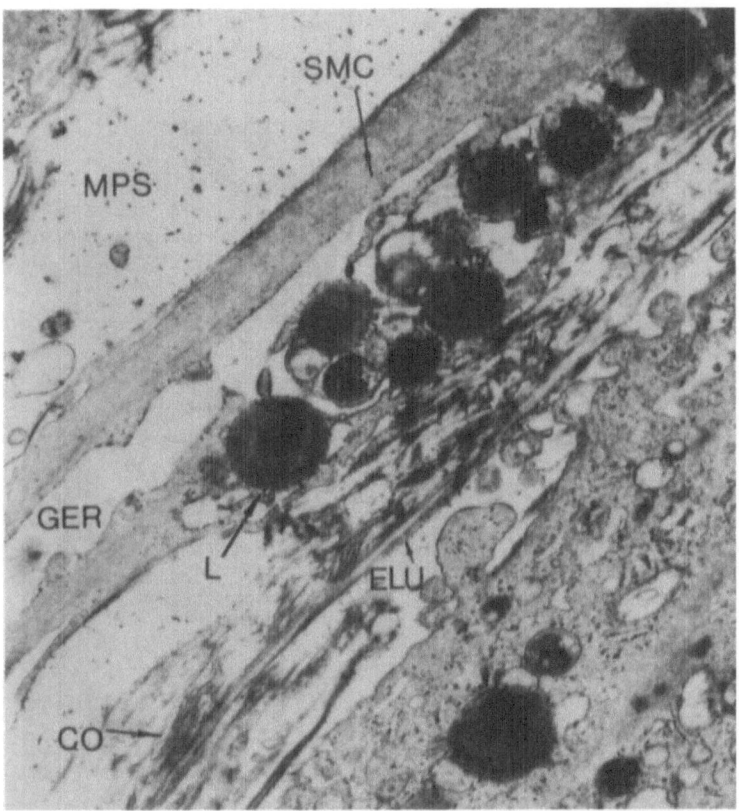

Fig. 4. Electron micrograph of a rather well differentiated smooth
muscle cell (SMC) from the peripheral growth of a 21 day explant.
The cell contains dilated granular endoplasmic reticulum (GER) and
lipid droplets. A less differentiated SMC is present at the bottom
of the picture. The extracellular space contains mucopolysaccharides (MPS), collagen fibers (CO) and elastic units (ELU)
(x 11,000).

and 21 days also showed a roughly circular structure composed of a
homogeneous clear or slightly electron dense center surrounded by
an electron-dense border (Figure 5). These structures were referred
to by Haust et al. (1965) as elastic units. The homogeneous
center, according to Haust, is composed of elastic matrix and the
periphery consists of elastic filaments. The size of the unit
varies from 40 to 300 mμ and the filament averages 10 mμ in
thickness. The elastic units were sometimes found singly, but in
general formed aggregates and sometimes fused with adjacent
elastic fibers and lamellae. When the units were cut longitudinally
(Figure 4), they were found to consist of a clear center and an
electron-opaque periphery composed of thin fibers.

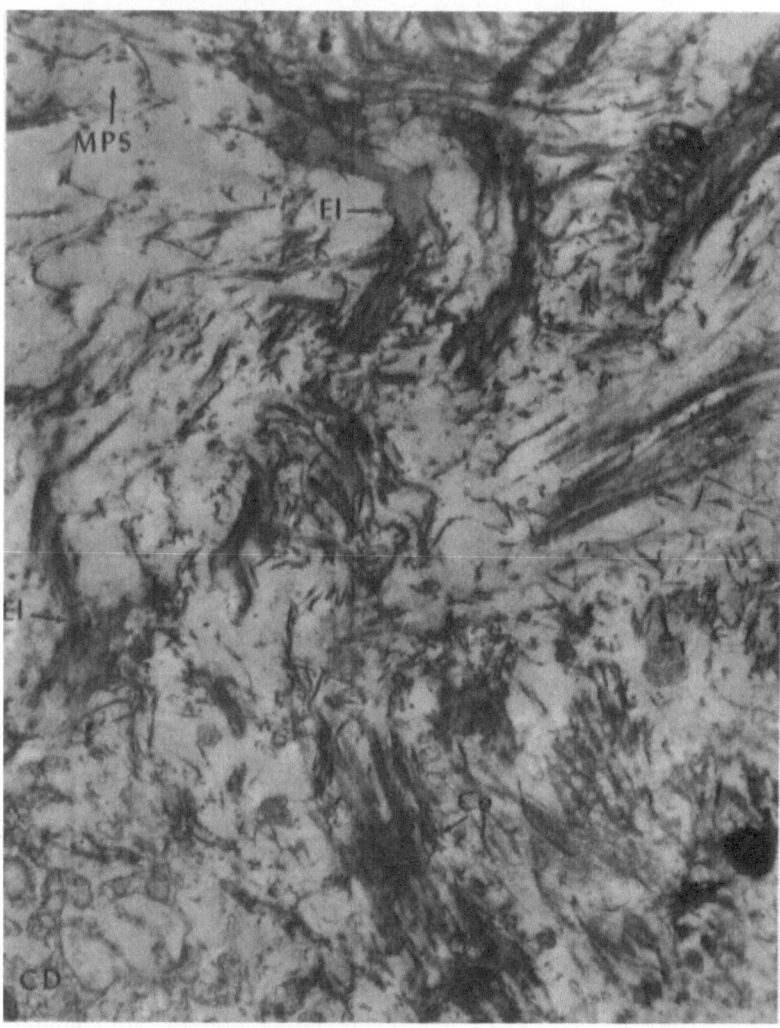

Fig. 5. Electron micrograph from the peripheral growth of a 21
day explant. The intercellular spaces contain mucopolysaccharides
(MPS), elastic fibers (EL), and collagen fibers (CO). At the
bottom of the picture cell debris (CD) suggestive of cell necrosis
is shown. (x 11,000). (Reproduced with permission from Jarmolych
et al., 1968 and Academic Press).

Experiment II

This experiment differed from the previous one in the amount
of extracellular substances in the peripheral growth. By light
microscopy, the peripheral growth was composed mainly of cells
piled on one another. Histochemical staining showed only minimal
amounts of mucopolysaccharides, collagen, and elastic tissue.
Collagen and elastic tissue were completely undetectable in large
areas. There were no qualitative differences between the explants
grown in the presence of human serum and those grown in swine serum.

Electron microscopic study revealed the presence of the same
types of cells demonstrated in the first experiment. However, here
the cells contained fewer myofilaments and more endoplasmic reticulum than in the previous experiment at 14 and 21 days. There
were many fibroblast-like cells, although some showed a basement
membrane, indicating SMC origin. Other cells showed no distinctive

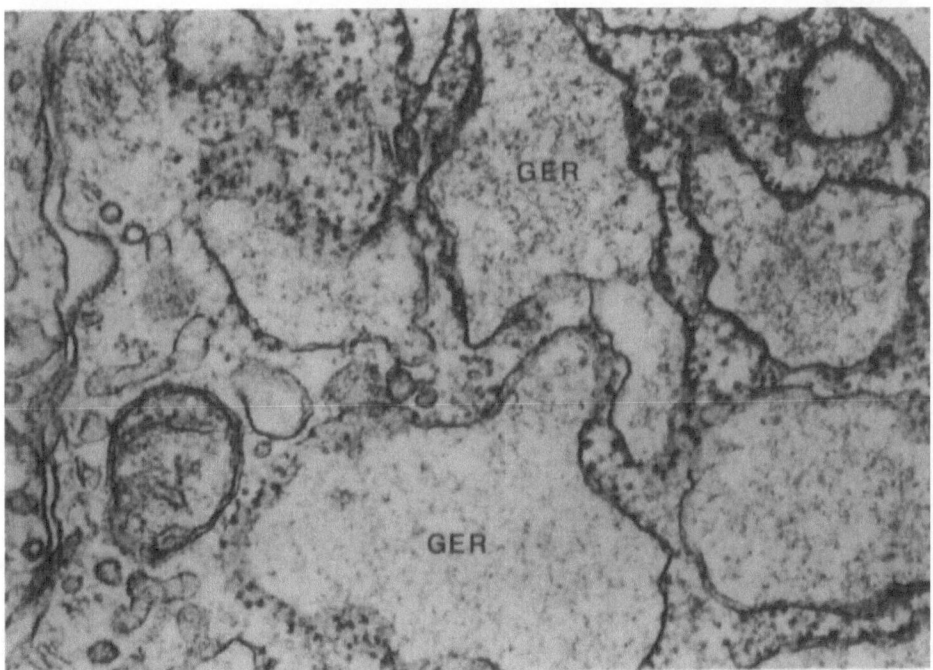

Fig. 6. Electron micrograph of a portion of a cell from peripheral
growth of an 18 day explant showing marked dilatation of the granular endoplasmic reticulum (GER) which contains flocculent electron
dense material. (x 70,000). (Reduced 15% for reproduction).

features and were classified as "primitive cells". The granular
endoplasmic reticulum was markedly dilated and contained a large
amount of flocculent electron-dense material (Figure 6). Many
cells revealed an accumulation of circular or elliptical electron
lucent structures in their cytoplasm, similar in shape and size to
the central part of elastic units (Figure 7). In the portions of
cells where these structures were found, the normal cytoplasmic
architecture appeared disrupted and only a few filaments and
vesicles were found. In some instances these structures were found
within a membrane-bound vesicle.

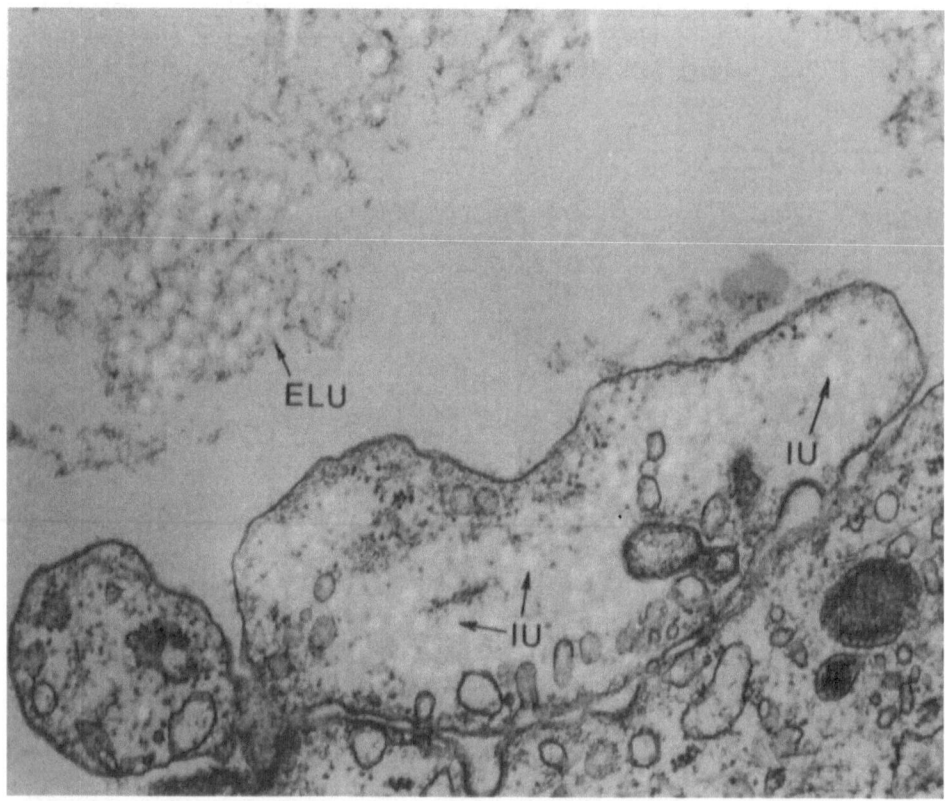

Fig. 7. Electron micrograph of the peripheral growth of an 18 day
explant showing the similarity between the electron lucent centers
of the elastic units (ELU) in the extracellular spaces and the
electron lucent intracellular structures (IU). Note the similarity
in shape and size. Both structures measure from 30-250 mμ. The
elastic units in the extracellular spaces are surrounded by microfibrils. (x 39,000).

In general, the extracellular spaces were narrowed and contained amorphous material similar to that found in the basement membrane and microfibrils of the same diameter and configuration as those described in the previous experiment (Figure 8). Mucopolysaccharides; elastic fibers; and, especially, collagen showing typical periodicity (Figure 9) were scarce in comparison with that found at 21 days in the previous experiment.

In several instances, the electron lucent intracellular structures and extracellular elastic units (Figure 7) and fibers could be seen side by side. The similarity between the intracellular structures and the central part of the elastic units was apparent. Measurements of the two structures showed them to be of the same size.

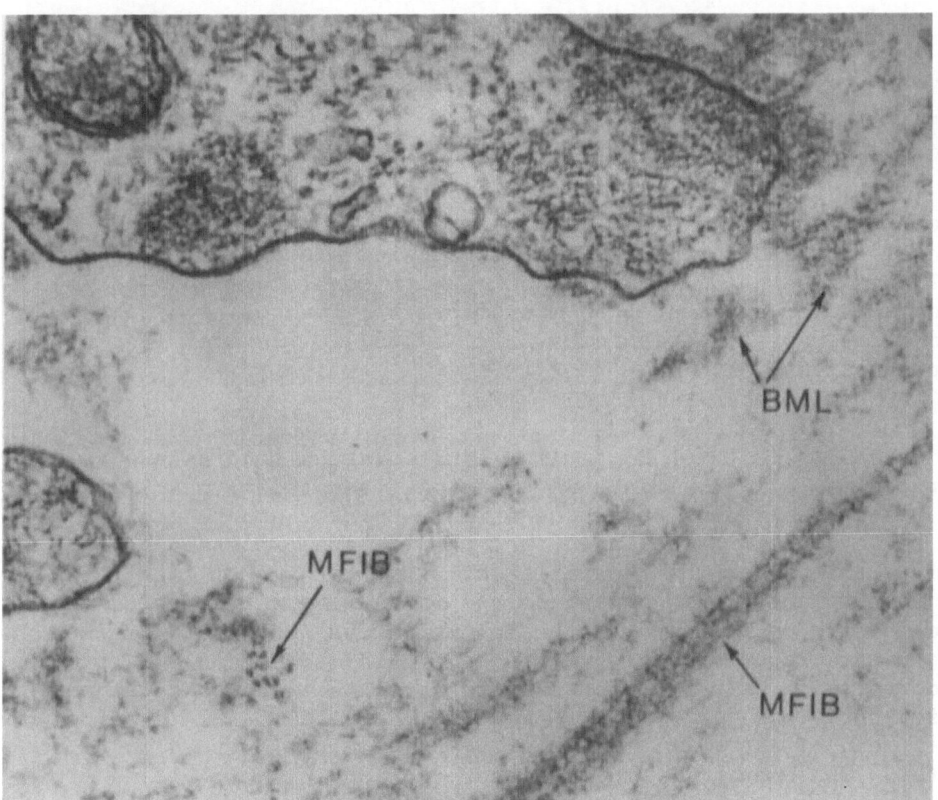

Fig. 8. An electron micrograph of the extracellular substances in the peripheral growth of an 18 day explant. Note the amorphous basement membrane-like material (BML) and the microfibrils (MFIB) cut longitudinally or transversely. (x 90,000).

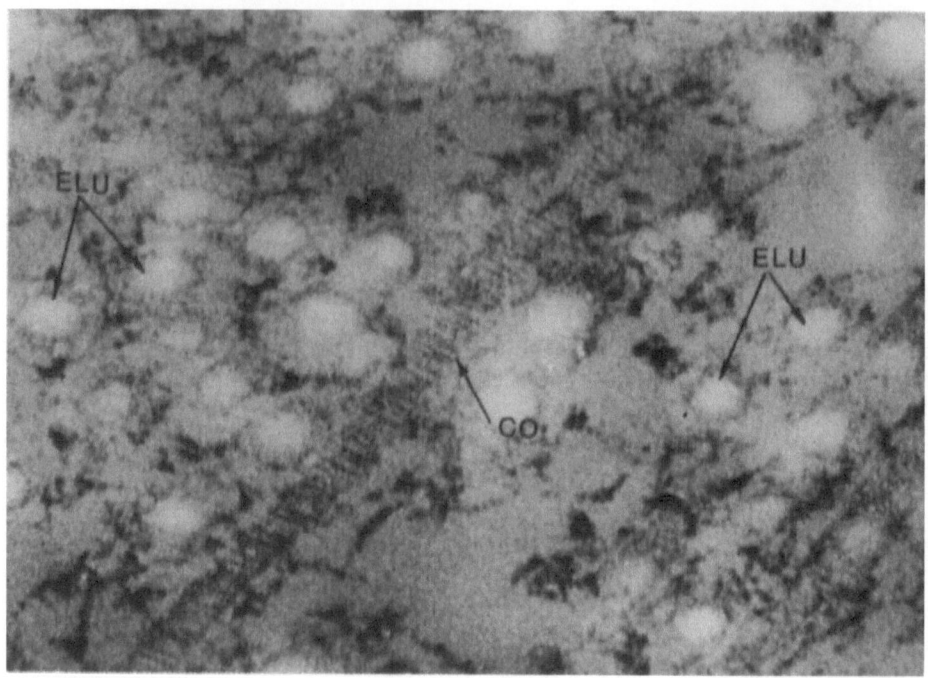

Fig. 9. Electron micrograph of extracellular spaces in the peripheral growth of an 18 day explant showing elastic units (ELU) and
collagen fibers (CO). The elastic units consist of an electron
lucent center surrounded by microfibrils. The collagen fiber
shows the typical periodicity. (x 180,000). (Reduced 15% for
reproduction).

Results of the [³H] proline incorporation studies are summarized in Table I. Since we questioned the relative activity
of the cells present under the stimulus of the growth medium
in the synthesis of collagen, the results are expressed as
dpm/μg DNA rather than specific activity in terms of total protein
of the explants. The number of dpm in hydroxyproline is taken as
the measure of collagen synthesis, while the number of dpm in
proline represents total protein synthesis. The mean [³H] proline
incorporation into protein as hydroxyproline in cultures grown in
swine serum was 119 dpm/μg DNA with a range of 54-221, as opposed
to a mean of 144 with a range of 54-847 for those grown in human
serum. The mean [³H] proline incorporation into protein as proline
in swine serum cultures was 10,771 dpm/μg DNA with a range of 5,079
to 15,531, compared to a mean of 10,762 with a range of 5,417 to
14,026 for human serum cultures. Of considerable interest is the
percent of total protein synthetic activity which is involved in
collagen synthesis, an estimate of which can be made by comparing
the radioactivity of the hydroxyproline to that of proline.

TABLE I

	Swine Sera			Human Sera		
	Number of Samples	dpm/µg DNA	SEM	Number of Samples	dpm/µg DNA	SEM
Hydroxyproline	17	.119	11	20	144	39
Proline	17	10771	692	20	10762	626

SEM: Standard Error of Mean

Human serum in the growth medium results in an average level of incorporation of ^{3}H into protein, either as hydroxyproline or as proline, similar to that resulting from swine serum.

TABLE II

	Swine Sera			Human Sera		
Number of Samples	$\frac{\text{OH-pro dpm}}{\text{pro dpm}}$ x 100		SEM	Number of Samples	$\frac{\text{OH-pro dpm}}{\text{pro dpm}}$ x 100		SEM
17	1.12		0.08	20	1.47		0.43

SEM: Standard Error of Mean

Human serum results in an average percentage of total protein synthesized as collagen, similar to that resulting from swine serum. However, the differences detected among human sera are much greater than are demonstrable among swine sera.

If $\dfrac{^3\text{H dpm/µg DNA OH-proline}}{^3\text{H dpm/µg DNA proline}}$ x 100 is calculated for each flask the mean value for the explants grown in swine serum is 1.12 with range of 0.75 to 2.1 as compared to a mean of 1.47 with range of 0.47 to 9.55 for those grown in human serum (Table II). There were no significant differences in these parameters between cultures grown in swine serum and in human serum, but there was a much greater variation in the percentage of the synthetic activity channeled into collagen synthesis among the human serum cultures than among the swine serum cultures.

DISCUSSION

Numerous published reports implicate the arterial cells, especially SMC, in the formation of collagen, elastic tissue and mucopolysaccharides. The evidence that these extracellular

substances are secreted by SMC is derived mainly from four major
sources: 1. from the study of the development of the atherosclerotic plaque (Haust et al., 1960; Parker and Odland, 1966; Imai
et al., 1966; Haust et al., 1965; Scott et al., 1967; and Wissler,
1968); 2. from the study of developing aorta in chick embryo
(Karrer, 1960), in newborn rat (Paule, 1963), and in prepubertal
rat (Ross and Klebanoff, 1971); 3. from the study of arterial
injury and repair (Murray et al., 1966); and 4. from tissue
culture studies. Ross (1971) reported that SMC derived from the
inner media and intima of immature guinea pig aortas grown in
cell culture for eight weeks maintained their morphological
characteristics. The cultured SMC were capable of producing
microfibrils and basement membrane-like material. Analysis of the
microfibrils showed that they had an amino acid composition similar
to that obtained from intact mature elastic fibers. Wissler (1973)
also reported that, using electron microscopy with ruthenium red
as an indicator, Rose Jones in his laboratory had produced evidence
for acid mucopolysaccharide production of cultured cells derived
from primary explants of arterial media obtained from rhesus monkey
aortas.

The results presented herein show that the medial explant
system develops a peripheral growth having many of the characteristics of the early atherosclerotic plaque. The electron microscopic classification of the cells in the peripheral growth
(primitive, fibroblast-like, and modified SMC) is that which we
have used previously in describing similar cells seen in the
atherosclerotic lesion in the monkey (Scott et al., 1967) and the
pig (Daoud et al., 1968). It is based on morphological criteria
and is not related to cell origin.

The fibroblast-like cells and the primitive cells in the
peripheral growth may originate either from mature smooth cells
by loss of myofilaments and the development of an extensive network of organelles, chiefly endoplasmic reticulum, or from some
rare cells in the swine aortic media which, under the conditions
of culture, overgrow the SMC. But, regardless of their origin,
their similarity to the cells in atherosclerotic lesions makes
them of potential importance in understanding atherogenesis.

At present the evidence favors SMC origin. Many of the
fibroblast-like cells and even the primitive cells show at least
a partial basement membrane or a few filaments in their cytoplasm.
Also, sequential electron microscopic studies of the mature SMC in
the explant proper (Fritz et al., 1970) showed that most cells
undergo a gradual decrease in the number of myofilaments and an
increase in granular endoplasmic reticulum. By the fourth day the
majority of the cells in the explant are morphologically similar
to primitive cells, fibroblast-like cells, or modified SMC. The

amount of cell proliferation, as determined autoradiographically by incorporation of $[^3H]$ thymidine into DNA, does not appear to be extensive enough at this early stage to account for such a drastic change in cell population. If, indeed, these cells are derived from SMC, these changes in the SMC may be an essential step in the transformation of these cells from contractile to secretory cells. This phenomenon may be present in the development of atherosclerotic lesions, where mature SMC may likewise undergo similar changes.

The relationship of the various cells to the individual extracellular substances cannot be inferred with certainty from the present work. Mucopolysaccharides appear to occur in all cultures regardless of the predominant cell type, while elastic tissue and collagen could be found only in older cultures in which the predominant cell was a modified SMC. This suggests the possibility that collagen and elastic tissue are secreted by the modified SMC, which often have a very dilated and elaborate endoplasmic reticulum network suggestive of synthetic activity. However, as demonstrated in Experiment II, the cytoplasm of cells from each of the three categories had structures resembling the central portions of the elastic units which indicates that at least elastic tissue can be produced by all of the three types of cells.

As we compared the results of the two experiments, the greater amount of extracellular components in the first, coupled with the large intracellular accumulation of elastin-like substance and of osmiophilic amorphous substance in the granular endoplasmic reticulum, raises the question of whether, rather than a difference in synthesis, there may possibly be a difference in secretory rate or an actual defect in secretory mechanism in the second experiment. Individual differences in sera or in tissues, the only variables between the two experiments, must be invoked to explain these phenomena, but the mechanism underlying them is completely obscure. Further study may shed light on a phenomenon, to our knowledge not previously defined but conceivably may be important in atherogenesis.

We have used extensively the explant system to study the influence of hyperlipemic serum (Daoud et al., 1970) and other serum factors (Fritz et al., 1972b) on cell proliferation. From the present experiments it appears that this same system lends itself advantageously to the study of extracellular substances produced under the influence of factors involved in atherogenesis. The quantitative studies reported herein revealed that both swine and human sera have the capacity of stimulating collagen synthesis to a level considerably above that resulting from culture in M199 alone. Previous studies have shown that normal human sera have significantly greater capacity to stimulate DNA synthesis in this system than do normal swine sera (Fritz et al., 1972a), but in the

current study no such significant difference, on the average,
between normal human and swine sera was demonstrated. This
observation suggests that the capacity to stimulate collagen
synthesis is separable from that influencing DNA synthesis.
Furthermore, although the swine sera resulted in remarkably
similar peripheral growth and collagen synthesis patterns,
striking differences among human sera were brought out by these
studies. These results suggest that we may have in our explant
culture a sensitive system for studying differences in collagen
synthesis-stimulating capacity among sera from individuals known
to have various risk factors such as hyperlipidemia and diabetes
mellitus, predisposing to atherosclerosis. Studies of the effect
of various lipoprotein fractions, or of different types of injury
on collagen synthesis, also should be feasible using this system
and are under consideration by this group for future research.
Furthermore, it is possible that analogous factors influencing
elastic tissue and mucopolysaccharide synthesis may be studied
profitably by this system.

SUMMARY

An explant system consisting of segments of swine aortic
medial tissue cultured in semi-synthetic medium develops a new
peripheral growth having many of the characteristics of the early
atherosclerotic plaque. The cells in the peripheral growth are
capable of secreting mucopolysaccharides, collagen, and elastic
tissue, whether the explants are grown in the presence of swine
or of human serum. Intracellular structures having the electron
microscopic appearance and dimensions of the central portions of
elastic units (elastin) were found in the cell cytoplasm, free
or in membrane-bound structures. Quantitative studies showed that
average collagen synthesis was equal in cultures exposed to human
serum or swine serum. However, differences from one serum to
another were detectable, with human sera showing a much wider
range of collagen synthesis-stimulating activity. Thus the system
appears to afford a sensitive indicator for the study of the
influence of external factors incriminated in atherogenesis as
well as sera from individuals with known risk factors on connective
tissue metabolism.

ACKNOWLEDGEMENTS

Supported by P.H.S. HL-14177 and VA Research Funds

REFERENCES

Daoud, A.S., Fritz, K.E., and Jarmolych, J. (1970). Exp. Mol. Pathol. 12, 354.

Daoud, A.S., Jarmolych, J., Zumbo, O., Fani, K., and Florentin, R. (1964). Exp. Mol. Pathol. 3, 475.

Daoud, A.S., Jones, R., and Scott, R.F. (1968). Exp. Mol. Pathol. 8, 263.

Fritz, K.E., Jarmolych, J., Bousvaros, G., and Daoud, A.S. (1972a). Circulation 46, II-263.

Fritz, K.E., Jarmolych, J., and Daoud, A.S. (1970). Exp. Mol. Pathol. 12, 354.

Fritz, K.E., Jarmolych, J., Daoud, A.S., and Peters, T., Jr. (1972b). Exp. Mol. Pathol. 16, 54.

Geer, J.C., McGill, H.C., Jr., and Strong, J.P. (1961). Amer. J. Pathol. 38, 263.

Goldberg, B., and Green, H. (1964). J. Cell Biol. 22, 227.

Haust, M.D., More, R.H., Bencosme, S.A., and Balis, J.U. (1965). Exp. Mol. Pathol. 4, 508.

Haust, M.D., More, R.H., and Movat, H.Z. (1960). Amer. J. Pathol. 37, 377.

Imai, H., Lee, K.T., Pastori, S., Panlilio, E., Florentin, R., and Thomas, W.A. (1966). Exp. Mol. Pathol. 5, 273.

Jarmolych, J., Daoud, A.S., Landau, J., Fritz, K.E., and McElevene, E. (1968). Exp. Mol. Pathol. 9, 171.

Karrer, H.E. (1960). J. Ultrastruct. Res. 4, 420.

Matukas, V.J., Panner, B.J., and Orbison, J.L. (1967). J. Cell Biol. 32, 365.

Murray, M., Schrodt, G.R., and Berg, H.F. (1966). Arch. Pathol. 82, 138.

Parker, F., and Odland, G.F. (1966). Amer. J. Pathol. 48, 451.

Paule, W.J. (1963). J. Ultrastruct. Res. 8, 219.

Ross, R. (1971). J. Cell Biol. 50, 172.

Ross, R., and Klebanoff, S.J. (1971). J. Cell Biol. 50, 159.

Scott, R.F., Jones, R., Daoud, A.S., Zumbo, O., Coulston, F., and
    Thomas, W.A. (1967). Exp. Mol. Pathol. 7, 34.

Wissler, R.W. (1973). Hospit. Pract. 8, 61.

Wissler, R.W. (1968). J. Atheroscler. Res. 8, 201.

DISCUSSION FOLLOWING THE PRESENTATION BY A.S. DAOUD

Dr. Kramsch: I agree with you that the electron microscopy
findings are logical and that what you have been growing is
probably elastic tissue, and it probably does contain elastin,
although there is no direct proof. One thing I would like to
caution you about, though, is to use the digestion of the elastica-
staining units in your tissue culture by elastase as evidence that
they are elastic tissue. Elastase is nonspecific, and if you
degrade these units with elastase, it does not really mean very
much. It might be more profitable to do it the other way around
by using enzymes that are known not to attack elastin, like
trypsin or collagenase. You might look at it that way. If the
elastica-staining units are not degraded by these enzymes, you
have some indirect evidence that they might be elastic tissue.

Dr. Kummerow: What was the age of the swine tissue? I
wonder how you can differentiate between cells without going into
specific staining techniques. Is there some way you can tell the
stage of your beginning tissue in relation to the later changes
in the cells?

Dr. Daoud: Tissues from the first experiment were aortas
from the slaughterhouse of Albany, and these were swine about six
months old, weighing about 150 pounds. In the second experiment
which we ran with the human sera, the swine were from our
laboratory. We know their age, their diet, and their blood
cholesterol levels. In general we know more about these swine
than we know about the human volunteers whose sera were used.

EFFECTS OF SERUM LIPOPROTEINS ON THE MORPHOLOGY, GROWTH, AND

METABOLISM OF ARTERIAL SMOOTH MUSCLE CELLS

Katti Fisher-Dzoga, Robert Chen, and Robert W. Wissler

Department of Pathology, University of Chicago

Chicago, Illinois

This paper summarizes some of the work we have been doing during the past five years to study the effects of hyperlipemia upon the growth, morphology and metabolism of arterial medial cells grown from primary explants. Although tissue culture methods have been used for over 70 years they were first introduced in the study of problems related to atherogenesis during the 1950's. Since this time there have been many studies of both experimentally induced and naturally occurring hyperlipemia and their effects on cultured cells, either of vascular origin or, more often, of established cell-lines unrelated to vascular tissue. Work has been reported on this subject by Rutstein and associates (1964), Robertson (1967), Rothblatt (1969), Baily and Keller (1971) and others. We have chosen to concentrate our efforts on medial cells, since more and more evidence has emphasized their importance in the pathogenesis of mammalian atherosclerosis (Haust et al., 1960; Wissler, 1968; Stary and McMillan, 1970; Thomas et al., 1971).

Our method of preparing the cultures is to carefully strip the intima and the adventitia off the thoracic aorta of normal young Rhesus monkeys or New Zealand rabbits. Single round explants, 2 mm in diameter, are punched out of the remaining media with a skin biopsy punch and placed individually in 30 ml plastic Falcon flasks containing 2.5 ml of Eagles basal medium, supplemented with 10% of calf serum or rabbit serum for the rabbit explants. The flasks are placed in an incubator at 37°C with 5% CO_2 in air. During the first few days they are turned upside down frequently until the explants are firmly attached to the bottom of the flask. The dormancy period varies from five days to three weeks, with

most of the explants showing outgrowth during the second week.
During the last five years, 50-70% of the explants have shown
outgrowth after three weeks under the described culture conditions.
In one experiment with 60 cultures, 42 (or 70%) showed growth,
34 of these within 15 days. If hyperlipemic serum is used as
medium supplement from the very beginning, the "take" (percentage
of explants growing to full size colonies) is increased to 90% or
over.

The round explants are clearly visible and measurable in the
flasks, often forming cords of dense cell growth. The slender cells
growing out from the explant are arranged in parallel fashion as
can be demonstrated by phase microscopy or by fixing the cells in
situ and staining with H & E. That they actively migrate is
illustrated by single detached cells found at the periphery of the
culture.

The cell colonies grow for a period of four to five weeks,
after which time they enter a more stationary phase with little
measurable increase in diameter. An average colony size is about
10-15 mm with a few cells in mitosis. Ultrastructural studies at
this time reveal the microfibrils and dense bodies characteristic
of mature smooth muscle cells.

To identify these cells further, we have used antibodies to
actomyosin, a smooth muscle cell protein, labeled with horseradish
peroxidase (HRP). Actomyosin is isolated from intestinal smooth
muscle of the rabbit or Rhesus monkey by extraction with 0.6 M KCl
and repeated precipitation with 0.05 M KCl. After testing its
potency and purity by measuring its ATP-ase activity and by gel
diffusion, the actomyosin is injected into rabbits or chickens and
the antisera is tested appropriately. Gamma globulin fractions
are prepared by ethanol fractionation according to Cohn, or for the
chicken serum by means of sodium sulfate precipitation. If not
pure as judged by immunoelectrophoresis, the fractions are further
purified by elution through a DEAE cellulose column using a 0.01 M
phosphate buffer at pH 7.4 as eluant.

Horseradish peroxidase, a histochemically demonstrable enzyme
of small molecular weight, is conjugated to these antibodies by
employing difluorodinitrophenyl sulfone (FNPS) or glutaraldehyde as
a coupling agent. The peroxidase activity then can be demonstrated
by Karnovsky's method using tetrachloridine as an oxidizable
substrate. The ensuing brown reaction product is strongly osmophi-
lic; when reacted with 2% osmium tetroxide solution, a distinct
dark reaction product is formed, indicating the antigenic sites.
The conjugates are tested to be immunologically pure and enzymati-
cally active before use.

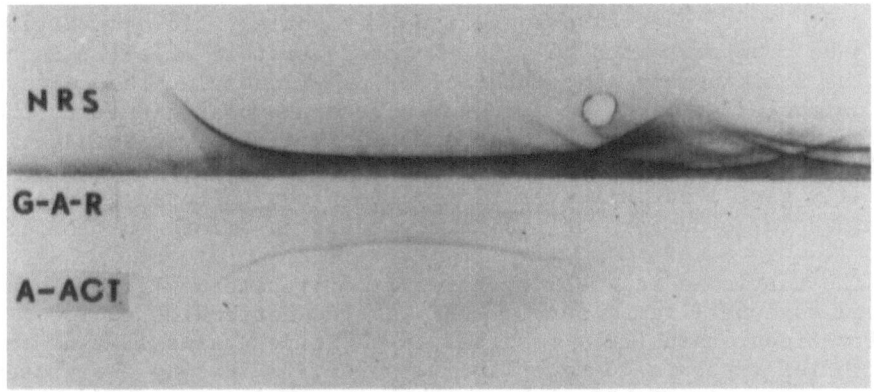

Fig. 1. Immunoelectrophoretic pattern of HRP-labeled anti-
actomyosin IgG as used for staining. Goat anti-rabbit serum
(G-A-R) was reacted against the HRP-labeled antibody (A-ACT).
Whole rabbit serum (NRS) was used as a control. For the antibody
only one line, the IgG, is visible, attesting to its purity. This
line was stained brown with the enzyme stain, demonstrating that
the HRP was firmly attached to the globulin. The other lines were
a light blue-green as stained with light green.

     In Figure 1, HRP-labeled anti-monkey-actomyosin-rabbit
globulin was placed in the lower well, normal rabbit serum as a
control, in the upper well and goat anti-whole rabbit serum, in the
trough. The whole slide was stained first for the enzyme and then
counterstained with light green, a protein stain. Only the conju-
gate, which appears to be a pure Ig-globulin, has taken up the
enzyme stain (e.g., is stained brown), indicating that the HRP is
firmly attached to the antibody.

     These preparations were used for histochemical staining of
the culture cells; they were stained in situ without previous
fixation, or after brief fixation with paraformaldehyde. After the
cells were washed with an appropriate buffer, the labeled antibody
was layered carefully over them and left to interact at least 45
minutes at room temperature or overnight in the cold. The cultures
were again washed extensively with buffer, treated for 15 minutes
with diaminobenzidrin, and washed again with buffer. In order to
avoid nonspecific staining of lipid droplets frequently present in
these cells, the final step of exposure to osmium was routinely
omitted. With this method, a brown stain at the site of antibody
localization was obtained against a yellow-tan background.

     When HRP-labeled antibody to actomyosin was used, the stain
was distributed evenly and often covered the whole surface of the
cell. When labeled normal rabbit IgG was used, no positive staining

occurred. These control preparations were pale yellow and often
had to be counterstained to make the cells visible at all. Such
negative staining was also obtained by pre-incubating the cultures
with unlabeled antibody to actomyosin before exposing them to the
labeled antibody. Cultures of the adventitia gave variable
results, cultures which appeared to consist mostly of fibroblasts
generally gave a negative reaction while other cultures evidently
contained large numbers of positively reacting smooth muscle cells.

The aortic medial cell cultures readily take up lipids when
exposed to hyperlipemic serum. HRP-labeled antibodies to low
density lipoprotein (LDL) resulted in positive stains in many cells
after brief exposure to hyperlipemic serum, indicating the presence
of the apoprotein of LDL although these antibodies stained the
cells in an uneven pattern. Not all of the cells were stained, and
there was an uneven distribution within any given cell. The stain
frequently appeared to be around vacuoles, giving the impression
of small droplets stained mostly on the outside (Figure 2).
Staining of cultures exposed to hyperlipemic serum with HRP-labeled
antibody to high density lipoprotein (HDL) gave negative results,

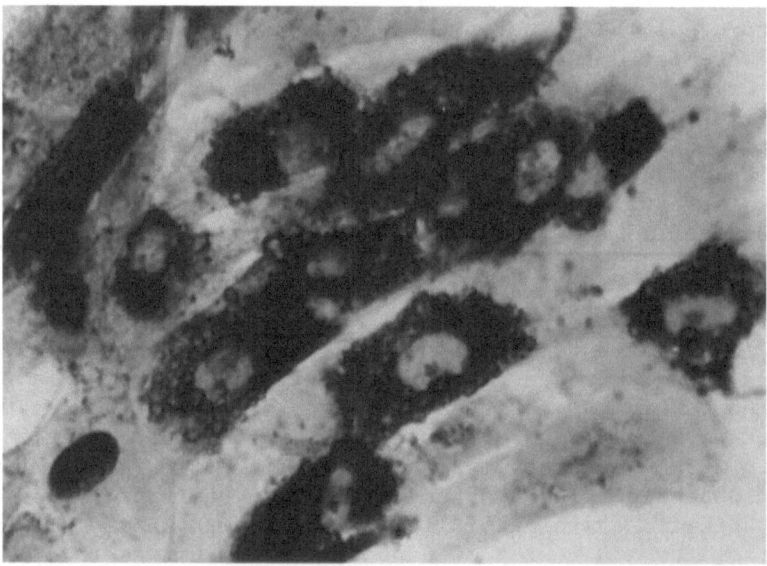

Fig. 2. Cells of four week old medial culture, incubated for 24
hours with hyperlipemic serum then stained with HRP-labeled antibody to LDL. Dark staining occurs in many of the cells indicating
the presence of the apoprotein of LDL. The stain is distributed
unevenly within the cells and is often seen around vacuoles -
seemingly staining the outside of droplets. (x 375).

as did cells stained with labeled normal rabbit globulin and cells
that were treated with unlabeled antibody to LDL prior to staining
with the HRP-labeled anti-LDL.

Staining these cells with Oil Red O, a neutral fat stain,
is another way to demonstrate that they readily take up lipids
even after brief exposure to hyperlipemic serum. The lipid droplets are clearly visible within the cells. Active division of
these lipid laden cells can be illustrated by autoradiography of
cultures exposed for 24 hours to hyperlipemic serum and then
pulse-labeled with tritium-labeled thymidine 12 hours before
fixation. A high percentage of nuclei show the presence of the
radioactive label, indicating DNA synthesis. When these cells
are five weeks old (that is, they have reached the stationary
growth phase when normally only a few cells are in mitosis), the
addition of hyperlipemic serum to the medium not only induces
lipid uptake, but also seems to trigger a second phase of proliferation resulting in another increase in colony diameter measurable usually after about five days.

In order to evaluate this phenomenon further we began systematically treating the cultures with homologous hyperlipemic serum
and its lipoprotein fractions. Hyperlipemic monkey serum was
obtained from animals that had been fed a monkey chow supplemented
with 2% cholesterol and 25% either coconut oil or peanut oil for
several months. Hyperlipemic rabbit serum was obtained from
rabbits that had been fed a diet containing 0.4% cholesterol and
10% sunflower oil.

Lipoprotein fractionation was accomplished according to the
method of Havel et al. (1955), by repeated ultracentrifugation
with increasing density of the solvent. Each fraction was characterized by solvent density; VLDL was spun up at density 1.019;
LDL, at 1.063; and the HDL, at 1.213. The immunological specifi-
cities of the LDL and HDL were verified by immunoelectrophoresis.

Cell colony size was evaluated by direct measurement of the
diameter along two perpendicular axes of the circular cell growth
and the average diameter was expressed in mm. Five to ten cultures
of comparable size were used for each study group. Treatment
periods lasted for ten days. Five percent of the test serum
replaced 5% of the calf serum in the medium. The lipoprotein
fractions were obtained from an equal amount of hyperlipemic serum
equivalent to 5% of the medium and this medium was changed three
times during the ten day experimental period. At the end of the
period the cultures were again measured, fixed in formalin, and
stained with Oil Red O to visualize lipid uptake.

The results of this experiment are outlined in Table I. It
is evident that the hyperlipemic serum has a strong proliferative

TABLE I.   STIMULATION OF GROWTH OF PRIMARY CULTURES OF AORTIC SMOOTH MUSCLE CELLS BY VARIOUS LIPOPROTEIN FRACTIONS

Group	Addition to Culture Medium	Average Diameter of Cultures (mm)		Average Increase In Surface Area (mm^2)
		Day 0	Day 10	
I	5% Normal Monkey Serum	13.8	15.7	15.4 $\pm$ 8.0
II	5% Hyperlipemic Monkey Serum	13.8	19.0	128.3 $\pm$ 34.6
III	VLDL from 5% Hyperlipemic Monkey Serum	13.8	15.8	35.9 $\pm$ 21.3
IV	LDL from 5% Hyperlipemic Monkey Serum	13.8	17.8	91.6 $\pm$ 12.2
V	HDL from 5% Hyperlipemic Monkey Serum	13.8	14.0	2.25 $\pm$ 2.1
VI	Protein Residue from 5% Hyperlipemic Monkey Serum	13.8	14.3	12.8 $\pm$ 4.5

effect on the cultures, as does the LDL from hyperlipemic serum. LDL seems to be the fraction mainly responsible for this phenomenon. HDL shows no effect and VLDL often produces a slight proliferative response. Simple measuring of the diameters of these cultures is admittedly a crude method, especially in view of the fact that these colonies often consist of two or three layers of cells, particularly near the explant.

To obtain another parameter of growth, the cultures were pulse-labeled with [^{3}H] thymidine at the beginning of the experiment, and autoradiographs were prepared and evaluated after the ten day experimental period. At least 500 cells were counted in each culture and the results were expressed in percentage of labeled cells. Results of this experiment are shown in Table II. It is evident that there is a much higher degree of labeling in the cultures receiving the hyperlipemic serum or its LDL fraction. Labeling of these two groups is over 30% as compared to less than 15% in the other groups. Lipid uptake is difficult to evaluate with accuracy by visual grading but we observed large variations within each group.

Autoradiographs also illustrate the fact that lipid uptake and proliferation do not necessarily occur together. Sometimes there is little cell division and little lipid uptake as observed in most cultures treated with HDL, or there is active cell division and active lipid uptake as is often found in cultures treated with

TABLE II. EFFECT OF VARIOUS LIPOPROTEIN FRACTIONS ON MITOSIS OF PRIMARY AORTIC SMOOTH MUSCLE CELL CULTURES

Test Serum 5% in Medium	Number of Cultures Counted	% of Cells Labeled with $[^3H]$ Thymidine
Normal Monkey Serum	15	8.7 ± 1.5
Hyperlipemic Monkey Serum	18	39.8 ± 5.2
Hyperlipemic VLDL	9	6.5 ± 1.6
Hyperlipemic LDL	12	39.2 ± 8.1
Hyperlipemic HDL	8	4.9 ± 0.7
Protein Residue	3	3.8 ± 1.0

TABLE III. EFFECTS OF VARIOUS QUANTITIES OF LDL ON GROWTH OF AORTIC MEDIAL CELLS IN TISSUE CULTURE

Composition of Culture Medium	Cholesterol Content of Test Serum (mg %)	Average Area of Growth (mm^2)		Average Growth Increase
		Day 0	Day 10	
5% Normal Monkey Serum	154	204.2	255.6	51.4
5% Hyperlipemic Monkey Serum	844	197.1	417.7	220.1
LDL from Normal Monkey Serum	64	204.2	247.7	47.6
LDL from Hyperlipemic Serum	584	199.1	372.3	173.2
LDL from Normal Serum Concentrated 2 x	128	198.5	216.1	17.6
LDL from Hyperlipemic Serum Diluted 1:4.5	129	205.4	364.6	159.3

hyperlipemic LDL. Some cultures show active cell division but little lipid uptake, or very few labeled cells but considerable lipid within the cells.

Since cholesterol is abundant in the low density lipoprotein fraction from monkey serum as compared to the other lipoprotein fractions, it is natural to speculate that it might be simply the increased level of cholesterol or cholesterol esters that stimulate the second wave of proliferation. Experiments designed to test this hypothesis contained a group of cultures (V) to which the normal low density lipoprotein was added, but in twice the usual (5%) concentration, and another group (VI) which was fed the hyperlipemic low density lipoprotein diluted 1:4.5. In this manner the cultures of groups V and VI received the same amount of cholesterol. Table III gives the results of this experiment. It is evident that there is little or no increase in growth in the groups receiving normal serum or normal LDL respectively (I and III) as compared to those treated with hyperlipemic serum and its LDL (II and IV). Hyperlipemic LDL is less effective after dilution but there is still substantial growth stimulation as compared to the normal LDL even when the latter is concentrated to the same cholesterol level as in group V.

These results are paralleled by a much higher percentage of cells labeled by [^{3}H] thymidine (Table IV). Again the values for groups V and VI are of particular interest. On several occasions, we used cultures of other organs of the same animal as controls (kidney, spleen, liver, peritoneum, subcutaneous tissue, skin, omentum, uterus, and another smooth muscle cell culture). Either very good proliferation was seen in all groups, including the ones receiving normal serum (indicating that these cultures were still in their growth phase) or, more often, the hyperlipemic serum in the concentrations used for arterial explants proved to be toxic and resulted in cell death. As control cultures explants of

TABLE IV.   STIMULATION OF GROWTH OF MEDIAL SMOOTH MUSCLE CELLS IN CULTURE BY HYPERLIPEMIC SERUM AND ITS LOW DENSITY LIPOPROTEIN

Addition to Culture Medium		Cholesterol Content (mg %)	% of Cells Labeled with [^{3}H] Thymidine Exp. A + B
I	Normal Monkey Serum	125	8.3 $\pm$ 4.0
II	Hyperlipemic Monkey Serum	900	36.0 $\pm$ 12.8
III	Normal LDL	65	6.6 $\pm$ 3.8
IV	Hyperlipemic LDL	600	27.8 $\pm$ 9.0
V	Normal LDL Concentrated	130	6.0 $\pm$ 4.4
VI	Hyperlipemic LDL Diluted	130	26.6 $\pm$ 10.6

adventitia from the same animal were used in most experiments. Results were inconsistent since in most cases we were probably dealing with a mixed culture of vessel fibroblasts and smooth muscle cells.

The experiments in which hyperlipemic serum was diluted show its effect on the medial smooth muscle cell cultures is not simply one of lipid concentration; even when the whole hyperlipemic serum or its LDL was diluted to near normal lipid values it still triggered a second phase of proliferation in stationary medial cultures. Primary cultures of aortic medial smooth muscle cells are peculiar inasmuch as they reach a stationary growth phase and can be maintained in this phase up to three months. Whatever the mode of action or nature of the factor(s) in hyperlipemic serum, it re-stimulates cells which have reached a phase of very low mitotic activity despite optimal nutritional conditions. The responsible factor(s) which trigger DNA synthesis is present predominantly in the LDL fraction. The apoprotein of LDL is demonstrable in the cells by immunohistochemical methods. Lipid

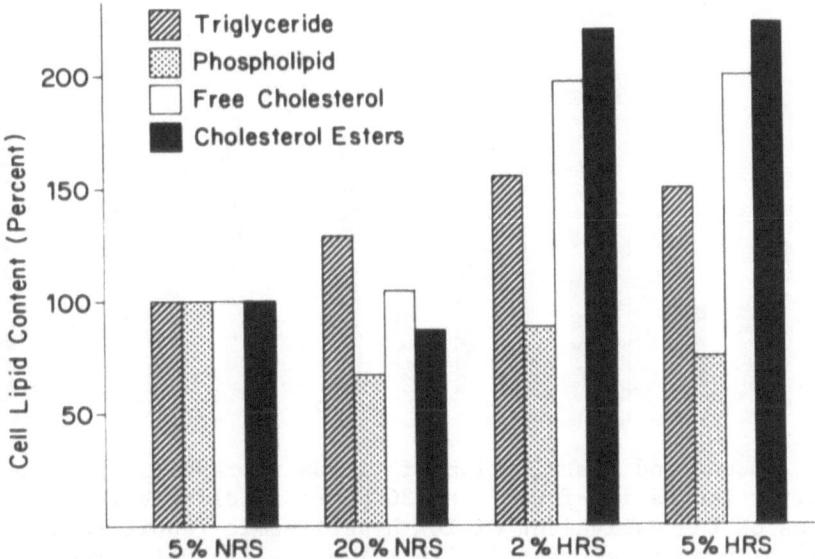

Fig. 3. Amount and distribution of lipids in rabbit aortic medial cells after exposure to different concentrations of normal rabbit serum (NRS) or hyperlipemic rabbit serum (HRS) for 40 hours.

accumulation occurs very rapidly after exposure to hyperlipemia;
however, it has been shown to be reversible.

Dr. Robert Chen has been studying the biochemical effects of
hyperlipemic serum and lipoprotein fractions on arterial medial
cells grown in subcultures obtained by trypsinizing the primary
cultures of explants of rabbit aortic medial cells. Biochemical
analysis of the lipid extracted from these cells has shown that
cells exposed to hyperlipemic serum accumulate much more lipid per
mg cell protein than cells grown in normal serum. The lipids were
extracted by a mixture of chloroform-ethanol and further separated
by thin layer chromatography.

After incubation in hyperlipemic serum for 40 hours there
was a twofold increase in free cholesterol and a two- to fourfold
increase in cholesterol ester as compared with cells exposed only
to normal serum. The type of serum seemed to be more important

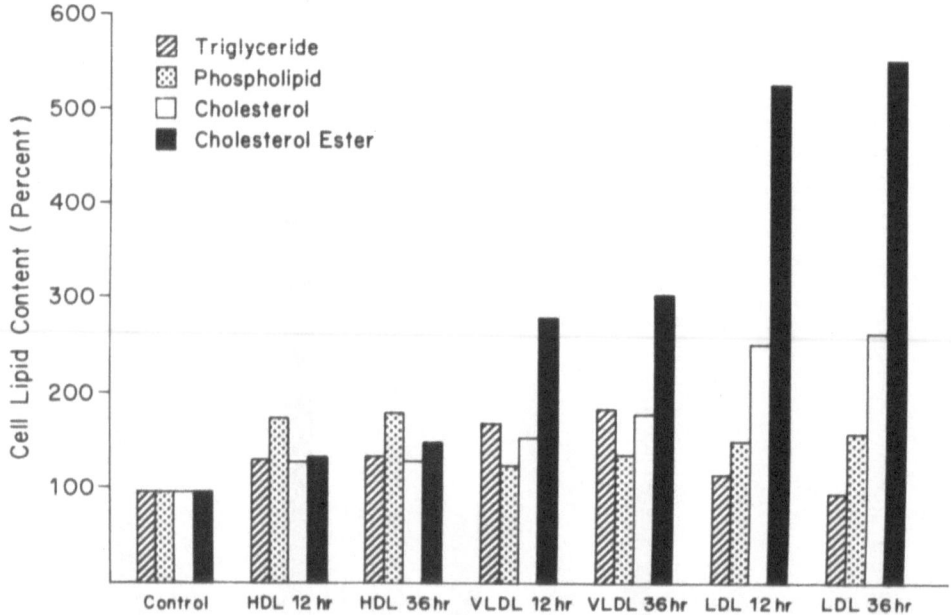

Fig. 4. Amount and distribution of lipids in rabbit aortic medial
cells after incubation for 12 and 36 hours in different lipoprotein
fractions of the equivalent of 10% hyperlipemic rabbit serum.
Control cultures were treated with 10% normal rabbit serum.

than the concentration or the amount of lipid in the medium. Cells incubated in 20 to 40% normal serum showed a lipid pattern similar to that of cells in 5% normal serum, while there was a significant increase in cholesterol and cholesterol ester in cells incubated in only 2% hyperlipemic serum (Figure 3). The hyperlipemic serum was then fractionated into its lipoprotein fractions by ultracentrifugation and the HDL, LDL, and VLDL fractions were added to the culture medium in amounts equivalent to 10% serum. The cells were incubated for 12 and 36 hours. As compared to the control group in 10% normal serum the LDL group had the largest increase in cholesterol and cholesterol ester. Cells exposed to the hyperlipemic VLDL showed some increase while the HDL group maintained near normal levels of total lipids (Figure 4).

SUMMARY

1. Cells of aortic media grow well in Eagle's Basal Medium supplemented with 10% normal serum.

2. The cells show morphological and immunohistochemical characteristics of smooth muscle cells.

3. LDL from hyperlipemic animals stimulates these cells to proliferate; whereas HDL or the lipid free serum does not; and VLDL has an intermediate effect.

4. LDL from normal serum does not affect the growth rate.

5. When exposed to hyperlipemic serum these cells readily take up lipid which is easily stainable with Oil Red O and reacts with antibodies to LDL-labeled with horseradish peroxidase.

6. Chemical analysis of the lipid accumulated in these cells after exposure to hyperlipemic serum shows an increase in cholesterol and cholesterol ester.

7. This lipid accumulation depends on the type of serum rather than the lipid concentration in the medium. Cells incubated in dilute (2%) hyperlipemic serum still show substantial lipid accumulation as compared to cells incubated in normal serum, even if the concentration of the latter is increased to 10% or 20%.

8. Cells incubated in hyperlipemic LDL show the largest increase in free cholesterol and cholesterol, VLDL shows some increase, while the effect of HDL is minimal.

ACKNOWLEDGEMENTS

Supported by USPHS grants HL 12358, HL 6894 and HL 15062.

REFERENCES

Bailey, P.J., and Keller, D. (1971). Atherosclerosis 13, 333.

Haust, M.D., More, R.H., and Movat, H.Z. (1960). Amer. J. Pathol. 37, 377.

Havel, R.J., Howard, A.E., and Bragdon, J.M. (1955). J. Clin. Invest. 34, 1345.

Robertson, A.L. (1967). In "Lipid Metabolism and Tissue Culture Cells" (G.M. Rothblatt and D. Kritchevsky, eds.), Wistar Institute Symposium Monograph 6, pp. 115-125.

Rothblatt, G.M. (1969). Advan. Lipid Res. 1, 135.

Rutstein, D.D., Costelli, W.P., Sullivan, J.C., Newell, J.M., and Nickerson, R.J. (1964). New Engl. J. Med. 271, 1.

Stary, H.C., and McMillan, G.C. (1970). Arch. Pathol. 89, 173.

Thomas, W.H., Florentin, R.A., Nam, S.C., Reiner, J.M., and Lee, K.T. (1971). Exp. Mol. Pathol. 15, 245.

Wissler, R.W. (1968). J. Atheroscler. Res. 8, 201.

DISCUSSION FOLLOWING THE PRESENTATION BY KATTI FISHER-DZOGA

Dr. Smith: Obviously, this is very exciting and provokes the question, what is the difference between the LDL from the hyperlipemic serum and the LDL from the normal serum? Can I ask first why were these animals hyperlipemic? Have you tried making them hyperlipemic using different regimens and seeing if this had any effect on the LDL in this respect?

Dr. Fisher-Dzoga: First of all, the animals were made hyperlipemic by adding 2% cholesterol and 25% lipid to the chow. The results I have shown today were induced by hyperlipemic serum after feeding peanut oil or coconut oil. This method gives a tremendous hyperlipemia, e.g., coconut oil produces hyperlipemia of about 900 mg% cholesterol. The rabbits were fed 0.4% cholesterol and 10% safflower oil, which again results in a hyperlipemia of over 1,000 mg% cholesterol. Comparison studies on the effect of hyperlipemic serum induced by different fats, e.g., corn oil, peanut oil or butterfat, did not give any significant difference; they all increased proliferation.

We completed one experiment where we did not add cholesterol to the diet. Unfortunately, since the induction period was very short in that particular experiment, there was hardly any hyperlipemia, and this serum did not show any effect on the growth of cells.

As far as the difference between hyperlipemic LDL and normal LDL is concerned, we are trying now to take this molecule apart.

Dr. Wissler: We are very fortunate in having Dr. Robert Chen[1] working with us on this problem at the present time. We hope to report further about the characteristics of these fractions of hyperlipemic sera that have such great effects on cells.

Dr. St. Clair: It appeared that when you labeled your LDL with horseradish peroxidase, the protein remained on the outer surface of the lipid droplet. Would you care to speculate as to whether you feel that the LDL is taken up as an intact complex? If this is so, then it would appear, wouldn't it, that the protein moiety of LDL is not readily catabolized.

Dr. Fisher-Dzoga: I really don't know if the LDL is taken up intact. We have tried to label the LDL apoproteins with [125]Iodine in order to localize them within the cells by autoradiography, but we didn't have much success.

Dr. Wissler: I think the answer is that at least in tissue culture[2] and probably in the artery[3], some LDL probably is taken up by the cells intact and is retained for a little while. We can not tell how much and how long by these methods.

---

[1]Chen, R., Dzoga, K., Borensztajn, J., and Wissler, R. W. (1972). Effect of hyperlipemic lipoproteins on the lipid accumulation of rabbit aortic medial cells in vitro. Circulation 46 (Suppl. II), 253.

[2]Fisher-Dzoga, K., Jones, R. M., Vesselinovitch, D., and Wissler, R. W. (1973). Ultrastructural and immunohistochemical studies of primary cultures of aortic medial cells. Exp. Mol. Pathol. 18, 162.

[3]Knieriem, H. J., Kao, V. C. Y., and Wissler, R. W. (1967). Actomyosin and myosin and the deposition of lipids and serum lipoproteins. AMA Arch. Pathol. 84, 118.

SECTION IV

PATHOLOGIC PROCESSES AND CONNECTIVE

TISSUE INTERACTIONS

THROMBOSIS AND CONNECTIVE TISSUE INTERRELATIONSHIPS IN ARTERIOSCLEROSIS

Michael B. Stemerman

Division of Hematology, Montefiore Hospital and Medical
Center, Albert Einstein College of Medicine, Bronx,
New York

The growth of a thrombus is determined by the combined
influences of blood flow, blood constituents, and blood vessel
(Virchow, 1860). Major attention has been given to the circulating elements of the blood which participate in thrombus formation.
Studies of these elements have led to a detailed in vitro description of blood coagulation in terms of the physiologic reactivity
of procoagulants and platelets. Recently, the biologic application
of numerous synthetic materials has brought those concerned with
thrombus formation to inquire in a detailed manner into the
influence of blood flow. The use of these materials has attracted
the expertise of bioengineers interested in the field of fluid
mechanics. The effect has been an emerging, comprehensive description of the behavior of physiologic fluids relating to the patho-
physiology of thrombus formation. Results from these disciplines
have underscored the need to consider the role of the remaining
affector of thrombogenesis - the vascular surface.

Under usual circumstances, circulating blood contacts a non-
thrombogenic surface, the vascular endothelium. These cells form
a continuous lining for the vascular tree, and appear to be non-
reactive even when injured (Stehbens and Biscoe, 1967). Thrombosis
is initiated when endothelial cells are dislodged, exposing the
underlying subendothelial connective tissue. The first event in
thrombosis is the adhering of platelets upon this surface, and the
disgorging of their intracytoplasmic materials. Subsequently,
coagulation reactions are generated which lead ultimately to the
generation of thrombin and fibrin (Marcus, 1969). It therefore
appears that the thrombogenic properties of the exposed subendothelium are closely related to the ultimate hemostatic potential of a
vessel. The following discussion will deal with recent developments

TABLE I.

COMPARISON OF VASCULAR CONNECTIVE TISSUE COMPONENTS

	Appearance On EM	Hydroxyproline Content	Hydrophilic Acidic Amino Acids	Hydrophilic Basic Amino Acids	Collagenase Digestible	Trypsin Digestible
Collagen fibers	Variable width, 640 Å periodicity	high (14%)	moderate	moderate	+	-
Vascular Basement Membrane	Moderate electron density. Tri-Laminar - Composed of filaments 50 Å and 100 Å wide	unknown but probably present	unknown	unknown	+	+
Microfibrils	Electron dense - 100 Å wide with 170 Å banding	absent	high	moderate	-	+
Elastin	Electron lucent	very low	low	low	-	-

in this area of blood vessel physiology and its relationship to
arteriosclerosis.

SUBENDOTHELIAL MORPHOLOGY

A detailed description of the subendothelium is not complete
at this time, but a number of recent reports have examined this
structure in different species and at different sites in the vasculature. The morphology of the material to which the endothelial
cell attaches varies according to the size and location of the
corresponding vessel.

In capillaries (Luft, 1963), small veins (Rhodin, 1968),
and heart valves (Kuhnel, 1966),the underlying structure is
generally called vascular basement membrane (BM), although its
chemical relation to BM of other cells is uncertain. The capillary BM is a meshwork of fine filaments varying from 50 Å to 100 Å
with the thicker filaments seen at the periphery (Bruns and Palade,
1968) (Table I). These filaments have none of the ultrastructural
characteristics of the more deeply located collagen fibers which
are easily identified on electron microscopy by a typical 640 Å
periodicity. The vascular BM does, however, share some antigenic
similarities (Krahower and Greenspon, 1964; Pierce, 1966) and other
properties with that of the collagen fiber (Table I).

Some larger vessels appear to have a subendothelium consisting
primarily of BM. Schwartz and Benditt (1972) have described a PAS-
positive reticulated BM of filaments interconnecting with electron
dense granules of approximately 150 Å. Gloster (1973) has described
the subendothelium of the human umbilical vein as consisting of a
moderately electron dense BM similar to capillary BM, as shown in
Figure 1.

The subendothelium of large arteries of the rabbit and other
mammals have an entirely different morphologic appearance (Figure
2). The subendothelium consists of a space beneath the endothelial cell from the vascular surface of the endothelial membrane to
the internal elastic lamina (IEL). This space varies considerably,
but is approximately 500 Å wide. Three distinct materials are
identifiable by electron microscopy: moderately electron dense BM,
electron dense microfibrils (MF) and electron lucent elastin
(Stemerman and Spaet, 1972). The BM of the arterial subendothelium appears to be morphologically similar to that in capillary
BM but, in contrast to that of the smaller vessel, it is irregularly distributed and fails to form a continuous lamella. The
content of BM in a given vessel may vary between abundance to
complete absence from one closely situated area to another. The
subendothelial elastin is continuous with the IEL and makes up a
small segment of the material contacting the endothelium   since it

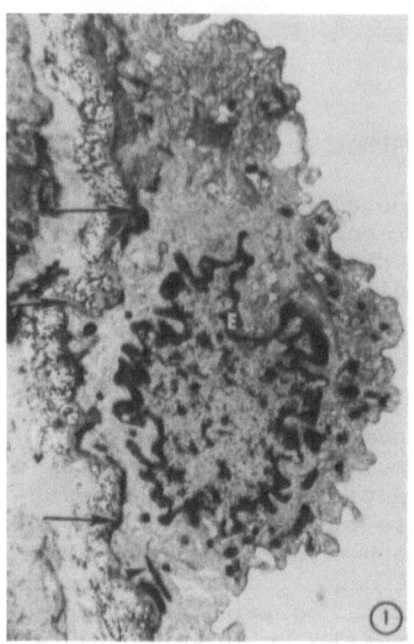 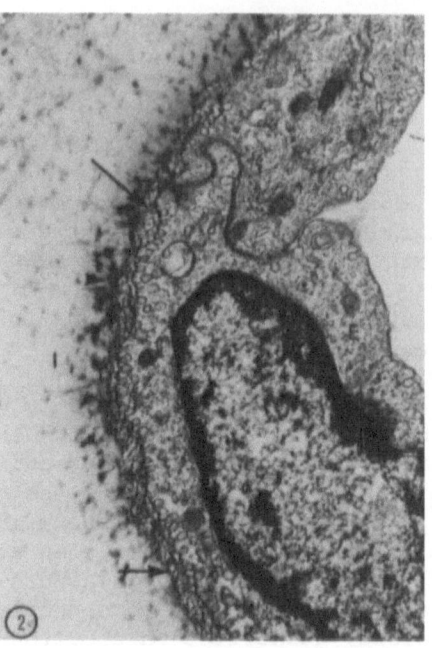

Fig. 1. The lumenal aspect of a human umbilical vein is shown in
this electron micrograph. The endothelia (E) form a continuous
lining for the vessel and rest on a moderately electron dense
basement lamella (arrows). The electron lucent material on the
vascular aspect of the basement membrane is elastin. The endothelial cell contains the usual organelles including a rod-shaped
tabular body (arrowhead). (x 20,000). (Reduced 4 % for reproduction).

Fig. 2. This is an electron micrograph of a rabbit iliac artery.
Shown in this view are the endothelium and the subjacent subendothelial region. This micrograph should be compared to Figure 1
for the contrast in the subintimal structures. The rabbit subendothelial region consists of elastin which is electron lucent
material in direct contact with the internal elastic lamina (I),
vascular basement membrane (arrows), and microfibrils (arrowhead).
(x 35,000). (Reduced 43% for reproduction).

is covered in most areas by the MF. The MF are 100 Å wide filaments embedded within the elastin and are similar to those
previously described which are associated with elastin in other
locations. The number of the MF differs from place to place in
the artery and may be diminished with aging and with testosterone
(Gaynor, 1973). The fibers are arranged longitudinally to the
long axis of the vessel, thus being seen on end when the vessel is

viewed in the cross-sectional plane. The high MF content of
arteries and the widespread distribution of these structures
make them a major material directly underlying the endothelium,
and one of the most abundant to which blood hemostatic elements
are exposed when endothelial cell detachment occurs.

Few collagen fibers are identifiable by electron microscopy
within the arterial intima (Karrer, 1961). Occasionally small
bundles of these fibers are present beneath the endothelial cells,
but this is a rare occurrence. Collagen is seen in abundance
within the media and adventitial layers of the vessel.

Bounameaux (1959) and Hugues (1960) observed that platelets
attached themselves to the connective tissue bundles at the cut
edge of severed vessels, and it was soon demonstrated that the
active material was collagen (Hovig and Holmsen, 1963). These
observations, coupled with the findings that collagen fibers were
capable of initiating blood coagulation by the activation of
Factor XII (Hageman Factor) (Wilner et al., 1968), led investigators to consider this material as the vascular substrate upon which
deposits accumulate. However, collagen fibers are an insignificant
component of the blood vessel subintima. To expose these fibers
to the hemostatic elements of the blood, penetration of the IEL is
necessary. This may occur in vessel severing (Kjaerheim and Hovig,
1962), crushing (Hoff and Gottlob, 1968) and other severe vascular
injuries (Studer, 1966). Whether this degree of penetration
occurs in spontaneous thrombotic disease is unknown; certainly the
first connective tissue layer to be uncovered following endothelial cell desquamation is the collagen fiber-poor subendothelium.
Accordingly, studies were undertaken to characterize the hemostatic
properties of this structure.

A necessary prerequisite in studying the hemostatic properties
of the subintima was a technique which selectively removed endothelium without disrupting the deeper layers of the vessel. Selective
removal was conveniently achieved in the intact animal by passage
of an intra-arterial balloon, inflated to a modest pressure, along
the lumen of the vessel (Baumgartner, 1963). Endothelial cells
were detached over the course of the balloon's transit, without
injury to the deeper structures of the vessel. Such denuded
vessels were suitable for perfusion of various reagents or blood
constituents.

The first observation derived from these stripped arteries
was that they were hemostatically active. Platelets adhered to
the subintima, providing an almost continuous cover, and subsequent
platelets aggregated to those which were adhering (Figure 3). The
appearance of the initial platelet layer was characteristic of the
adhering process. The platelets spread upon the surface in dendritic fashion and underwent degranulation. In the absence of

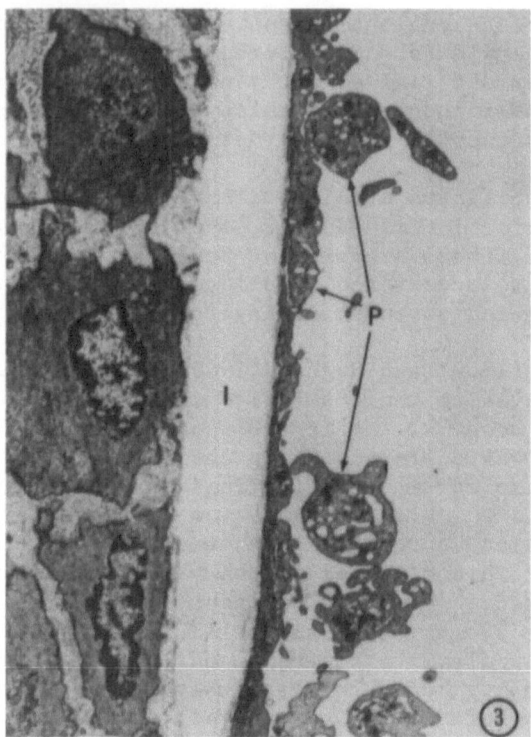

Fig. 3. Shown here is a rabbit artery in which the endothelial
cover was removed by an intra-arterial balloon catheter and fixed
by perfusion ten minutes after denudation. Platelets (P) cover
the de-endothelialized surface, spreading with loss of intracytoplasmic granules. Other platelets are closely associated with
the adhering layer but have not lost their intracytoplasmic granules. It should be noted that no fibrin is present and that the
medial tissue beneath the internal elastic lamina (I) shows no
evidence of trauma. (x 8,000). (Reduced 30% for reproduction).

demonstrable collagen fibers, two questions arise: The first concerns the material to which the platelets stick. MF, elastin, and
vascular BM are all candidates based upon morphological considerations alone. The second concerns the nature of the adhesion
reaction and whether the observations previously derived from
studies with collagen are applicable here as well.

To examine the qualities of the subendothelium and to compare
them with collagen reactions, an isolated rabbit arterial segment
was prepared and freed of its endothelium without allowing contact
with the blood (Baumgartner et al., 1971). This vessel segment

was then perfused with various blood constituents and the platelet deposits graded. Heparinized whole blood and platelet-rich-plasma (PRP) and citrated whole blood produced a rich accumulation of platelets, while citrated PRP gave a reduction in deposition and EDTA whole blood produced no adhesion (Baumgartner et al., 1971) (Table II). This indicated that calcium ion was necessary for platelet accretion upon the subendothelium, and that red cells or leukocytes facilitated the reaction as well. The reactivity of the subendothelium clearly differed from collagen fibers to which platelets adhered in the absence of calcium, and the presence of other cells evidently had no effect on this reaction (Owren, 1964). The factors influencing the reaction of platelets with the subendothelium were reminiscent of those observed with platelet-glass interaction, where divalent cation was required (Hellem et al., 1961), and red cells produce an enhanced effect. This latter phenomena may be related to a material such as adenosine diphosphate supplied by the erythrocytes, or it may be related to the action of red cell motion which augment platelet movement to the surface (Goldsmith, 1972).

Although it is clear from these experiments that the subendothelium was not collagen, it was not clear what the active component or components might be. The vascular BM, although irregularly distributed, should act as a nidus for platelet adhesion if it does represent an extension to larger vessels of capillary BM. Investigators have shown that platelets stick to capillary BM which had been exposed by various maneuvers that cause endothelial cell separation (Majno and Palade, 1961; Tranzer and Baumgartner, 1967). The vascular BM does appear to bear some relationship with collagen (Krahower and Greenspon, 1964), but platelets adhering to this structure show a lesser degree of alteration and little degranulation (Tranzer and Baumgartner, 1967), in contrast to the profound changes which follow adhesion to collagen fibers. Although vascular

TABLE II.   RELATIVE AFFINITY OF CONNECTIVE TISSUE COMPONENTS FOR
            PLATELETS

Collagen Fibers	Highly Reactive
Intact Subendothelium	Reactive _in vivo_: Require erythrocytes and divalent cation
Subendothelial Microfibrils	Reactive with native whole blood
Vascular Basement Membrane	Low Reactivity: _in vitro_
Subendothelial Elastin	Little Reactivity: Poorly accessible

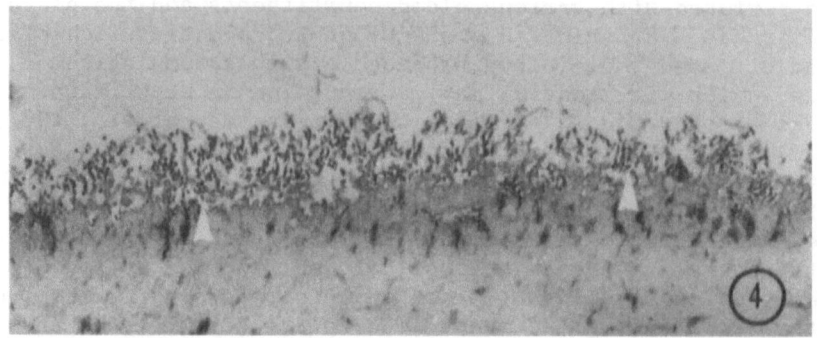

Fig. 4. A section from a rabbit artery digested with collagenase
for twenty-four hours is shown in this electron micrograph. The
vascular basement membrane is no longer present, but the microfibrils seen here in cross-section (arrowheads) and the electron
lucent elastin remain. (x 40,000).

BM may be active in arteries, it does not appear to be necessary
for platelet adhesion. This has been demonstrated by the use of
the isolated vessel segments described previously. Perfusion of
these segments with a collagenase solution causes disappearance of
morphologically demonstrable vascular BM as well as the collagen
fibers that lie beneath the IEL (Stemerman et al., 1971). The
remaining surface consists of MF and elastin as shown in Figure 4.
Perfusion of these digested vessels with native whole blood was
followed by formation of a layer of degranulated platelets with
accompanying aggregation as shown in Figure 5. The reaction was
identical to that with undigested preparations, indicating that the
digested material was not essential for platelet deposition.

     The affinity of platelets for the vascular BM remains uncertain
at this time. Baumgartner and Haudenschild (1972), using a flow
chamber in which citrated PRP was perfused over rabbit subendothelium before and after collagenase digestion, were able to detect a
decrease in platelet accumulation in the absence of vascular BM.
Gloster (1973) demonstrated that human platelets adhere to the
BM of human umbilical veins. In his experiments there was adhesion
of platelets to the surface with little tendency to aggregation.
Suresh et al. (1973) also attempted to demonstrate platelet
affinity for vascular BM. In their preparations rabbit heart
valves which are lined with BM were freed of their endothelium
by both mild trypsin digestion and mechanical means. Repeated
attempts to cause platelet adhesion to this surface, including
multiple centrifugations of platelets upon the surface, were unsuc-
cessful. Platelet thrombi were detected at peripheral areas of the
valves in which collagen fibers were available at the cut surface.
These experiments indicate that while the BM may be available as a

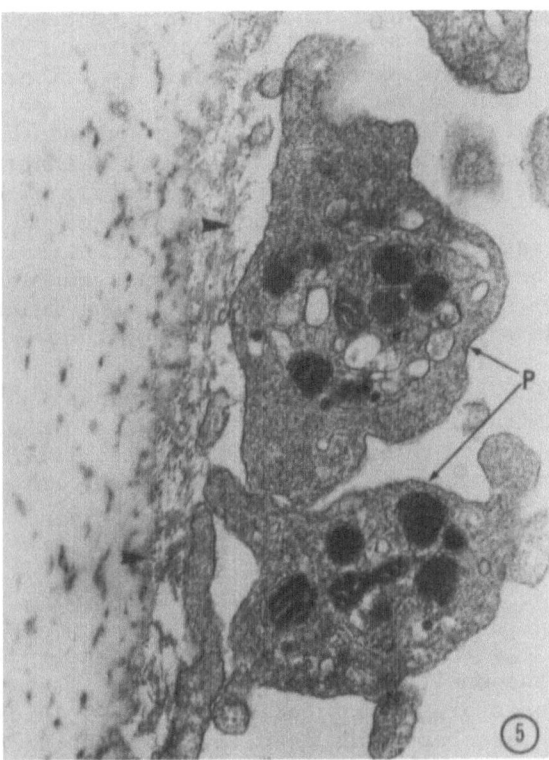

Fig. 5. This is an electron micrograph of a vessel infused with
collagenase and then perfused with native whole blood for ten
minutes prior to fixation. Platelets (P) are shown in the process
of spreading upon the digested surface. The subintimal region
shows an absence of vascular basement membrane while the microfibrils (arrowheads) appear morphologically unaltered. (x 35,000).
(Reduced 30% for reproduction).

reactive surface, it does not appear to be a subendothelial component essential for platelet adhesion; furthermore, it appears to
be a material of low platelet affinity.

Components of the subintima remaining after collagenase
digestion are elastin and the MF, and some evidence indicates
activity to reside with the latter structures. Earlier findings
of Spaet and Erichson (1966) showed failure of purified elastin
to react with platelets in vitro. Moreover, little elastin is
available for hemostatic reactions, since it is largely overlaid
with MF. In vessels digested with collagenase, morphological
evidence points to the MF as the main site of adhesion.

The MF resist prolonged digestion with collagenase, while they are readily destroyed by the action of trypsin. This contrasts with the enzymatic characteristics of collagen fibers, which are digested by collagenase but are unaffected by trypsin (Table I). The electron microscopic appearance of the subendothelial MF as well as the enzymatic characteristics indicate that these are similar to the MF of elastin described in detail by Ross and Bornstein (1969). The amino acid composition of these MF differs markedly from that of both collagen and elastin (Ross and Bornstein, 1969), and can be considered as an additional species of connective tissue (Table I). It appears that at least one function of the MF is to provide a hemostatically active surface.

In discussing the subendothelial components and their thrombogenicity, consideration has been given only to those substances recognized by electron microscopy. Other materials may be both active and electron lucent. In particular, the role of subendothelial proteoglycans remains unexplored.

ALTERED SUBENDOTHELIUM

The morphology and properties of the subendothelium described above apply to the unaltered artery. However, many diseases such as arteriosclerosis are associated with intimal thickening. The manner in which thrombogenesis is altered following such an intimal change is pertinent to the natural history of vascular disease.

As mentioned previously, selected removal of the endothelial covering of an artery produces a carpet of platelets. This initial layer is first the site of a polymorphonuclear leukocytic and then a mononuclear leukocytic reaction which appears to be involved in the removal of the platelets (Baumgartner and Spaet, 1970). After several days, smooth muscle cells are seen migrating through the fenestrae of the IEL, and by seven to ten days the entire surface has been covered by cells similar to endothelial cells (Stemerman and Ross, 1972). The intima is not stable at this point, but continues to grow, forming a dense layer of cicatricial material on the luminal side of the original IEL (Figure 6). The original IEL remains intact and no leukocytes are seen beneath it; no medial damage can be distinguished by electron microscopy. Smooth muscle cell migration has been noted to occur as late as two weeks following injury. After four weeks, the thickness of the injured vessel has almost doubled, with the neointima approximating the media in thickness. The neointima is covered by cells recognized as endothelial cells. Beneath the endothelial cells the neointima consists of smooth muscle cells intermixed with connective tissue elements (Stemerman, 1973). This cellular proliferation appears similar to the early arterial fibromusculoelastic intimal thickening considered by some to precede atherosclerotic change (Movat et al.,

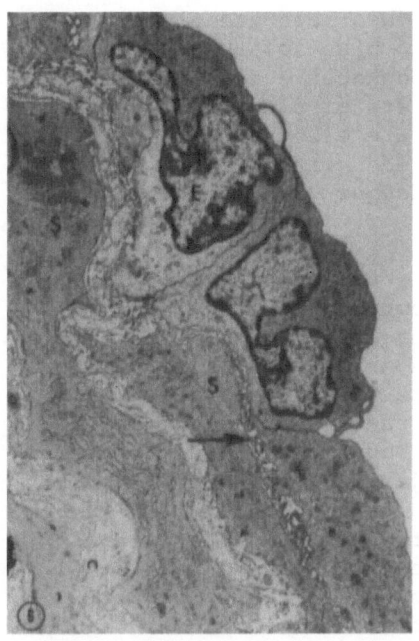 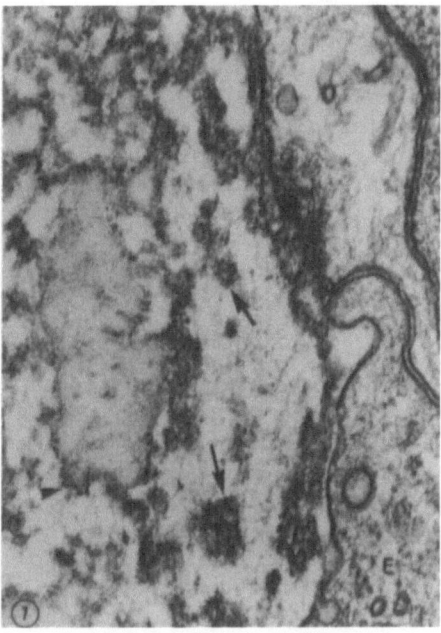

Fig. 6. This electron micrograph shows a section from a rabbit artery injured by balloon catheter and allowed to heal for four weeks; it should be compared to Figure 2 for the alteration in the subendothelium. The endothelia (E) appear more cuboidal than in the non-injured artery, but otherwise retain the usual characteristics. The subendothelium is composed of a variety of connective tissues in random distribution. The elements of the subintima are vascular basement membrane (arrow) and elastin fragments with associated microfibrils; smooth muscle cells (S) are seen in abundance within the neointima, and collagen fibers (C) are seen beneath the neo-subintima. (x 7,500). (Reduced 45% for reproduction).

Fig. 7. This is a higher magnification of the subintimal region from a vessel similar to that shown in Figure 6. The endothelial cells (E) are shown in close contact with the subintima which consists of vascular basement membrane (arrows) and elastin filaments with associated microfibrils (arrowhead). The basement membrane appears to be a granular-material interconnected by a reticulated meshwork. (x 104,000). (Reduced 45% for reproduction).

1958). The thickening is diffuse over the course of the de-endothelialization and has been reproduced in rabbits (Stemerman, 1973), rats (Schwartz et al., in preparation), and primates (Stemerman and Ross, 1972).

The structure of the subintima also has been greatly altered
by this process as shown in Figure 7. In place of the continuous
band of the IEL, there is a complex of connective tissue fragments
and cells. The new subendothelium consists of elastin fragments
with associated MF and material of moderate electron density
similar to BM. Collagen fibers are not seen within the subendothelial area but are found located in the deeper layers of the
experimental plaque (Stemerman, 1973).

Removal of the endothelium from this plaque by balloon
catheter produces a greatly altered thrombogenic response when
compared to a vessel not previously injured and allowed to heal
(Stemerman, 1973). Ten minutes after injury, there is far greater
accumulation of hemostatic material on the plaque vessel. In both
cases, there is a cover of platelets on the denuded surface, but
when cross-sections of the once-injured and plaque-injured vessels
are compared for thrombi, the plaque-injured vessels consistently
exhibit a much greater thrombotic accumulation (Table III). This
heightened thrombogenicity continues for at least three hours.
At this point, thrombi are no longer present on the once-injured
surface, while they persist in reduced numbers in the doubly-
injured vessel. An electron microscopic examination shows that
there is also evidence of an enhanced hemostatic reaction. The
thrombotic mass no longer is composed strictly of platelets;
fibrin strands are present both within the platelet thrombi
and occasionally as a layer interposed between the platelets
and the subendothelium or are buried within the subendothelium
(Figure 8). The configuration of the platelets in relation
to the adhering surface is also altered. Where platelets which
were previously spread in dendritic fashion conform to the
continuous sheath of the IEL, platelet pseudopods now are found to

TABLE III. COMPARISON OF THE THROMBOGENIC RESPONSE OF THE SUB-
            ENDOTHELIUM

	Thrombi at 10 Minutes	Thrombi at 3 Hours	Fibrin	Platelet Adhesion
Once-Injured	Present	Absent	Absent at Subendothelial Surface	Spread and conform to IEL
Healed Re-injured (Plaque)	Very plentiful (three times as plentiful as once-injured vessel)	Present	Present at Subendothelial Surface	Penetrate into the Subendothelium

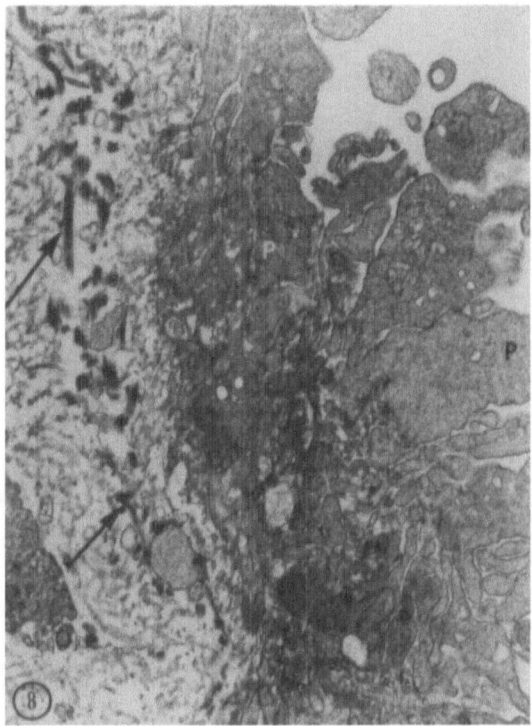

Fig. 8. This rabbit artery has been allowed to heal and was then
de-endothelialized for a second time by balloon catheter. The
vessel was fixed ten minutes after the fresh injury. Platelets (P)
accumulate at the denuded surface and degranulate. Fibrin (arrows)
is found to penetrate the subintima. This electron micrograph
should be compared to Figure 3 for the change in thrombus formation.
(x 20,000). (Reduced 30% for reproduction).

penetrate the plaque's subintima; at times entire platelets are
buried within it (Figure 9). After re-endothelialization the
experimental plaque appears to produce a highly altered, more
intense, and persistent thrombogenicity.

The cause for this alteration in thrombosis is unclear, but
may be related to the following, acting alone or in concert:

1. Alteration of the flow pattern at the surface
2. Ready access to tissue factor
3. Porosity of the altered subendothelium
4. Blood contact with a highly reactive connective tissue
component, hitherto unidentified by electron microscopy.

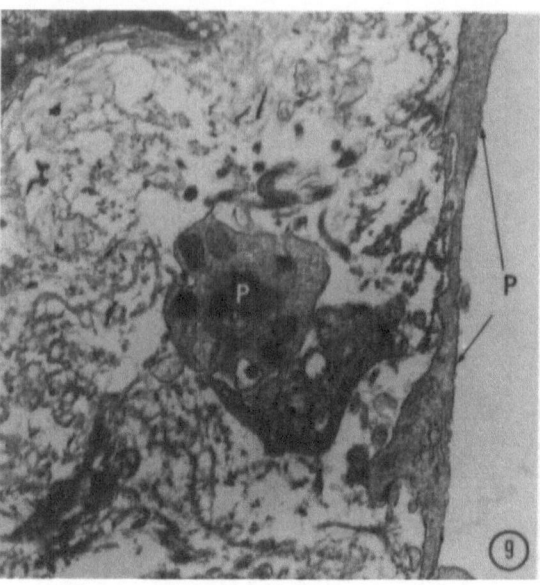

Fig. 9. Platelets (P) cover the subintima. The marked porosity of this region is demonstrated by the platelets which have lodged within the subintima. (x 22,000). (Reduced 30% for reproduction).

Under certain circumstances alteration of intravascular flow appears to enhance the deposition of thrombotic material (Goldsmith, 1972). Arterial flow in the unaltered vessel is streamlined; luminal changes may disrupt streamlining and create an area of low flow known as a captured vortex (Goldsmith, 1972). Disruption of the endothelial cover in the doubly-injured vessel uncovers a highly irregular surface which might modify streamlining and produce such areas of diminished flow. These relatively static regions would hamper the scouring effect of high flow in arterial vessels and thus promote a greater thrombotic mass.

The tendency for platelets to penetrate through and fibrin to form within the subendothelium appears to be related to the highly porous nature of the altered subendothelium. The relationship of this change in platelet conformability to the development of the thrombus is unclear. The porous nature may also provide ready accessibility of tissue clotting constituents that are unavailable in a vessel with an intimal IEL. There is also the possibility that neointimal connective tissue is not detectable by electron microscopy under usual staining techniques. This material may be an uncharacterized proteoglycan and from the standpoint of platelet adhesion might act as a nidus for thrombus formation. The data for the reactivity of proteoglycans with platelets comes from _in vitro_

studies that at times appear contradictory. Muir and Mustard
(1968) showed that digests of proteoglycans had variable effects
on platelet aggregation. Legrand et al. (1967) presented evidence
implying an inhibitory effect by proteoglycans, in contrast with the
data of Spaet (personal communication), which suggests that hyaluronidase or trypsin digestion of human connective tissue fragments
increased their platelet reactivity in vitro.

SUMMARY

Ultrastructurally and biochemically, the subendothelium is a
highly complex structure which, when contacted by blood, provides a
precursor for thrombosis. The connective tissue lining beneath the
endothelium displays a remarkable degree of variability throughout
the vascular tree. This diversity is apparent when the morphologic
entities constituting the subintima (basement membrane, subendothelial microfibrils, and elastin) are listed. These materials each
have a unique enzymatic, biochemical, and thrombotic endowment, properties which are perhaps highly relevant to the thrombogenic
capacity of a vessel involved in a hemostatic process.

The subendothelium also clearly distinguishes itself from collagen fibers by a structural reactive dissimilarity, even though a
collagen-like material may be present. This does not deny the importance of collagen fibers in hemostatic processes not restricted
to the vascular intima, but does limit its importance at the vascular surface. The definition of the role of the various subendothelial constituents continues to unfold, and may remain imprecise
until purified materials can be examined under conditions simulating
the vessel's lumen. In this respect, materials influencing the ability of platelets to aggregate or adhere in vitro may be of minor
consequence in vivo, as readily demonstrated in studies of platelet
suppressant drugs (Harker and Slichter, 1970). This would, of
course, imply that in vitro methods may not be suitable for extrapo-
lation to in vivo conditions.

The arrangement of the reactive ingredients adds to the ultrastructural, as well as the biochemical complexity of the subendothelium. This is best illustrated by the altered thrombogenic response
produced by injury to the rabbit plaque. It appears that the influence of this multifaceted parameter, as well as changes of flow and
blood constituents, produces variability of thrombogenesis within
the arterial vasculature that may be as specific as the difference
between venous and arterial thrombi. The consequences for the
arterial vessel's patency and its embolic potential may be profound.

This discussion implies a heterogeneity of thrombotic disease
which depends upon the location in the vasculature and the condition
of the subendothelium. With this background, a more varied approach
toward the treatment and control of this disease process may emerge.

ACKNOWLEDGEMENTS

These studies were supported by NIH Grant HL 05415. Dr.
Stemerman is a recipient of a Research Career Development Award
(HL 70564-01) from the National Heart and Lung Institute.

The author would like to express his appreciation to Mary Jo
Sweeny for her help in preparing this manuscript.

REFERENCES

Baumgartner, H.R. (1963). Eine Neue Methode zur Erzeugung von
    Thromben durch gezielte Überdehnung der Gefässwand.
    Z. Ges. Exp. Med. 137, 227.

Baumgartner, H.R., and Haudenschild, C. (1972). Adhesion of
    platelets to subendothelium. Ann. N.Y. Acad. Sci. 201, 22.

Baumgartner, H.R., and Spaet, T.H. (1970). Endothelial replacement
    in rabbit arteries. Fed. Proc. 29, 710.

Baumgartner, H.R., Stemerman, M.B., and Spaet, T.H. (1971).
    Adhesion of blood platelets to the subendothelial surface:
    Distinct from adhesion to collagen. Experientia 27, 282.

Bounameaux, Y. (1959). Accolement des plaquettes aux fibres
    sous endotheliales. C.R. Soc. Biol. 153, 865.

Bruns, R.R.,and Palade, G. (1968). Studies on blood capillaries.
    I. General organization of blood capillaries in muscle.
    J. Cell Biol. 37, 244.

Gaynor, E. (1973). (Personal communication).

Gloster, S. (1973). (Personal communication).

Goldsmith, H.L. (1972). The flow of model particles in blood
    cells and its relation to thrombogenesis. In "Progress in
    Hemostasis and Thrombosis" (T.H. Spaet, ed.), Vol. I, p. 97-
    139. Grune and Stratton, New York.

Harker, L.A., and Slichter, S.J. (1970). Studies of platelet and
    fibrinogen kinetics in patients with prosthetic heart valves.
    New Engl. J. Med. 283, 1302.

Hellem, A.J., Borchgrevink, C.F., and Ames, S.B. (1961).
    The role of red cells in hemostasis: The relationship
    between hematocrit, bleeding time and platelet adhesiveness.
    Brit. J. Haematol. 7, 42.

Hoff, H.F., and Gottlob, R. (1968). Ultrastructural changes of large rabbit blood vessels following mild mechanical trauma. Virchows Arch. Abt. A. 345, 93.

Hovig, T., and Holmsen, H. (1963). Release of platelet aggregation substance (adenosine diphosphate) from rabbit blood platelets induced by saline "extracts" of tendons. Thromb. Diath. Haemorrh. 9, 264.

Hugues, J. (1960). Accolement des plaquettes au collagene. C.R. Soc. Biol. 154, 866.

Karrer, H.E. (1961). An electron microscopic study of the aorta in young and in aging mice. J. Ultrastruct. Res. 5, 1.

Kjaerheim, A., and Hovig, T. (1962). The ultrastructure of haemostatic blood platelet plugs in rabbit mesenterium. Thromb. Diath. Haemorrh. 7, 1.

Krakower, C.A., and Greenspon, S.A. (1964). The antigen of capillary venular basement membranes elucidated by the use of lens capsule. In "Small Blood Vessel Involvement in Diabetes Mellitus." Proceedings of the Conference on Small Vessel Involvement in Diabetes Mellitus Held at Airlie House, Warrenton, Virginia, 1963. (M.D. Siperstein et al., eds.), p. 161. Amer. Inst. Biol. Sci. Publ., Washington, D.C.

Kuhnel, W. (1966). Electronenmikroskopische Untersuchungen über den unterschiedlichen Bau der Herzklappen. I. Mitteilung, Mitralis und Aortenklappe. Z. Zellforsch. 69, 452.

Legrand, Y., Caen, J., and Robert, L. (1967). Collagens purifies et plaquettes sanguines(effet de certains "usides" sur l'adhesion et l'aggregation plaquettaire). Nouv. Rev. Fr. Hematol. 7, 879.

Luft, J.H. (1963). Fine structure of the vascular wall. In Evolution of the Atherosclerotic Plaque" (R.J. Jones, ed.), p. 3. University of Chicago Press, Chicago, Illinois.

Majno, G., and Palade, G.E. (1961). Studies on inflammation. I. The effect of histamine and serotonin on vascular permeability. An electron microscopic study. J. Biophys. Biochem. Cytol. 11, 571.

Marcus, A. (1969). Platelet function. New Engl. J. Med. 280, 1330.

Movat, H.A., More, R.H., and Haust, M.D. (1958). The diffuse intimal thickening of the human aorta with aging. Amer. J. Pathol. 34, 1023.

Muir, H., and Mustard, J.F. (1968). Enhancement of platelet
    aggregation by glucosaminoglycans (mucopolysaccharides).
    In "Le Role de la Paroi Arterielle dans l'Atherogenese,"
    p. 589. Centre National de la Recherche Scientifique,
    Paris. Colloques internationaux, No. 169.

Owren, P.A. (1964). Nutrition and thrombosing atherosclerosis.
    Bibl. Nutr. Dieta. 6, 156.

Pierce, G.B. (1966). The development of basement membranes of
    the mouse embryo. Develop. Biol. 13, 231.

Rhodini, J.A.G. (1968). Ultrastructure of mammalian venous
    capillaries, venules and small collecting veins. J.
    Ultrastruct. Res. 24, 425.

Ross, R., and Bornstein, P. (1969). The elastic fiber.
    I. The separation and partial characterization of its
    macromolecular components. J. Cell Biol. 40, 366.

Schwartz, S.M., and Benditt, E.P. (1972). Studies on aortic
    intima. I. Structure and permeability of rat thoracic
    aortic intima. Amer. J. Pathol. 241, 66.

Schwartz, S.M., Stemerman, M.B., and Benditt. (In preparation).
    The aortic intima. II. Cells of regeneration of the rat
    aortic intima.

Spaet, T.H. (1973). (Personal communication).

Spaet, T.H., and Erichson, R.B. (1966). The vascular wall in the
    pathogenesis of thrombosis. Thromb. Diath. Haemorrh.
    Suppl. 21, 67.

Stehbens, W.E., and Biscoe, T.J. (1967). The ultrastructure of
    early platelet aggregation in vivo. Amer. J. Pathol. 50, 219.

Stemerman, M.B. (1973). Thrombogenesis of the rabbit arterial
    plaque: An electron microscopic study. Amer. J. Path 73, 7.

Stemerman, M.B., Baumgartner, H.R., and Spaet, T.H. (1971).
    The subendothelial microfibril and platelet adhesion.
    Lab. Invest. 24, 179.

Stemerman, M.B., and Ross, R. (1972). Experimental arteriosclerosis.
    I. Fibrous plaque formation in primates, an electron
    microscopic study. J. Exp. Med. 136, 769.

Stemerman, M.B., and Spaet, T.H. (1972). The subendothelium and
    thrombogenesis. Bull. N.Y. Acad. Med. 48; 2, 289.

Studer, A. (1966). Experimental platelet thrombus. Thromb. Diath. Haemorrh. Suppl. 21, 109.

Suresh, A., Stemerman, M.B., and Spaet, T.H. (1973). Thrombogenicity of rabbit heart valves: Low platelet reactivity. Blood 41, 359.

Tranzer, J.P., and Baumgartner, H.R. (1967). Filling gaps in the vascular endothelium with blood platelets. Nature 216, 1126.

Virchow, R.L.K. (1860). In "Cellular Pathology," p. 230. Robert M. De Witt, New York.

Wilner, G.D., Nossel, H.L., and Le-Roy, E.C. (1968). Activation of Hageman factor by collagen. J. Clin. Invest. 47, 2608.

DISCUSSION FOLLOWING THE PRESENTATION BY MICHAEL B. STEMERMAN

Dr. Wissler: I think this is a beautiful demonstration of how to use the experimental method and the electron microscope. It may help to explain a puzzling observation that Dr. Kao[1] made in our laboratory a number of years ago when he first started using immunofluorescent techniques to trace various proteins in the vessel wall. He found not only that LDL seemed to be trapped in the intima some way or other, but he very frequently found small amounts of fibrin or fibrinogen that did not seem to be in the correct pattern or correct place to represent organizing mural thrombi. These little clumps were present more often than almost anything else except low density lipoprotein as far as we could tell. I wonder if he was seeing the evidence in human arteries of the kind of reactions that you have described. I suppose if one wanted to define injury in terms of natural disease, the developing atherosclerotic plaque is really an injured area, and that something happens to produce small areas where the process that you have described could take place.

Dr. Stemerman: There is some evidence that there may be a supply of tissue factor available in these areas, and this may account for the polymerization of fibrin.

Dr. Gross: In the repair tissue, does collagen appear in the subendothelium?

---

[1]Kao, V. and Wissler, R. W. (1965). A study of the immuno-histochemical localization of serum lipoproteins and other plasma proteins in human atherosclerotic lesions. Exp. Mol. Pathol. 4, 465.

Dr. Stemerman: In the nonlipid treated animals that we looked at, we did not see any identifiable collagen at the sub-endothelial region at four weeks. These are all four week preparations. If you allow this process to continue, the intimal thickening does regress, and there is almost a reduplication of the injured elastic lamina by about six months. The subendothelial region in these older lesions does contain identifiable collagen fibers.

Dr. Robert: I would like also to congratulate you on these very nice findings. It might be significant in this respect to investigate the chemical nature of the subendothelial "micro-fibrils." We did study in some detail the microfibrils of aortic media which could not be distinguished from the structural glyco-protein preparations.[2,3] Purified structural glycoproteins preparations obtained by the urea-mercaptoethanol procedure[4] were shown to give under the electron microscope "microfibrillar" patterns indistinguishable from those seen in native elastic tissue.[5] Therefore, we undertook recently, in collaboration with Prof. J. Caen and Dr. Y. Legrand, the study of interaction between structural glycoproteins of different tissues and blood platelets.

Dr. Stemerman: When the calcium is removed, the platelet accumulations drop off dramatically. When you remove red cells, again platelet accretions drop dramatically. This latter phenomenon may be related to the availability of ADP. Red cells also may catalyze platelet accumulation by bringing more platelets to the surface.

Dr. Rodbard: This is a beautiful demonstration. Does normal endothelium inhibit subendothelial proliferation of connective tissue?

Dr. Stemerman: I think that is a very good question. I can not give you an answer, but it is something we are investigating. I think that you need some kind of endothelial damage to alter intimal structure. At least it appears that way, and when you let these rabbits age, they appear to change their intima in a manner similar to the intimal changes following injury. These phenomena may be related to some type of endothelial leakage.

---

[2]Atherosclerosis 11, 7-25, (1970).

[3]Eur. J. Biochem. 21, 507-516, (1971).

[4]C. R. Acad. Sci. [D] (Paris) 256, 323-325, (1963).

[5]Kadon, Robert, Robert. Pathol. Biol. (In Print).

IMMUNOLOGICAL PROPERTIES OF CONNECTIVE TISSUE AND SMOOTH MUSCLE CELLS

J. Renais, P. Hadjiisky, and L. Scebat

Centre de Recherches Cardiologiques

Hopital Boucicaut, Paris, France

Previous data from our laboratory have suggested the hypothesis that injury to the arterial wall precedes experimental arterial lesions which closely mimic human atherosclerosis. In order to test this hypothesis we attempted to injure the rat aorta by injections of rabbit antiserum antirat aorta (Scebat et al., 1964a). We found that injections of rat aorta homogenates led to a generalized arteriosclerosis in sensitized rabbits (Scebat et al., 1964b). This finding prompted us to further investigations, the results of which are the subject of this report.

METHODS

Rat, pig, dog, horse, bovine, human, rabbit, chicken, and goose aortas were used. Each vessel was opened longitudinally and divided into segments. After the adventitia was removed, the aortas were homogenized in saline by means of an "ultraturax" homogenizer. The homogenates were distributed for lyophilization in vials containing 10 mg of aorta protein (microkjeldahl). A mixture of 0.5 mg of aorta proteins (using indifferently the whole homogenate or its supernatant) and 0.5 ml of Freund complete adjuvant (FCA) was injected three times a week for five weeks (Renais et al., 1968). In each experiment there was an equal number of control and sensitized animals. In some experiments FCA was omitted. All animals were fed on commercial diets.

Rabbits (New Zealand, Fauves de Bourgone) were immunized with rat, pig, dog, horse (Scebat et al., 1967a), bovine, human, and rabbit aortas (Scebat et al., 1966a), chickens (Patterson) with chicken and goose aortas (Hadjiisky et al., 1972), and mongrel dogs with rat aortas. Tanned cell hemagglutination tests, double diffusion gel precipitation test, complement binding, and delayed hypersensitivity reactions were used as previously described (Scebat et al., 1966b; Renais et al., 1968).

ARTERIAL LESIONS

Macroscopic lesions were observed in rabbits, sometimes as early as the sixth week but usually after the sixth month of study. Lesions were present in 65 percent of the immunized animals, and involved the whole arterial system including visceral arteries and particularly the coronary arteries. The aorta was enlarged both in length and width and was sinuous, rigid and obviously calcified (Figure 1). Aneurysms were scattered along the aortic wall. In most animals normal endothelium was barely visible. Although lesions were widespread, grossly normal areas were apparent and were used for histological and histochemical studies.

Spontaneous macroscopic lesions were seen within the range of 5 to 90 percent of control rabbits. They were almost always restricted to the aortic arch, consequently, only the lesions located below the implantation of ductus arteriosus were considered to have resulted from immunization.

HISTOGENESIS OF THE LESIONS

Rabbit Lesions

In rabbits, lesion morphogenesis was studied in serially killed animals (Tsonev et al., 1972a). Early lesions consisted of edematous foci on both sides of the internal elastic lamina, extending into the media and intima. They were stained with Alcian Blue and were metachromatic. These alterations had been described previously by Szigeti et al. (1960) in rabbits immunized against homologous aorta.

Parallel to the development of metachromatic swelling, changes appeared in the internal elastic membrane and elastic layers of the media. The elastic tissue stained poorly, and elastic fibers were fragmented, resulting in gaps in the elastic membrane. Finally the whole elastic network was disrupted (Figure 2). This association of alcianophilic edema and ruptured elastic fibers is a nonspecific response of mesenchymatous tissues to most aggressions (Hauss et al., 1968).

It was not possible to assess whether the elastic changes or the edema was the first lesion.   Indeed, although muscle cells seemed normal on conventional microscopic examination, histochemistry disclosed enzymatic modifications which perhaps could have triggered elastic changes and/or alcianophilic edema.

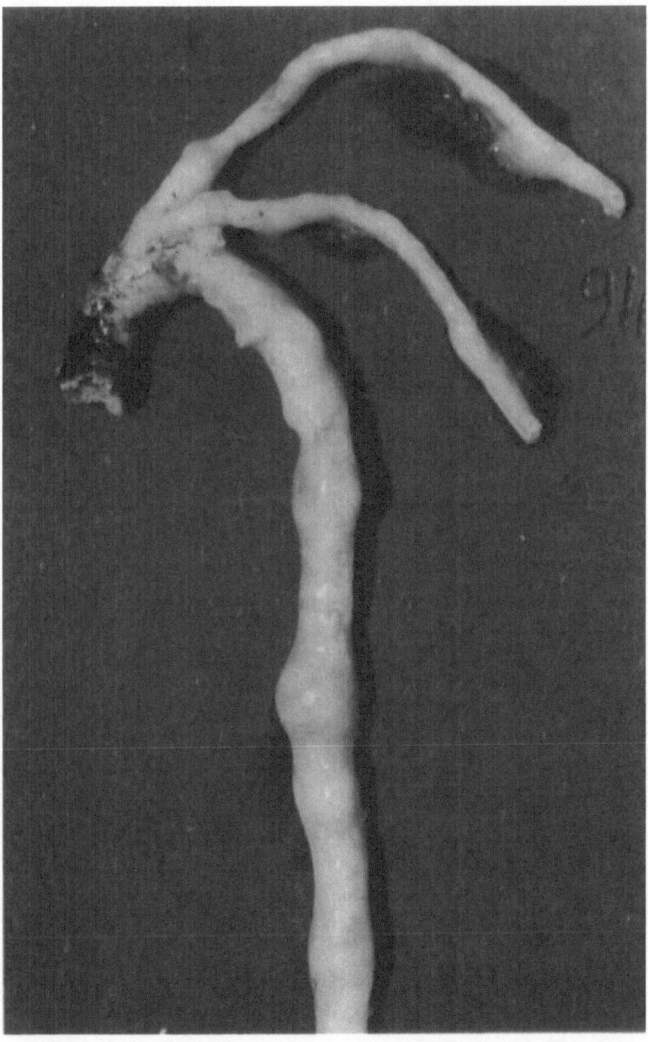

Fig. 1.   Rabbit aorta six months after immunization against bovine aortic media.

Structural changes of muscle cells appeared a little later. Cells
became rounded and radially or longitudinally oriented. In certain
areas they proliferated, stained normally, or became lighter.
Collagen and elastic fibers were destroyed and disappeared within
the areas of cell proliferation, whereas connective tissue fibers
multiplied and crowded around them.

    The early lesion complex resulted in two types of lesions.
In some areas of proliferating cells or metachromatic edema,
smooth muscle cells necrotized, beginning from the inner third of

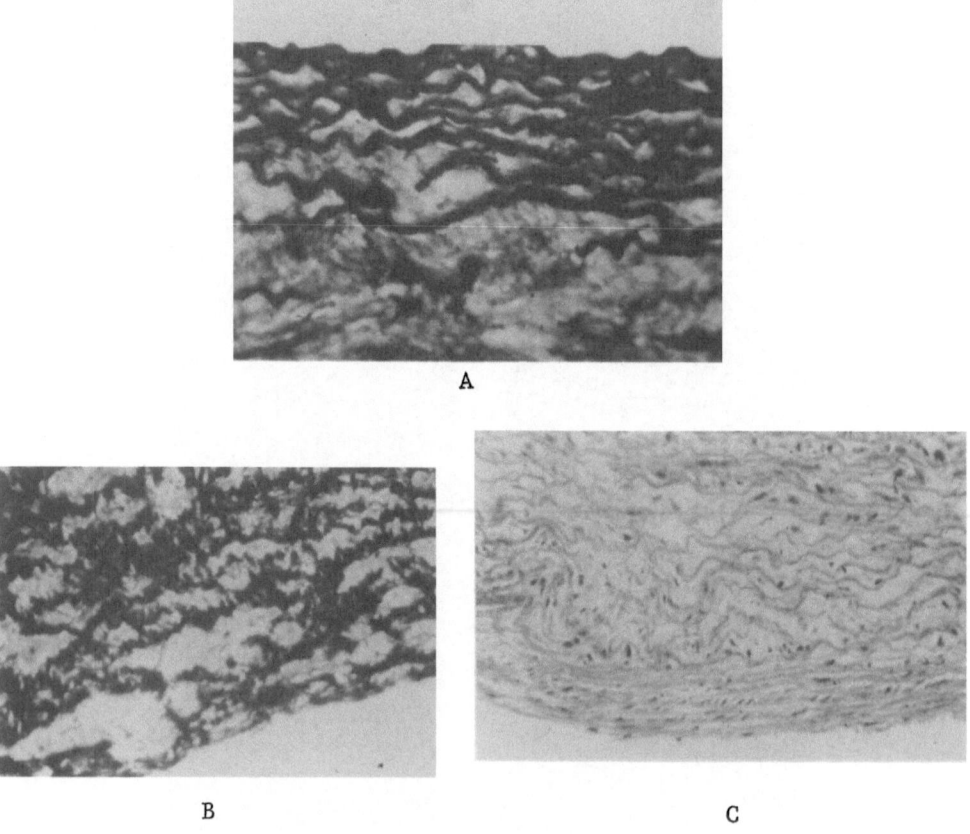

A

B   C

Fig. 2. Alterations of elastic fibers in animal aortas immunized
against heterologous aorta homogenates a) chicken aorta, b) dog
aorta, c) rabbit aorta.

the media (Figure 3). These necrotic foci involved the external
third of the media and/or the intima and at times affected the
whole circumference of the aorta, spreading along the length of the
vessel. At a later stage their center broke down, forming irregular
cavities surrounded by material staining very positively for mucopolysaccharides. In this metachromatic boundary, collagen fibers
proliferated. Medial changes allowed outpouching in the arterial

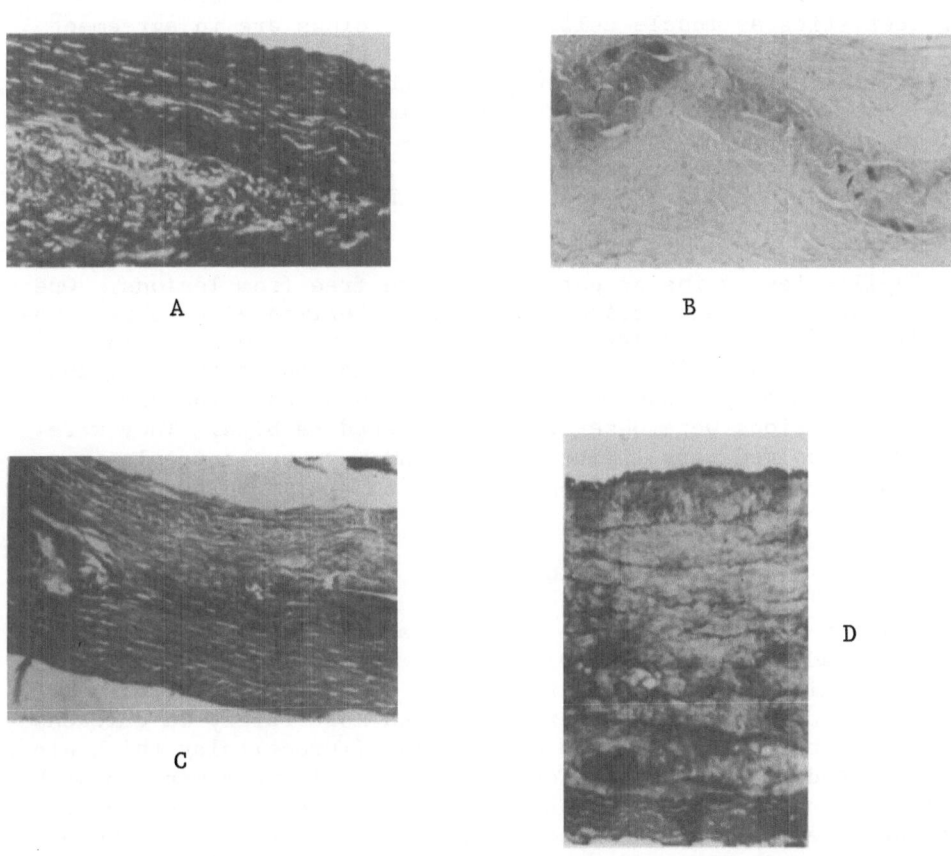

A

B

C

D

Fig. 3. Alterations of smooth muscle cells in animal aortas
immunized against heterologous aorta homogenates a) disorientation
of muscle cells in the middle media (rabbit), b) necrosis in the
middle media of a rabbit immunized six months previously against
rat aorta, c) necrosis with collagen fibers proliferation (rabbit),
d) necrosis near the adventitia in a chicken immunized 10 months
previously against goose aorta.

walls, leading to aneurysm formation. These lesions were repaired
by fibrosis and dystrophic calcification. Sometimes at this stage,
staining with Oil Red O demonstrated secondary deposits of lipid
material in degenerated foci. Not infrequently cell degeneration
developed slowly; cellular elements were reduced in number, became
rounded, and connective fibers multiplied, leading to atrophic
sclerosis with eventual cartilaginous metaplasia and often metamorphosis into bone. Within a given distance of the necrotic
lesions or just close to them a fibrocellular thickening of the
intima occurred. Cells became rounded, disoriented, perpendicular
to the internal elastic lamina, and had the same metabolic
characteristics as muscle cells. These findings are in agreement
with those of Parker (1960) who identified these cells as modified
muscle cells by electron microscopy and those of Knieriem et al.
(1967), who used antimyosin fluorescent immune serum for muscle
cell identification. However, some cells of intimal thickenings
have enzymatic characteristics of endothelial cells, suggesting
that these cells could originate from both endothelial and muscle
cells.

Capillaries, veins or parenchyma were free from lesions. One
of the most outstanding features of this experimental arteritis was
that the whole range of lesions was seen on the same aorta in
rabbits killed 10 to 12 months after immunization, suggesting that
this experimental process is a self-maintained one. The same
elementary lesions were observed in untreated rabbits. They were
discrete, involved very limited areas, and were present only in a
few cross-sections. Only exceptionally did they result in necrosis.

Chicken Lesions

Similar lesions that were seen in rabbits were present in
chickens (Hadjiisky et al., 1972), i.e., metachromatic edema,
broken elastic fibers, and necrosis (not observed in control
animals). However, this pattern was found more rarely in chickens
(16%) than in rabbits. On the other hand, fibrocellular thickenings
of intima and radialized bundles of muscle cells intermingled with
elastic fibers similarly in both. At times when these lesion
patterns were seen in untreated chickens, they were sparse and of
small size in one year old control chickens, while in immunized
chickens of the same age, they were as extensive and advanced as
in untreated four year old chickens.

Dog Lesions

In mongrel dogs, metachromatic edema and disruption of
elastic layers were more advanced than in control animals, yet no
necrosis was ever seen.

IMMUNOLOGICAL TESTS

During sensitization of each of the three animal species, circulating antibodies appeared binding complement, precipitating and giving passive hemagglutination against supernatants of aorta homogenates. The levels, expressed as the reciprocal of the highest dilution that still gave hemagglutination, varied according to species and individuals from 20 to 500 in chickens, from 600 to 20,000 in rabbits, and from 2,000 to 20,000 in dogs.

Using the double diffusion or the passive hemagglutination tests, cross-reactions were observed with serum or tissue homogenates (heart, kidney, liver) of the species of the aorta donor, and with supernatants of aorta homogenates of various species (dog, horse, ox, man, guinea pig, pig, goat, sheep) (Table I). With rabbit aorta the results of passive hemagglutination tests were variable and the levels were low (20 to 80). Nevertheless, the double diffusion test gave always positive results against rabbit aorta. No cross-reactions were observed with serum or tissue homogenates of the species which were not used as aorta donors. Finally, a delayed hypersensitivity test was obtained with heterologous or homologous aorta homogenates; in this case the strongest reactions were usually observed with rabbit aorta (Table I).

TABLE I. CROSS-REACTIONS STUDIED THROUGH PASSIVE HEMAGGLUTINATION AND DELAYED HYPERSENSITIVITY TESTS IN RABBITS SENSITIZED AGAINST RAT AORTA.

PASSIVE HEMAGGLUTINATION   CROSS-REACTIONS

	Rat				Pig/Human or Bovine				Rabbit
	Aorta	Serum	Heart	Liver	Aorta	Serum	Heart	Liver	Aorta
Rabbit Anti-Rat Aorta Anti Serum	10.000	10.000	250	250	1.000	0	0	0	80

DELAYED HYPERSENSITIVITY IN RABBIT SENSITIZED WITH RAT AORTA

	Rat	Horse	Human	Dog	Guinea-Pig	Rabbit
Aorta	+ +	+	+	±	+	+ + +
Heart	+	0	0	0	0	0
Serum	+ +	0	0	0	0	0

SIDE EFFECTS

In addition to developing arteriosclerosis, immunized rabbits
developed hyperlipemia and hypertension. The level of cholesterol,
triglycerides, and beta-lipoproteins increased in rabbits but not
in chickens or dogs. The cholesterol increase was usually moderate
(150 mg/100 ml) and sometimes more intense (250 to 350 mg/100 ml)
(Figure 4). It was generally transient and increased again after
booster injections. Sometimes hypercholesterolemia lasted until
the end of the experiment. These facts were confirmed by Beaumont
and Beaumont (1968); Bricaud et al. (personal communication); and
Robert et al. (1971).

A moderate arterial hypertension was found in 20 percent of
the rabbits in which the blood pressure was measured both before
and during the experiment.

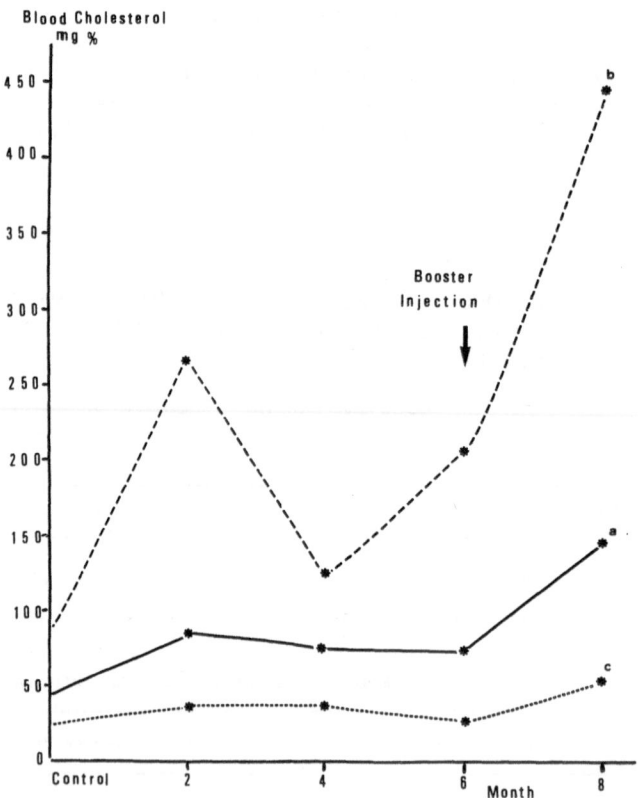

Fig. 4. Serum cholesterol variations in rabbits immunized against
rat aorta a) mean values for the whole group of 20 rabbits, b) maximum variation, c) minimum variation.

NATURE OF ANTIGEN(S)

Immunological Analysis

Rabbit immune serum against pig or human aortas was successively absorbed with 200 mg/ml of lyophilized homologous plasma and
200 mg/ml of homologous liver extract. The absorbed immune serum
no longer reacted against pig or human organ homogenates or plasma.
It gave four precipitation lines by double diffusion tests against
pig or human aortas and these four lines were considered as specific
constituents of aortic tissue. Three of the four lines stained with
Sudan Black and two of these restained with Schiff reagent. Therefore, it seems that these three aortic specific antigens may be
lipoproteins or lipoglycoproteins different from those of serum.
Investigations in progress in our laboratory suggest that these
aortic lipoproteins, studied by electrophoresis or ultracentrifugation, behave like serum lipoproteins.

Using horse aortas, we tried to distinguish the pathogenic
properties of intima from media (Scebat et al., 1967a). Dissection
by means of a sharp knife made it possible to collect most of the
intima. Fragments of media alone were easily removed from the very
large media of horse aorta. Two groups of twenty-four rabbits each
were immunized, one against intima and the other against media
homogenates. Twenty-one percent of the animals immunized against
media and 65 percent of those immunized against intima had aortic
lesions. There were cross-reactions between each of the two immune
sera and each of the two antigens. Antiserum against intima absorbed with horse plasma and liver extract again produced four
lines by the double diffusion test against aortic intima homogenates.
Absorption of this previously absorbed immune serum with horse aorta
media left one single line stained with Sudan Black which might have
been one of the lipoproteins already identified. These data are
similar to those reported by Milgrom et al. (1967) who used bovine
aorta.

Biochemical Analysis

Robert et al. (1968) separated various aortic components,
specifically structural glycoproteins and elastin, by using biochemical dissections. Immunizing rabbits against these components,
they observed aortic lesions; Szigeti et al. (1968) obtained similar
results. Immunization of rabbits with kappa 2 elastin (highly
reticulated) isolated from pig aorta (Moschetto et al., 1969) produced aortic lesions in 100 percent of rabbits sacrificed after the
sixth month of the experiment (Figure 5). On microscopic examination, lesions were similar to those already described. Anti-elastin
immune serum gave one precipitation arc against the supernatant of
pig aorta homogenate by the double diffusion test. This suggests
that the supernatant contains either some protoelastin or some

elastin degradation product (Tsonev et al., 1972b). These findings
make it clear that there are specific components of aortic tissue;
but their true nature and their respective pathogenic power require
further investigations.

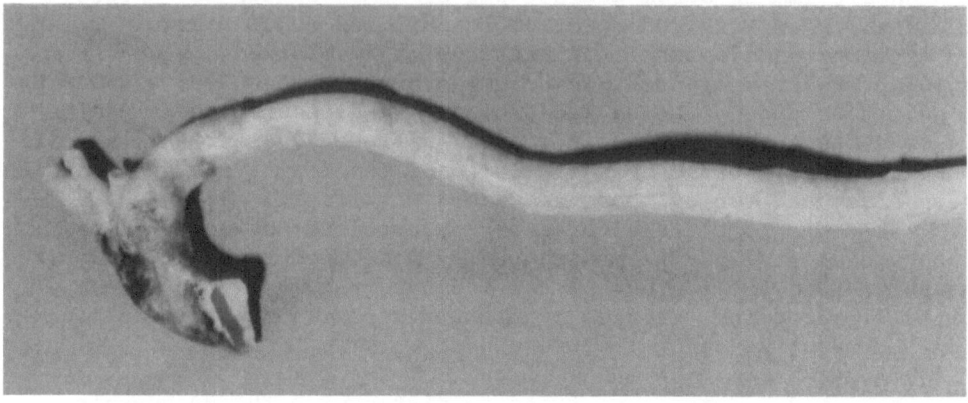

Fig. 5. Rabbit aorta six months after immunization against pig
aorta elastin.

MECHANISMS OF ARTERIAL LESIONS

It was not possible to establish any definite correlation
between the occurrence or severity of the arterial lesions on
the one hand, and the level of circulating antibodies or the
intensity of delayed hypersensitivity reaction on the other hand.
Mild lesions sometimes coincided with a high level of antibodies
or an intensive response to the delayed hypersensitivity test.
Inversely, severe lesions sometimes coincided with very weak
immune reactions. These findings suggest that this immunological
aggression does not act directly on the arterial wall but through
intermediary mechanisms.

Arterial hypertension (by means of a renal mechanism) was
postulated by Wegelius et al. (1970) as the mechanism that produced arterial lesions after immunization of rabbits against
bovine heart homogenate. However, in one of our experiments,
renal lesions were present in only 18 percent and hypertension
in 20 percent of animals at a time when arterial lesions were
observed in 65 percent of the animals. Unquestionably, all hypertensive rabbits had arterial lesions; but, the most severe injuries
affected equally the hyper- and normotensive animals. Therefore
the hypertension hypothesis can no longer be held.

Arterial wall hypoxia could be the intermediary link between immune injury and arterial lesions. As a matter of fact, before any histological change was noted, enzymatic modifications were located in roughly triangular areas with an adventitial base. In these highly metachromatic areas, adenosinetriphosphatase activities were missing. The enzymatic activities of the Kreb's cycle were reduced, whereas, there was an increase in glycolytic (lactic dehydrogenase and aldolase) and lysosomal activities (acid phosphatase). All these findings indicate chronic hypoxia (Adams et al., 1967) and cell sufferance. The topography of these areas suggests constriction of the vasa vasorum which are sometimes surrounded by lymphoid cells. Indeed, such hypoxia is observed in most cases of wall aggressions such as atherosclerosis (Wegmann and Fouquet, 1961), arterial hypertension (Postnov, 1966), and vitamin D intoxication (Lojda, 1965). Many investigators consider hypoxia to be a nonspecific response to various aggressions (Lojda, 1965; Zemplenyi, 1968).

The hypothesis of direct affects on arterial wall of immunization to aortic tissue is supported by the following arguments.

The incidence and severity of the lesions depend upon the intensity of sensitization. Injections of aorta homogenates without FCA during five weeks or with FCA during two weeks induced lesions in only 30 to 35 percent of rabbits, whereas injections of aorta homogenates with FCA during five weeks produced lesions in 65 percent of animals (Renais et al., 1968).

Attempts at proving the immune nature of the process in question gave different results according to the immunosuppressor used. Cortisone given in doses of 2.5 mg/day, one week before sensitization to the end of the experiment reduced the incidence of lesions to 15 percent although this might have been caused by the drug's anti-inflammatory effect. Sheep immunoglobulins against rabbit lymphocytes resulted in septicemia and all animals died within two months. Methotrexate given in doses of 100 mg/day, one week before sensitization to the end of the experiment did not reduce the incidence of lesions. Control experiments showed that, whereas injection of FCA or methotrexate alone produced no lesion, simultaneous injections of both drugs without aortic homogenates produced arterial lesions in 60 to 70 percent of rabbits. Infiltration of adventitia with lymphocyte-like cells were seen in some aortas (Figure 6). Finally, Bricaud et al. (personal communication) stained aortas with sheep anti-rabbit-immunoglobulin and observed fluorescence localized along the elastic fibers. Comparable investigations using peroxidase are in progress in our laboratory.

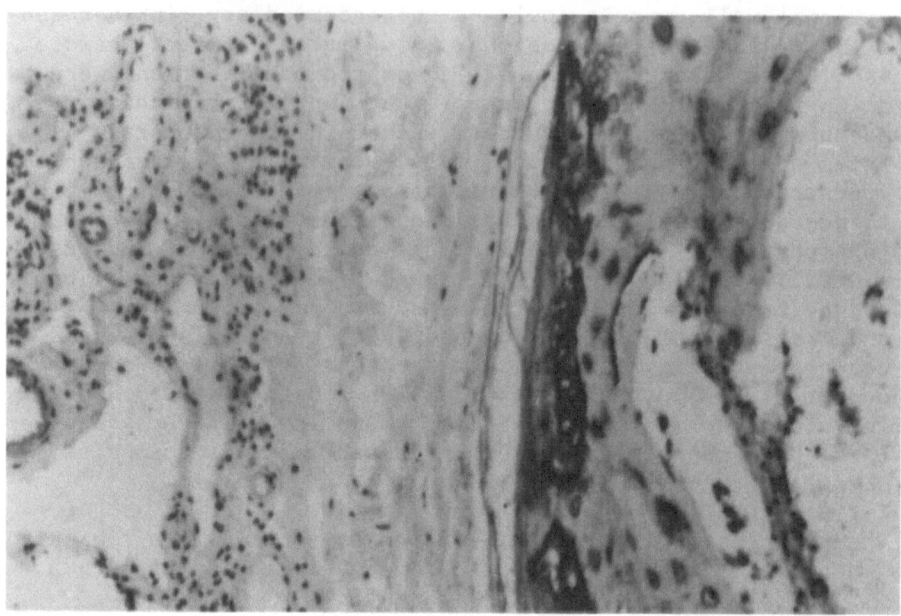

Fig. 6. Accumulation of lymphocyte-like cells in the adventitia
of a rabbit immunized against rat aorta.

NATURE OF THE IMMUNE PROCESS

Assuming the immune nature of this arteriopathy, we have
attempted to define the nature of the immune process under investigation. It might be a nonspecific arterial aggression like
that of serum sickness known for a long time. Dixon (1963)
demonstrated in animals the presence of circulating immune-
complexes which could be transported to the target tissue through
increased permeability of arterial wall (Cochrane, 1971). Robertson
(1967) observed deposits of immunoglobulins in muscle and endothelial aortic cells of rabbits injected with heterologous serum.
On the other hand, immune-complexes-arteritis is characterized by
massive accumulations of polymorphonuclear neutrophil leukocytes
in the intima, together with lesions of the elastic lamina, penetration into the media, and necrosis. However, no neutrophils were
ever seen at any stage during the present experiments. Other
findings are in disagreement with such a mechanism. This arterial
disease was preferentially produced by injecting aortic tissue or
one of its components. Indeed, injecting various tissue antigens
(heart, kidney, liver) serum, or serum components (bovine albumin,
human gamma globulin) with FCA (Scebat et al., 1967b) might produce
in 10 to 20 percent of animals exactly the same arteriopathy

as that described.   Injecting the whole aorta homogenate or
its supernatant induced lesions in 65 percent of rabbits, whereas
when kappa 2 elastin was used the incidence of lesions amounted to
100 percent of the animals sacrificed six months after immunization.
These findings are at variance with those of Wegelius et al. (1970)
who observed aortic lesions in 80 percent of rabbits immunized
against bovine heart, although in rabbits immunized against heterologous aortic tissue the incidence was 10 to 20 percent.   The methodology used by these authors was quite different from ours; e.g. they
injected 200 mg of the homogenate three times a week during three
periods of three weeks each without Freund adjuvant.

The arterial origin of antigens bears a relationship to the
incidence of lesions, and suggests a specific aggression through a
specific antiaortic antibody, perhaps an experimental autoimmune
disease.   This thesis is supported by (1) the presence in sensitized
rabbits of circulating antibodies and delayed hypersensitivity test
against rabbit aorta ("autoimmune" antibodies), (2) the presence in
sensitized chickens of circulating antibodies against chicken aorta,
and (3) the presence of the whole range of lesions of different ages
in aortas of rabbits sacrificed more than one year after priming
injection suggesting "autoimmune" disease (Tsonev et al., 1972a).

An attempt was made to test the possibility of inducing
experimental autoimmune arteritis by changing some aortic component
through a localized aortic trauma.   In this manner, "neoantigens"
may be produced.   Sixty rabbits were divided into three groups.
Two groups were injected with 0.5 ml FCA during two successive days.
On the third day the abdominal aorta was surgically exposed.   A
mechanical, biochemical, or physical trauma was applied on the aorta
below the origin of the left renal artery.   On each of the two
successive days FCA was reinjected again.   In addition, the second
group received methotrexate injections (100 mg/day) beginning one
week before and during the whole experiment.   The third group was
used as a control, undergoing aortic trauma without either FCA or
methotrexate.   All rabbits were sacrificed six months after the
aortic trauma.   In the control animals, lesions were strictly
localized to the injured area.   Sixty-five percent of the adjuvant
injected rabbits had generalized lesions, and in the group treated
with methotrexate the incidence of lesions was reduced to 5 percent
(Scebat et al., 1968).   In this experiment, the immunosuppressive
effect of methotrexate seemed to indicate an immunological nature
of the arteriopathy thus produced.   The results apparently differ
from those obtained in the previously mentioned experiment in
which injection of both methotrexate and FCA induced arteritis.
It seems that the different doses of FCA used might account for
the differences in results.

POSSIBLE APPLICATIONS TO HUMAN ARTERIAL CHANGES

Arterial Lesions in Transplanted Organs

It is well known that during transplant rejection, arteries of the transplants may be affected by diffuse intimal thickening, sometimes circumferential and obstructive. These changes were described in relation to transplanted kidneys (Porter et al., 1963; Hamburger et al., 1967). They were observed in transplanted hearts in dogs (Leandri et al., 1967) and man (Thomson, 1969). The intimal build-up was attributed to various mechanisms such as surgical trauma, transitory wall hypoxia, and thrombi production. Rossen et al. (1971), using immunofluorescent methods, displayed immunoglobulins in thickened intimas. The conclusive experiment of the antigenic properties of aortic components suggests to us the theory of specific arterial tissue rejection; and the demonstration of lymphoid cells in the thickened intima of coronary arteries in rejected heart transplants supports the theory (Hadjiisky et al., 1971).

Aging of Arterial Wall

Some authors (Burnet, 1959; Comfort, 1961; Walford, 1969) set forth the hypothesis that aging may be related to immunological processes. Data supporting this theory have been analyzed by Walford (1969). The following observations made during this experiment in question provide arguments for this assumption with regard to the arterial wall. Thus, a previously mentioned, immunized one year old chickens had intimal and medial changes of the same extent as the lesions naturally occurring in four year old chickens.

In sensitized young rabbits, staining with Alcian Blue demonstrated that intimal thickening appeared rather early and increased with the course of time. In untreated rabbits of the same age such lesions were quite rare, while in three to four year old control rabbits these changes were equally extensive. They stained poorly with Alcian Blue, demonstrating their chronic development. Moreover, in immunized rabbits, certain areas of arterial wall became atrophic; cells were rare and smaller in size and sometimes absent. The bulk of the connective tissue was increased with rupture of elastic fibers and metachromasia. These lesions could be the after-effects of slowly evolutive degeneration. Their histologic patterns resembled those described in man (Rottino, 1940; Carlson et al., 1970) and are probably related to age. Finally, quantitative analysis of acid mucopolysaccharides in aortas of immunized young rabbits showed a reduction of hyaluronic acid/chondroitin sulfate B ratio (Hillion et al., 1969) as in normal old rabbits. All the above findings are interpreted as meaning that immune processes may accelerate the aging of arterial wall.

Role of Immune Processes in Human Arterial Diseases

It has been suggested that immune processes may play a role in the development of some human arterial diseases such as polyarteritis nodosa or Takayasu's disease. However, our current research theme revolves around the hypothesis that in certain patients the accelerated course of atherosclerosis may be related to an immune or autoimmune process.

Indeed, arterial hypertension, increased circulating catecholamines in relation with psychial behavior, thrombogenic disease (Duguid, 1946) and decreased arterial wall fibrinolytic power (Astrup, 1968) have been described as agents accelerating the course of human atherosclerosis.

Furthermore, we assume that both immune and autoimmune mechanisms may accelerate the course of atherosclerosis as well. During life, arteries undergo various type of aggressions (toxic, toxinic, allergic, etc.) which may change the structure of the tissue components, resulting in unmasking of concealed antigenic sites. These fragments behave like "neoantigens," inducing antibody production.

In agreement with Szigeti et al. (1968), in some patients we found circulating antibodies at levels reaching 250, positive delayed hypersensitivity test, and positive lymphoblastic transformation test against human aortas. Obviously, these antibodies are just evidence of arterial lesions. It may also happen that in some patients repeated aggressions or a change in the antibody forming system may transform these antibodies into pathogenic ones. Moreover, Mitchell and Schwartz (1965) noted round cell infiltration of adventitia in relation with human atherosclerotic plaques.

Thus the autoimmune process by injurying undamaged areas of arterial tissue would precipitate the development of atherosclerosis if one accepts, as we do, that changes in the arterial wall do precede the build-up of atherosclerosis.

REFERENCES

Adams, C.W.M., Bayliss, O.B., and Orton, C.C. (1967). J. Atheroscler. Res. 7, 567.

Astrup, T. (1968). In "Le Rôle de la Paroi Artérielle dans l'Athérogénèse." p. 535. C.N.R.S., Paris.

Beaumont, V., and Beaumont, J.L. (1968). Pathol. Biol. 16, 869.

Bricaud, H. (Personal Communication).

Burnet, M. (1959). Brit. Med. J. 2, 720.

Carlson, R.G., Lillehei, C.W., and Edwards, J.E. (1970). Amer.
    J. Cardiol. 25, 411.

Cochrane, C.C. (1971). J. Exp. Med. 134, 75.

Comfort, A. (1961). Amer. Heart J. 62, 293.

Dixon, F. (1963). Harvey Lecture 58, 21.

Duguid, J.B. (1946). J. Pathol. Bact. 58, 207.

Hadjiisky, P., Scebat, L., Renais, J., Cachera, J.P., Dubost, C.,
    and Lenegre, J. (1971). Revue Europ. Etud. Clin. Biol. 16,
    596.

Hadjiisky, P., Renais, J., and Scebat, L. (1972). Pathol. Europ.
    7, 131.

Hamburger, J., Crosnier, J., and Dormont, J. (1967). Ann. N.Y.
    Acad. Sci. 120, 538.

Hauss, W.H., Junge-Hulsing, G., and Gerlach, U. (1968). In
    "Le Rôle de la Paroi Artérielle dans l'Athérogénèse."
    p. 745, C.N.R.S. Paris.

Hillion, P., Renais, J., Hadjiisky, P., Maurice, P., and Scebat,
    L. (1969). Revue l'Athérosclér. Arteriopathies Peripheriques
    11, 58.

Knieriem, H.J., Kaov, C.Y., and Wissler, R.W. (1967). Arch.
    Pathol. 84, 118.

Leandri, J., Cachera, J.P., Locombe, M., Bui-Mong-Hung, Vigano, M.,
    and Haradas, S. (1967). Pathol. Biol. 15, 501.

Lojda, Z. (1965). In "Morphology and Histochemistry of the
    Vascular Wall." International Symposium, Fribourg, 1965.
    (Comel, M., and Laszt, L., eds.) Vol. II., Karger, Basel,
    N. Y.

Milgrom, F., Intorp, H.N., and Witebsky, T. (1967). J. Immunol.
    99, 164.

Mitchell, J.R.A., and Schwartz, C.J. (1965). In "Arterial
    Disease." Blackwell, Oxford.

Moschetto, Y., Davril, M., and Biserte, G. (1969). Revue
l'Athéroscler. Arteriopathies Peripheriques 11, 44.

Porter, K.A., Owen, K., Mowbray, J.F., Thomson, W.F., Kenyon, J.R.,
and Peart, W.S. (1963). Brit. Med. J. 14, 639.

Parker, F. (1960). Amer. J. Pathol. 36, 19.

Postnov, J.W. (1966). Virchow. Arch. Pathol. Anat. Physiol. 341,
237.

Renais, J., Groult, N., Scebat, L., and Lenegre, J. (1968). In
"Le Rôle de la Paroi Artérielle dans l"Athérogénèse." p. 323.
C.N.R.S., Paris.

Robert, L., Robert, M., Moczar, M., and Moczar, E. (1968). In
"Le Rôle de la Paroi Artérielle dans l'Athérogénèse." p. 395.
C.N.R.S., Paris.

Robert, A.M., Grosgogeat, Y., Reverdy, V., Robert, B., and Robert,
L. (1971). Atherosclerosis 13, 427.

Robertson, A.L. (1967). In "Lipid Metabolism in Tissue Culture
Cells." Wistar Institute Symposium, Philadelphia, 1966.
(Rothblat, G.H., and Kritchevsky, D. eds.) Vol. 6, 115.

Rossen, R.D., Butler, W.T., Reisberg, M.A., Brooks, D.K., Leachman,
R.D., Milam, J.D., Mittal, K.K., Montgomery, J.R., Nora, J.J.,
and Rochelle, D.G. (1971). J. Immunol. 106, 171.

Rottino, A. (1940). Amer. Heart J. 19, 330.

Scebat, L., Renais, J., Groult, N., Iris, L., and Lenegre, J. In
"Enzymologie et Immunologie dans l'Athérosclérose." Colloque
International Bordeaux. (1964a). p. 247; J.B. Bailliere,
Paris, 1967.

Scebat, L., Renais, J., Groult, N., Iris, L., and Lenegre, J. In
"Enzymologie et Immunologie dans l'Athérosclérose." Colloque
International Bordeaux. (1964b). p. 249; J.B. Bailliere,
Paris.

Scebat, L., Renais, J., Iris, L., Groult, N., and Lenegre, J.
(1966a). Revue l'Athérosclér. Arteriopathies Peripheriques
8, 56.

Scebat, L., Renais, J., Groult, N., Iris, L., and Lenegre, J.
(1966b). Revue Fr. Etud. Clin. Biol. 11, 806.

Scebat, L., Renais, J., and Groult, N.   (1967a).   Revue l'Athéro-
    scler. Arteriopathies Peripheriques 9, 50.

Scebat, L., Renais, J., Groult, N., and Lenegre, J.   (1967b).   In
    "The Reticuloendothelial System and Atherosclerosis." (DiLuzio
    N. R. and Paoletti, R. eds.), p. 451.   Plenum Press, New York.

Scebat, L., Renais, J., Iris, L., Groult, N., and Lenegre, J.   (1968).
    In "Le Rôle de la Paroi Artérielle dans l'Athérogénèse." p. 425,
    C.N.R.S., Paris.

Szigeti, L., Ormos, J., Jako, J., and Toszegi, A.   (1960).   Acta
    Allergol. Suppl. VII, 374.

Szigeti, L., Piko, C., and Doman, J.   (1968).   In "Le Rôle de la Paroi
    Arteriélle dans l'Athérogénèse." p. 493.   C.N.R.S., Paris.

Thomson, J.C.   (1969).   Lancet 2, 1297.

Tsonev, I., Hadjiisky, P., Renais, J., and Scebat, L.   (1972a).
    Pathol. Biol. 20, 383.

Tsonev, I., Hadjiisky, P., Renais, J., and Scebat, L.   (1972b).
    Z. Forsch.Mikrosk. Anat. 86, 177.

Walford, R.L.   (1969).   "The Immunologic Theory of Aging."
    Munksgaard, Copenhagen.

Wegelius, O., Jokinen, E.J., Vonknorring, J., and Friman, C.
    (1970).   Ann. Med. Exp. Biol. Fenn. 48, 3.

Wegmann, R., and Fouquet, J.P.   (1961).   Ann. Histochim. 6, 61.

Zemplenyi, T.   (1968).   In "Enzyme Chemistry of the Arterial Wall."
    p. 145.   Lloyd-Luke, London.

DISCUSSION FOLLOWING THE PRESENTATION BY J. RENAIS

Dr. Chobanian: Have you ever seen arterial changes with
immunological injury in those animals that became hypertensive?
Furthermore, do you think that the hypertension is due to renal
damage from immunological injury or is there some other mechanism
involved?

Dr. Renais: I don't know the mechanism of this hypertension.
Some rabbits had nephrocalcinosis with intrarenal arterial alterations. On the other hand, all the hypertensive rabbits had calcified lesions of the whole arterial tree, perhaps accounting for an
increase in systemic resistance.

Dr. Wissler: I would like to pay tribute to this immense amount of very interesting work and extend a little further the question asked by Dr. Chobanian. The hypercholesterolemia that you describe occurred, I assume, without cholesterol in the diet. It does seem that renal injury with some degree of nephrosis and perhaps some degree of hypertension would be compatible. I just wondered if you had another explanation for the hypercholesterolemia that the rabbits showed?

The second question I would like to ask is how firm do you think your evidence is that autoantibodies are producing the damage to the arteries versus cellular immunity or "killer" lymphocytes.

Dr. Renais: I don't know the cause of the hyperlipemia in the immunized animals. This hyperlipemia was observed during immunization against other antigens, particularly tissue. But it was stronger when the antigen was arterial tissue. I have no sure evidence of an autoimmune process. However, there were cross-reactions with rabbit arterial tissue, and in our experiments cellular immunity is demonstrated, I think, by the positivity of delayed hypersensitivity tests. But this fact does not exclude the hypothesis of an autoimmune mechanism. Finally it is not, I think, an immune complex disease because of the absence of lymphocytic infiltration in the intima.

Dr. Robert: Immunoglobulins have been demonstrated by immunofluorescence in the sclerotic human lesion (Exp. Geront. 5, 339-356, 1970). Nobody, to my knowledge at least, has as yet demonstrated systematically appearing lymphocytic infiltrates in the arteriosclerotic plaques. Passive transfer of anti-aorta immune-sera to unimmunized animals also induced sclerotic lesions (Renais et al. (1968). In "Le Role de la Paroi Arterielle dans l'Atherogenese." Colloque C.N.R.S., Paris. p. 323). These are the main arguments in favor of a humoral mechanism.

Dr. Berenson: Have you used any specific glycoprotein fractions that are isolated from aortas and are capable of producing antibodies to see if they will produce arterial injury?

Dr. Renais: The immunization with specific aorta glycoproteins is in progress in our laboratory. There are anti-glycoprotein antibodies, but we still have not sacrificed the immunized rabbits.

Dr. Robert: Similar lesions to those obtained with elastin were produced by immunizing rabbits with urea-mercaptoethanol extracted structural glycoproteins of the aorta. The frequency of the lesions was however lower than with elastin (Atherosclerosis 13, 427-449, 1971).

IMMUNOLOGIC INJURY AND ATHEROSCLEROSIS

C. Richard Minick and George E. Murphy

Department of Pathology

The New York Hospital-Cornell Medical Center, New York

Injury to the arterial wall is probably a primary causative factor in arteriosclerosis (Anitschkow, 1933; Duff, 1935; Rössle, 1944; Hass, 1955; Taylor, 1955; Waters, 1955; Constantinides, 1965; Minick et al., 1966; Haust, 1971; Minick and Murphy, 1973). Injury, the resulting inflammation, and subsequent repair may favor the deposition and accumulation of blood-borne lipid at the site of injury. Therefore, it is essential for our understanding of human arteriosclerosis to discover the causes of injury and the nature of the local reactive changes that may be important in man. In this regard Dr. McMillan (this publication) reminded us earlier that the reaction of arterial mesenchyme to syphilitic injury could lead to atherosclerosis. Moreover, rheumatic injury to the aorta, heart valves, and coronary arteries can lead to atherosclerosis of these structures (Zeek, 1932; Murphy, unpublished observations, 1973). Data obtained from clinical observations and from experiments indicate that immunological injury plays an important role in the pathogenesis of rheumatic cardiovascular disease (Murphy, 1960) and also may be important in the pathogenesis of syphilitic cardiovascular disease (Chesney, 1926). Finally, immunological reactions are known to cause release of vasoactive substances that may alter vascular permeability and thereby favor deposition of blood-borne lipid in the arterial wall (Kniker and Cochrane, 1965; Cochrane, 1971). Thus, an immunological response to many antigens including those in infecting microorganisms, vaccines, antibiotics, and other drugs, foods, and tobacco, as well as immunological response to substances in one's own tissues may be an important causative factor in an even greater amount of arterial disease in man, some of which may evolve as athero-arteriosclerosis.

For several years we have investigated the role that arterial

355

changes caused by immunological injury might play in the production
of atherosclerosis. Results of our experiments demonstrate that
the synergy of immunological injury to arteries and hypercholesterolemia can lead to atherosclerosis in rabbits. In many instances
the arterial lesions bear close resemblance to atherosclerosis in
man (Minick et al., 1966; Alonso et al., 1970; Minick and Murphy,
1973; Hardin et al., 1973). The purpose of this communication is
to report on results of these experiments.

    Immunological injury to arteries was induced by repeated
injections of foreign serum protein or graft rejection. Hypercholesterolemia was induced by feeding cholesterol-supplemented
or semi-synthetic lipid-rich, cholesterol-poor diets. Aortas,
pulmonary arteries, and cardiac valves were examined grossly at
the time of autopsy and visible atherosclerotic change quantitated.
Hearts were cut into approximately twelve blocks and sections of
coronary arteries in each block were examined microscopically.
In some experiments, sections of splenic, gastric, mesenteric,
femoral, subclavian, hepatic, renal, carotid, cerebral, and pulmonary
arteries and aortas were also examined microscopically. Arterial
lesions were tabulated as to the size of the artery involved and the
histologic character of the lesion. In this report we will discuss
changes in aortas and coronary arteries in detail. The changes
in coronary arteries will be emphasized because of the predilection
of immunological injury to involve coronary arteries and the special
importance of coronary atherosclerosis as a cause of morbidity and
mortality in man.

    In the initial experiments (Minick et al., 1966), immunological
injury to arteries was induced in 55 rabbits by four intravenous
injections of 10 ml horse serum/kg body weight at intervals of 16
to 18 days. To assess the effect of immunological injury alone,
17 of the serum injected rabbits were fed commercial rabbit ration
low in lipid (Group II). To investigate the possible synergistic
effect of immunological injury and hypercholesterolemia, the
remaining 38 rabbits were injected with foreign serum and concomitantly fed a diet supplemented with 0.5% cholesterol by weight
(Group III). To assess the effect of hypercholesterolemia alone,
25 rabbits were fed the cholesterol-supplemented diet for a period
of approximately 80 days but were not injected with horse serum
(Group I). Feeding the cholesterol-supplemented diet resulted in
an increase in the average serum cholesterol to approximately 700
mg% in both groups of rabbits (Groups I and III). Serum cholesterol levels remained normal in rabbits of Group II.

    At autopsy no grossly visible changes were seen in the linings
of the aortas from rabbits of Group II. Rabbits of Groups I and
III developed grossly visible yellow-white fatty streaks and

plaques in the aortas. There was a greater amount of fatty change
in aortas of rabbits that received the dietary supplement of
cholesterol and concomitant injections of foreign serum (Group
III) than in the group that received the cholesterol supplement and
no foreign serum (Group I). The greatest difference between the
two groups was in the thoracic aorta. Thus, of the 16 thoracic
aortas examined of Group I, a marked amount of fatty change was
present in four, or 25%; an intermediate amount in five, or 31%;
and a slight amount in seven, or 44%. In contrast, of the 21
thoracic aortas examined of Group III, a marked amount of fatty
change was present in 15, or 71%; an intermediate amount in five,
or 24%; and a slight amount in one, or 5%.

Lesions of the coronary arteries in rabbits of Group I were
confined almost solely to the small arteries. Ninety-six percent
of the lesions occurred in small vessels and the remaining 4%
were in medium-sized arteries. Microscopically these were fatty
lesions comprised of lipid laden intimal and medial cells with
little or no proliferative change (Figure 1). In rabbits of Group
II changes were present throughout the arterial tree; 22% of
lesions in large arteries, 36% in medium-sized arteries, and 42%
in small arteries. Microscopically these were proliferative
lesions without fatty change; they comprised musculoelastic hyper-
plastic intimal changes, focal fragmentation and/or reduplication
of the internal elastic membrane, degenerative changes in the
media, focal thinning and scarring of the media and cellular proliferative and infiltrative change and fibrosis in the adventitia
(Figure 2). In rabbits of Group III changes were also present
throughout the coronary arterial tree with 29% in large arteries,
33% in medium-sized arteries, and 38% in small arteries. These
changes were of three types - fatty, proliferative, and fatty-
proliferative. The vast majority were fatty-proliferative; they
accounted for 90% of the arterial lesions. These lesions were
similar to the proliferative changes but principally differed from
them by the presence of lipid in intimal and medial cells and by
fatty-hyaline intimal change, sometimes with lack of or little
elastification. Some of the fatty-proliferative lesions resembled
human atherosclerosis (Figures 3 and 4). Changes in the renal,
mesenteric, and splenic arteries of Groups II and III were similar
to those in the coronary arteries. In rabbits of Group I, however,
only very occasional fatty lesions in small arteries were found
in vascular beds other than the coronaries.

Thus, both with respect to their proliferative character and
their distribution in the coronary arterial tree, the lesions
in rabbits of Group III were unlike those in Group I, but similar
to those in Group II. Since rabbits in both Groups II and III
were similarly injected with horse serum, it is reasonable to infer

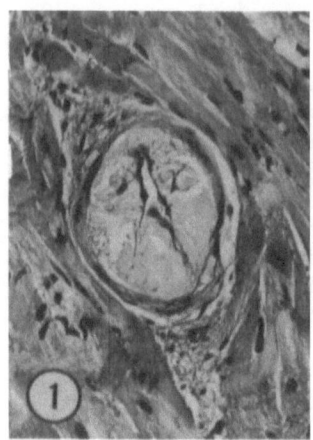 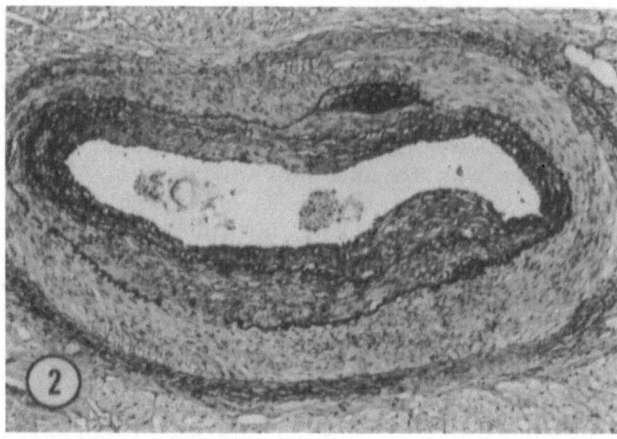

Fig. 1.   Fatty, virtually acellular lesion in small myocardial
artery of a rabbit fed cholesterol-rich diet for 80 days.   This
is the characteristic arterial lesion induced in the hearts of
rabbits by cholesterol-rich diet or semi-synthetic lipid-rich,
cholesterol-poor diet alone.   H & E. (x 200).   (Reproduced with
permission from Hardin et al., 1973, and the American Journal of
Pathology).

Fig. 2.   Characteristic musculoelastic intimal thickening induced
in a main coronary artery of a rabbit by repeated injections of
foreign serum over many months.   H & E. (x 78).   (Reproduced with
permission from Minick and Murphy, 1973, and the American Journal
of Pathology).

that in Group II, in the absence of a large amount of lipid in the
blood, proliferative lesions without fatty change developed at sites
of immunological injury; whereas in Group III, in the presence of
a large amount of lipid in the blood, fatty-proliferative lesions
evolved at some sites of immunological injury.   The inference is
supported by the observation that in Group I elevation of serum
lipids similar to that in Group III induced in the absence of
immunological injury arterial lesions that were only fatty and
limited almost solely to small arteries, never large arteries.

     In the experiments outlined above, rabbits were injected
repeatedly with foreign protein at intervals of two to three weeks
and concomitantly fed a dietary cholesterol supplement for as long
as 80 days.   The average serum cholesterol level was approximately
700 mg%.   In man, the amount of hypercholesterolemia is rarely this
great; and, as compared with the arterial injuries induced in those
rabbits, arterial injuries in man are likely to be more protracted
or recurrent at longer intervals over a much longer period of time.

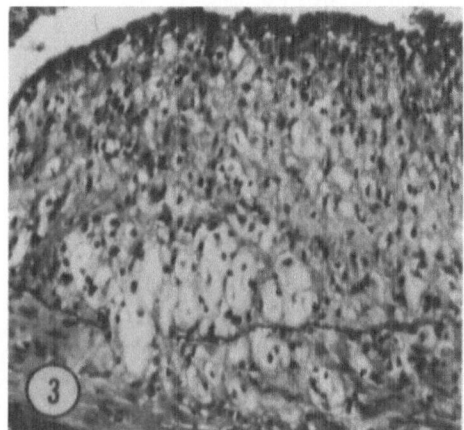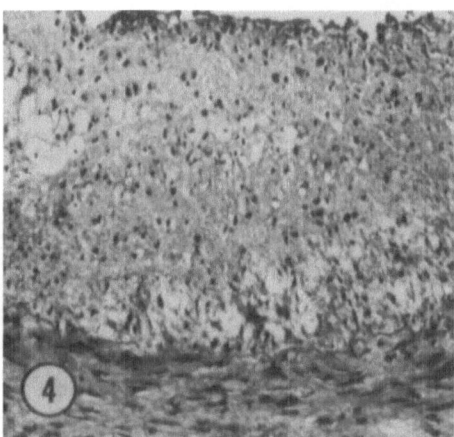

Fig. 3. Fatty-proliferative changes induced in a main coronary
artery of a rabbit by repeated injections of foreign serum and concomitant feeding of cholesterol-rich diet over a period of 82 days.
Elastic stain. (x 153). (Reproduced with permission from Minick
et al., 1966, and the Journal of Experimental Medicine).

Fig. 4. Fatty-proliferative changes in a main coronary artery of a
35 year old man with mitral and aortic stenosis and marked coronary
atherosclerosis. H & E. (x 120). (Reproduced with permission
from Minick et al., 1966, and the Journal of Experimental Medicine).

        Accordingly, it appeared reasonable to hypothesize that athero-
sclerosis even more closely resembling that in man could be induced
in rabbits by more chronic arterial injury in combination with a
lipid-rich diet, resulting in an amount of blood cholesterol of the
same magnitude as that in man. In more recently completed long-
term experiments (Minick and Murphy, 1973), chronic atherosclerosis
bearing marked similarity to that in man was induced in rabbits by
the combined action of foreign protein injected repeatedly at intervals of four to eight weeks and semi-synthetic lipid-rich, cholesterol-poor diets fed concomitantly for as long as 17 months. One
diet contained 16 to 22% hydrogenated coconut oil and 3% corn oil,
and the other contained 24% lard. By actual analysis the cholesterol content of these diets was 0.003% and 0.016%, respectively.

        Feeding the semi-synthetic lipid-rich diets to rabbits of
Groups I and III resulted in an increase of blood cholesterol from
the normal range of 50 to 80 mg% for rabbits to values averaging
between 200 to 250 mg% throughout the course of the experiment (Text-
Figure 1). This latter value is the average concentration for blood
cholesterol in adult humans in the United States. The average level
of serum cholesterol for the 66 rabbits fed lipid-rich diet alone
(Group I) did not differ from that for the rabbits fed the lipid-

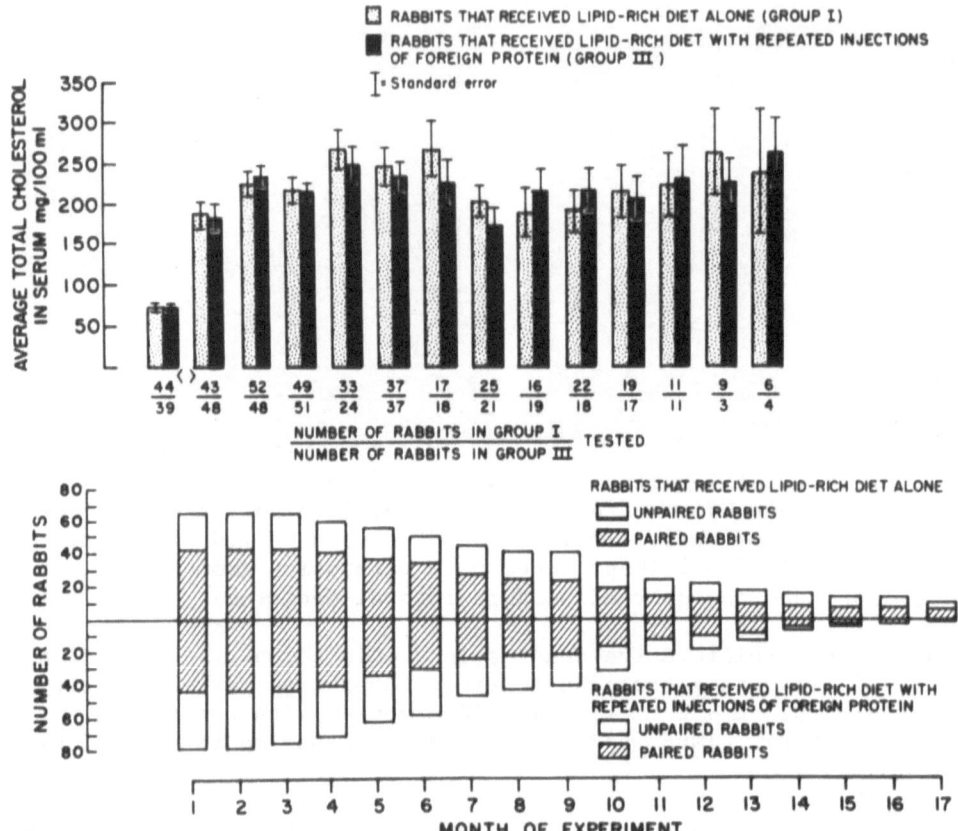

Text Fig. 1. Upper portion of figure shows average total cholesterol in serum of rabbits in Groups I and III. Lower portion shows
that the number of rabbits in Groups I and III was similar throughout the experiment. (Reproduced with permission from Minick and
Murphy, 1973, and the American Journal of Pathology).

rich diet and injected with foreign serum protein (Group III).
Serum cholesterol levels remained normal in 29 rabbits (Group II)
fed lipid-poor, commercial rabbit ration.

As in the experiment reported above, aortas of rabbits fed a
lipid-rich, cholesterol-poor diet and concomitantly injected with
foreign serum protein (Group III) exhibited significantly greater
atherosclerotic change in the ascending thoracic, descending thoracic, and abdominal portions than did those of animals fed the same
diet (Group I) but without injections of foreign serum protein
(Text-Figure 2). In the fatty-proliferative lesions of Group III,
there were degenerative changes including fatty change and necrosis
of sub-intimal smooth muscle, fragmented elastic lamellae, and proliferated intimal and sub-intimal cells. In some rabbits of Group III

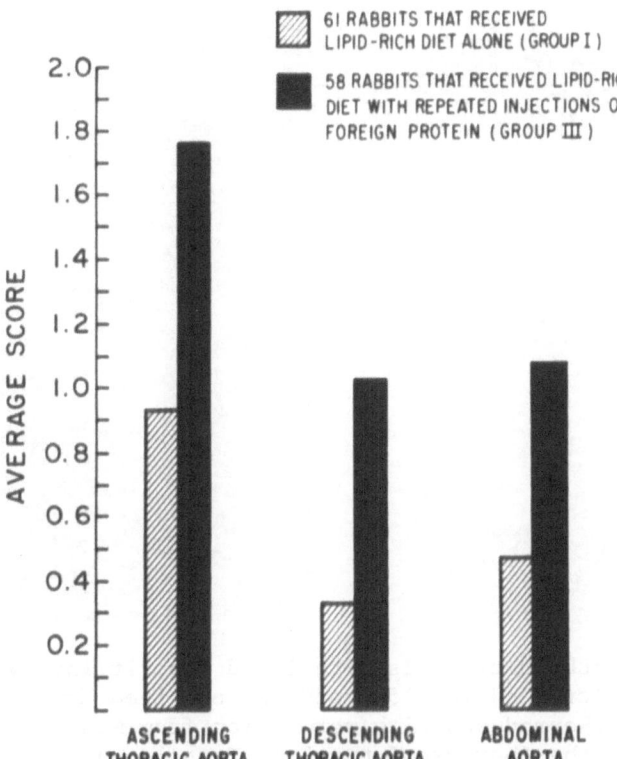

Text-Fig. 2. Average score is an index of the amount of grossly visible streaks and plaques in all three segments of aortas of rabbits in Groups I and III. (Reproduced with permission from Minick and Murphy, 1973, and the American Journal of Pathology).

even more advanced fatty-proliferative atherosclerosis of the aorta with fatty-hyaline intimal and medial change, and pools of lipid deep in the arterial wall was encountered. These changes strikingly resembled aortic atherosclerosis in man (Figures 5 and 6).

As in the previous experiments, rabbits of Group III that were repeatedly injected with foreign serum protein and concomitantly fed a lipid-rich, cholesterol-poor diet, developed coronary arterial lesions that were different both in quality and distribution from those in rabbits fed the same lipid-rich diet but not injected with foreign protein (Group I), and similar in distribution and proliferative character to those in rabbits injected with foreign protein and fed a lipid-poor diet (Group II). Thus, as in the previous experiments there was strong evidence that the lesions of Group III represented immunologically induced lesions that had acquired lipid to evolve as atherosclerosis. Results of these experiments differed from those described earlier, in that the fatty-proliferative lesions of Group III in the latter experiments

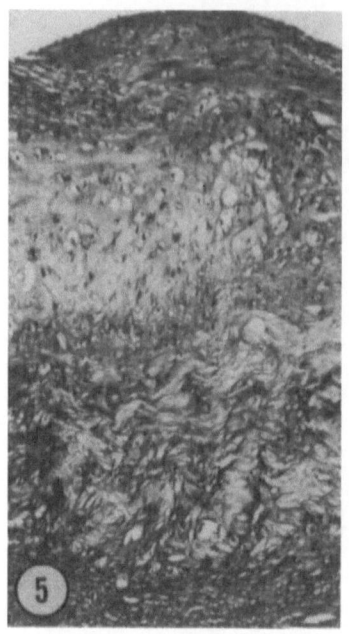 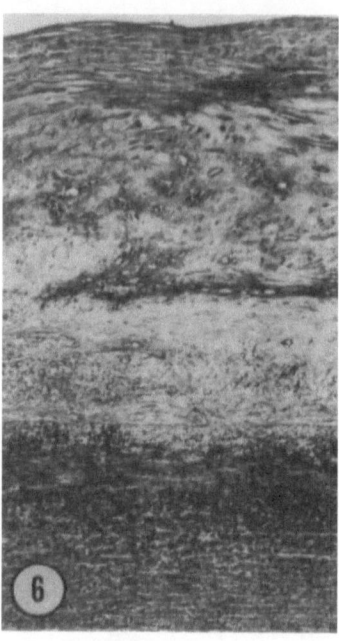

Fig. 5.   Aortic atherosclerosis with lipid deposit involving media in a rabbit treated for 15 months as outlined for Figure 8. H & E. (x 75). (Reproduced with permission from Minick and Murphy, 1973, and the American Journal of Pathology).

Fig. 6.   Aortic atherosclerosis with lipid deposit involving media in a 62 year old man. Note close resemblance to rabbit aortic atherosclerosis in Figure 5. H & E. (x 60). (Reproduced with permission from Minick and Murphy, 1973, and the American Journal of Pathology).

bore closer, often marked, resemblance to chronic human atherosclerosis (Figures 7-12). Among the many characteristics shared with human atherosclerosis were: Lipid filled foam cells clustered deep in the intima, fatty-hyaline change with little or no elastification, pooled lipid and cholesterol clefts deep in the intima and media with overlying fibromuscular caps or jackets, vascularization, occasional focal calcification of intima, and rarely an overlying recent thrombus. Other changes in the rabbit arteries that were similar to human atherosclerosis included segmental medial degenerative change, scarring, and thinning, and cellular proliferative and infiltrative change and fibrosis in the adventitia. In Group III, changes like those in coronary arteries occurred in arteries at many other sites. In contrast, the arterial lesions of Group I which occurred primarily in small myocardial arteries and only rarely in large coronary arteries bore little resemblance to human coronary atherosclerosis.

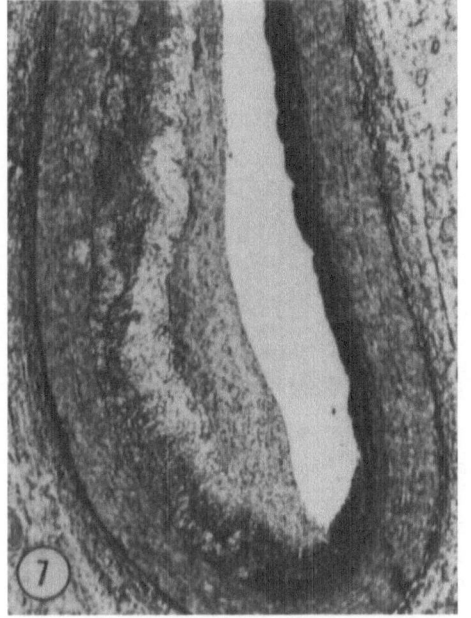 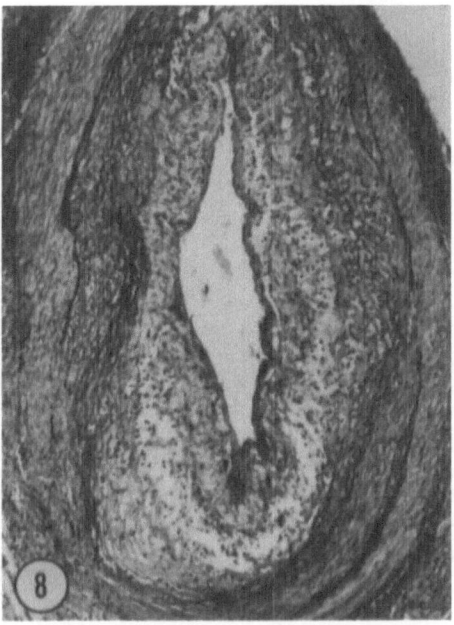

Fig. 7. Coronary atherosclerosis in man referred to in Figure 4
closely resembling rabbit atherosclerosis in Figures 8,9, and 11.
Elastic stain. (x 30). (Reproduced with permission from Minick
and Murphy, 1973, and the American Journal of Pathology).

Fig. 8. Coronary atherosclerosis induced in a rabbit by repeated
injections of foreign serum and concomitant feeding of semi-
synthetic, lipid-rich, cholesterol-poor diet for 9 months. Elastic
stain. (x 96). (Reproduced with permission from Minick and
Murphy, 1973, and the American Journal of Pathology).

     Thus, in testing the hypothesis that the synergy of immuno-
logical injury and hypercholesterolemia can lead to atherosclerosis,
we have produced by means of repeated and protracted immunologic
injury and lipid-rich diet an animal model of atherosclerosis
which in several important respects resembles atherosclerosis in
man. First of all, immunologic reactions commonly occur in the
human population. Secondly, the hypercholesterolemia of the
animal model is of the same order of magnitude as that of adult
humans in the United States. Thirdly, arterial lesions induced
by repeated injections of foreign serum protein in rabbits concomitantly fed a lipid-rich diet are histologically very similar
to those of human arteriosclerosis. Finally, marked involvement
of the major coronary arteries is often a prominent feature of
both atherosclerosis in man and in the rabbits that received the
lipid-rich diet and repeated injections of foreign serum.

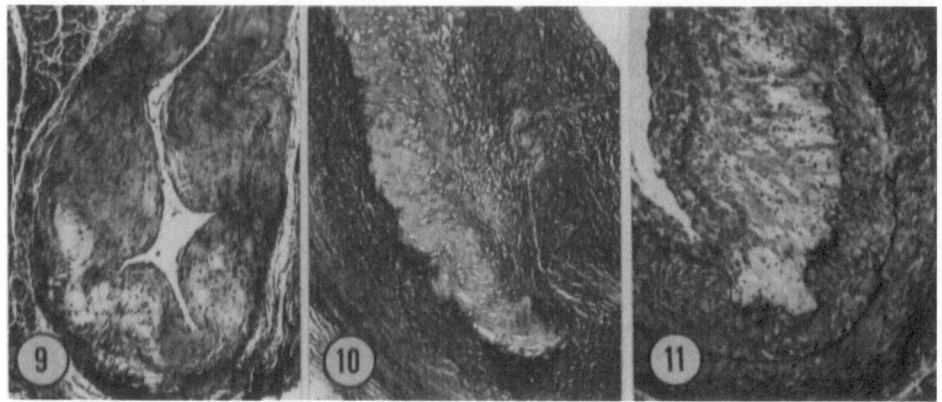

Fig. 9. Coronary atherosclerosis in a rabbit treated for 10 months as outlined in Figure 8. Elastic stain. (x 64).

Fig. 10. Coronary atherosclerosis in a 19 year old man with systemic lupus erythematosus closely resembling rabbit atherosclerosis in Figures 8, 9, and 11. Elastic stain. (x 40).

Figure 11. Coronary atherosclerosis in a rabbit treated for 13 months as outlined for Figure 8. (x 80). (Figures 9, 10, and 11 are reproduced with permission from Minick and Murphy, 1973, and the American Journal of Pathology).

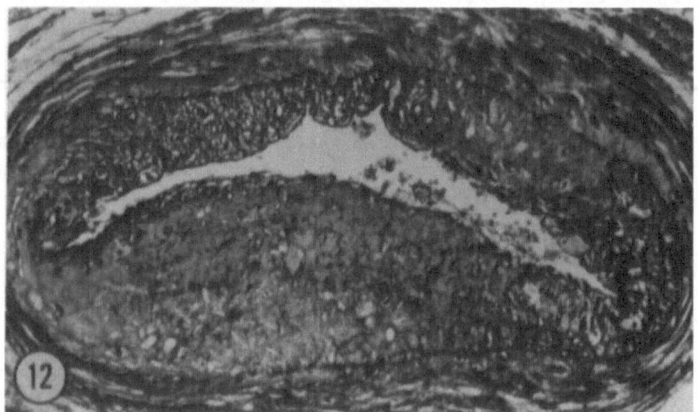

Fig. 12. Coronary atherosclerosis with cholesterol clefts in a rabbit treated for 16 months as outlined for Figure 8. Elastic stain. (x 192). (Reproduced with permission from Minick and Murphy, 1973, and the American Journal of Pathology).

During the past several years unexpectedly severe and apparently
rapidly developing atherosclerotic changes in coronary arteries
have been found to occur in some human cardiac homografts (Thompson,
1969; Bieber et al., 1970; Murphy and Minick, 1973), and it has
been suggested that alterations of lipid metabolism or immunological
injury resulting from graft rejection may be causative in the development of such atherosclerotic change (Thompson, 1969). It is
noteworthy that these coronary arterial changes bear a striking
resemblance to the coronary atherosclerosis induced by the synergy
of immunological injury and hypercholesterolemia. In those experiments, arterial intimal thickening, which resulted from repeated
injections of foreign serum protein, accumulated lipid and evolved
as atherosclerosis. Since arterial lesions similar to those induced
by foreign serum injections and probably likewise resulting from
immunological injury occur in graft rejection, it seemed reasonable
to expect that arterial intimal thickening induced by graft rejection might also accumulate lipid and evolve as atherosclerosis.

Accordingly, we (Alonso et al., 1970) performed experiments
designed to test the hypothesis that the synergy of immunologic
injury to coronary arteries, due to cardiac homograft rejection,
and hypercholesterolemia can result in coronary atherosclerosis.
Heterotopic cardiac homotransplants were performed in the necks
of 41 rabbits. Twenty-three rabbits (Groups I and II) were fed
a diet supplemented with 0.4% cholesterol by weight, and the
remaining 18 rabbits (Groups III and IV) were fed a lipid-poor
diet. In addition, Groups II and IV were injected with immunosuppressive drugs, methyl prednisolone and azathioprine, (3 mg/kg/
day).

Most rabbits fed lipid-poor diets had no grossly visible
lesions in the transplanted segment of the aorta. Rabbits fed
cholesterol supplement had grossly visible fatty change in the
transplanted segment of the ascending aorta, and in some aortas
almost the entire surface was so affected. Invariably, this
atherosclerotic change stopped abruptly at the anastomosis of the
transplanted ascending aorta with the recipient's carotid artery.
Either no fatty change or only slight fatty change was present in
aortas of recipients.

In transplanted hearts, coronary arterial lesions developed
that were different in quality, quantity, and distribution from
arterial lesions found in the recipient hearts. In rabbits fed
a lipid-poor diet, arterial lesions were mainly proliferative
without fatty change and arteries of all sizes were affected. In
rabbits fed a cholesterol supplement, some lesions likewise were
proliferative without fatty change, but the majority were fatty-
proliferative. Some fatty-proliferative arterial lesions bore
close resemblance to human coronary atherosclerosis. In contrast,

in hearts of the recipient rabbits fed a lipid-poor diet, no
arterial lesions developed; and in hearts of the recipient rabbits
fed cholesterol-rich diets only occasional fatty lesions developed
in small intramyocardial arteries.

Results of experiments discussed earlier in this paper demonstrated that lipid accumulated at sites of immunologic injury to
arteries and led to atherosclerosis, which in some instances
closely resembled that in man. In the same experiments we found
that immunologic injury without hypercholesterolemia led to fibromuscular intimal thickening without lipid. This latter change
closely resembled the fibromuscular intimal thickening without
manifest lipid that often occurs in man's arteries and is frequently
referred to as diffuse intimal thickening. It could not be determined in these experiments whether lipid had accumulated only
acutely at sites of recent immunologic injury to arteries, or
whether previously induced fibromuscular intimal thickening preferentially accumulated lipid and led to atherosclerosis.

Although observations in man and other animals suggest the
possibility that earlier acquired fibromuscular intimal thickening
without evident lipid may predispose to later developing atherosclerosis (Dock, 1946; Wilens, 1951; Movat et al., 1958; French,
1966; Andrus and Portman, 1966; Moss and Benditt, 1970), there is
little direct experimental evidence to support this hypothesis.
In fact, some investigators have shown that under certain experimental conditions fibromuscular intimal thickening may be resistant
to later developing atherosclerosis (Ssolowjew, 1930; Hass et al.,
1961; Taylor et al., 1963; Gore and Goodman, 1967).

Experiments now to be described were designed to determine
whether immunologically induced fibromuscular intimal thickening
in rabbits, closely resembling diffuse intimal thickening in man,
would preferentially accumulate lipid and lead to atherosclerosis.
In these experiments 65 rabbits were fed a lipid-poor diet, and
concomitant immunologic arterial injury was induced by multiple
intravenous injections of horse serum (Text-Figure 3). The
resulting arterial lesions were allowed to heal for either 40 days
(Groups IIA and IIIA) or 80 days (Groups IIB and IIIB) following
the last serum injection. In order to assess arterial changes at
sites of immune injury, 23 of the rabbits were sacrificed at
various intervals during an 8 to 21 week period following the last
serum injection. In order to determine whether lipid would preferentially accumulate at such sites of intimal thickening, the
remaining 42 rabbits were then fed cholesterol-supplemented diet
for 80 days, commencing either 40 days (Group IIIA) or 80 days
(Group IIIB) after the last serum injection. To assess the effect

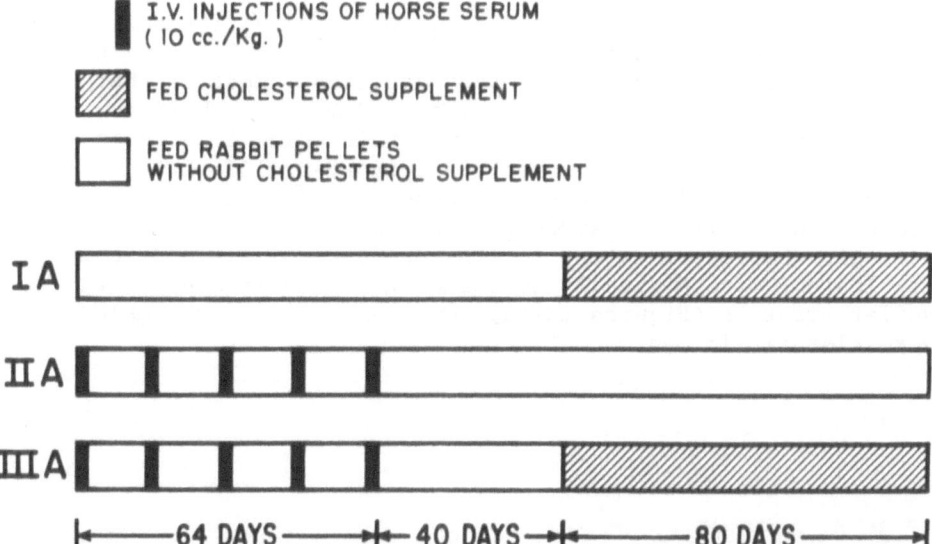

Text-Fig. 3. Design of Experiment A. Arteriosclerosis without manifest lipid was induced immunologically in Groups IIA and IIIA by repeated horse serum injections. Group IIIA was subsequently fed cholesterol-rich diet, to determine whether the serum-induced arterial lesions could later and preferentially accumulate lipid. Concurrently, Group IA was also fed cholesterol-rich diet to determine the effect of this diet on uninjured arteries. Experiment B was similar but the delay period between the last serum injection and the onset of cholesterol feeding was extended from 40 to 80 days. (Reproduced with permission from Hardin et al., 1973, and the American Journal of Pathology).

of cholesterol feeding alone, two other groups (Groups IA and IB) were fed the cholesterol diet for 80 days.

As in the previously described experiments, cholesterol feeding alone induced fatty lesions in the small intramyocardial coronary arteries. The lesions did not resemble human coronary arteriosclerosis. Rabbits that received four injections of horse serum and were then sacrificed at intervals ranging from 8 to 21 weeks after the last serum injection had coronary arterial lesions equally distributed among large, medium, and small arteries. The lesions were characterized by fibromuscular intimal thickening with no lipid. These proliferative lesions resembled the fibromuscular intimal thickening or so-called diffuse intimal thickening commonly found in man's arteries. Rabbits that received injections of horse serum and a cholesterol-supplemented diet after an interval of 40 or 80 days (Group III) had coronary arterial lesions distributed like those in Group II, i.e., in approximately equal numbers in large, medium, and small coronary arteries. Most of the lesions in Group III were of two types. Some were characterized by proliferative fibromuscular intimal thickening like those in Group II. The majority, however, were fatty-proliferative. The lesions were similar to the serum-induced proliferative arterial lesions of Group II in distribution and also with respect to histologic character, except for the presence of lipid deposits. These lesions were virtually identical to those in other large muscular arteries (Figures 13-16), and many closely resembled atherosclerosis in man.

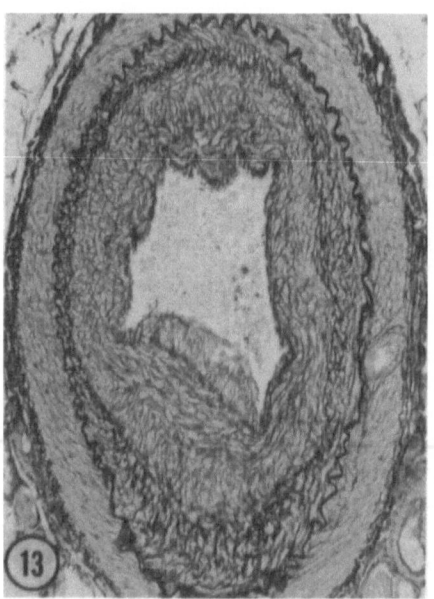 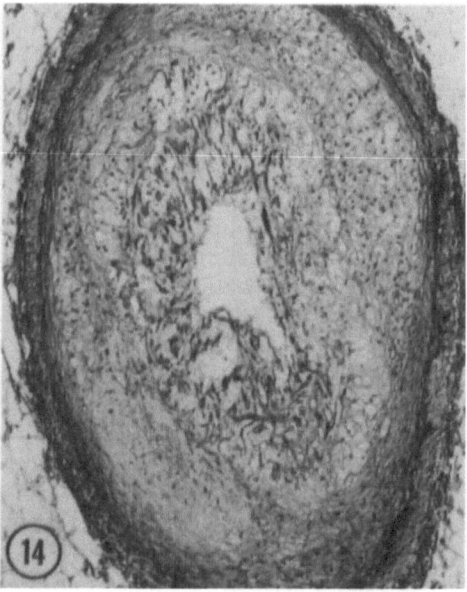

Fig. 13. Mesenteric arteriosclerosis in a rabbit repeatedly injected with foreign serum over several months, followed in 40 days by cholesterol-rich diet fed for 80 days. In other segments of this thickened artery, there was atheromatous change, as shown in Figure 14. Elastic stain.(x 120). (Reproduced with permission from Hardin et al., 1973, and the American Journal of Pathology).

Fig. 14. Atherosclerosis of a segment of the artery shown in Figure 13. Elastic stain. (x 78). (Reproduced with permission from Hardin et al., 1973, and the American Journal of Pathology).

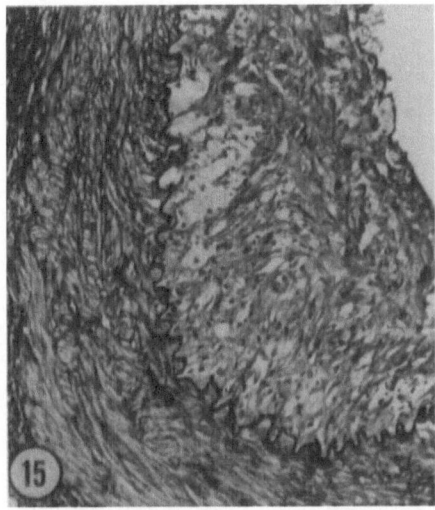 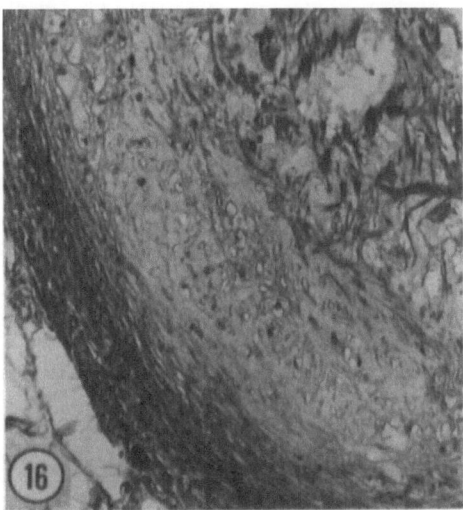

Fig. 15. Atherosclerosis of splenic artery of a rabbit treated
as outlined for Figure 13. Elastic stain. (x 120). (Reproduced
with permission from Hardin et al., 1973, and the American Journal
of Pathology).

Fig. 16. Higher magnification of left lower portion of atheromatous artery shown in Figure 14. Elastic stain. (x 153). (Reproduced with permission from Hardin et al., 1973, and the American
Journal of Pathology).

Both the morphology and distribution of the fatty-proliferative
lesions provide strong evidence that they were serum-induced proliferative changes that subsequently accumulated lipid. The data
for other large muscular arteries were similar and support the
conclusion that fatty-proliferative lesions were serum-induced
proliferative lesions which subsequently accumulated lipid.
Certain sites of the thickened intima of one arterial segment
contained no lipid deposit, whereas in thickened intima of another
segment of the same artery there was atheromatous change (Figures
13 and 14).

In this latter experiment, the extent of grossly visible
atherosclerotic change was greatly increased in all segments of
the aorta in rabbits which had received prior injections of horse
serum and were then subsequently fed a cholesterol supplemented
diet (Group III) as compared to rabbits that received the cholesterol-supplemented diet alone (Group I). Moreover, the thickness
of fat containing lesions was significantly greater in cholesterol
fed rabbits which had received prior injections of horse serum.

MICROSCOPIC ANALYSIS OF AORTAS

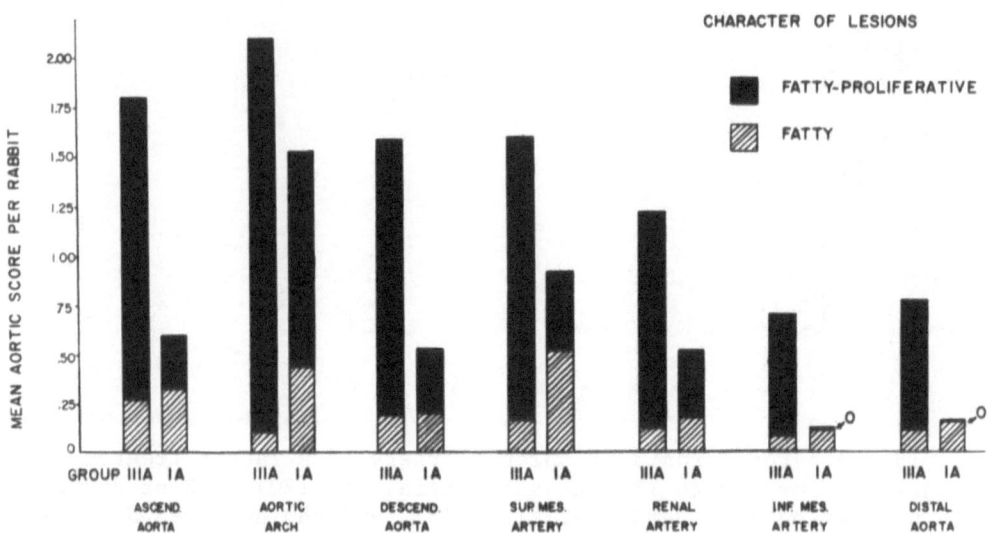

Text-Fig. 4. Experiment A. Mean aortic score is an index of the
thickness of fat-containing intimal lesions in aortas of cholesterol
fed rabbits. Those previously injected with foreign serum protein
(Group IIIA) subsequently developed more severe atherosclerosis
than controls (Group IA) in all segments of the aorta (all t-tests,
p < 0.05); and specifically, Group IIIA developed significantly
greater fatty-proliferative change (all t-tests, p < 0.02).
(Reproduced with permission from Hardin et al., 1973, and the
American Journal of Pathology).

When the histologic type of fat containing lesion was considered,
it was evident that the thickness of fatty lesions was only slight
and not significantly greater in Group III than Group I, whereas
the thickness of fatty-proliferative lesions was significantly
greater in Group III than in Group I. Results for Groups IA and
IIIA are shown in Text-Figure 4. Results for Groups IB and IIIB
were similar. Thus, in aortas as in muscular arteries, previous
immunological injury enhanced the subsequent accumulation of
lipid. In contrast to muscular arteries, however, previous immunological injury alone did not consistently produce any evident intimal thickening or other appreciable structural alteration of the
aortic wall. This finding suggests that the pathogenesis of the
enhanced atherosclerosis may be different in the musculoelastic
aorta than in muscular arteries.

CONCLUSION

The results of experiments described here demonstrate that
the synergy of immunological injury and hypercholesterolemia
can lead to atherosclerosis in rabbits which shares many characteristics with human atherosclerosis. The synergy of modest dietary
hypercholesterolemia like that in Western man (average serum
cholesterol concentrations between 200 and 250 mg%) and recurrent
immune injury protracted over a period of many months led to atherosclerosis in rabbits that bore striking resemblance to human
atherosclerosis. In other experiments, the synergy of arterial
injury due to homograft rejection and hypercholesterolemia led to
atherosclerosis, suggesting that the unexpectedly severe coronary
atherosclerosis in human cardiac homografts may have evolved from
lipid deposition at sites of intimal thickening resulting from
graft rejection. In still other experiments immunologically
induced fibromuscular intimal thickening without evident lipid
later accumulated lipid preferentially in the presence of hypercholesterolemia. Results of these latter experiments support the
hypothesis that in man similar intimal thickening acquired earlier
in life can predispose to later developing atherosclerosis.

ACKNOWLEDGMENTS

This investigation was supported by research grant HL-01803
of the National Heart Institute of the National Institutes of
Health, by grants from The Cross Foundation and The John Polachek
Foundation for Medical Research, and by grant 5T 1GM 78 of the
Division of General Medical Sciences of the United States Public
Health Service.

REFERENCES

Alonso, D.R., Starek, P., and Minick, C.R. (1970). Induction of
atherosclerosis in transplanted rabbit hearts by the synergy
of graft rejection and cholesterol-rich diet. (Abstract).
Circulation 42, Suppl. III -5.

Andrus, S.B., and Portman, O.W. (1966). Comparative studies of
spontaneous and experimental atherosclerosis in primates.
In "Some recent developments in comparative medicine."
(R.N. T-W-Fiennes, ed.). Zool. Soc., London 17, 161.
Academic Press, London.

Anitschkow, N.N. (1933). Experimental arteriosclerosis in animals.
In "Arteriosclerosis: A Survey of the Problem" (E.V.
Cowdry, ed.), MacMillan, New York, 271.

Bieber, C.P., Stinson, E.B., Shumway, N.E., Payne, R., and Kosek, J. (1970). Cardiac transplantation in man. VII. Cardiac allograft pathology. Circulation 41, 753.

Chesney, A.M. (1926). Immunity in syphilis. Medicine 5, 537.

Cochrane, C.G. (1971). Mechanisms involved in the deposition of immune complexes in tissues. J. Exp. Med. 134, 75.

Constantinides, P. (1965). "Experimental Atherosclerosis." Elsevier Publishing, Amsterdam.

Dock, W. (1946). The predilection of atherosclerosis for the coronary arteries. J. Amer. Med. Ass. 131, 875.

Duff, G.L. (1935). Experimental cholesterol arteriosclerosis and its relationship to human arteriosclerosis. Arch. Pathol. 20, 81; 259.

French, J.E. (1966). Atherosclerosis in relation to the structure and function of the arterial intima, with special reference to the endothelium. Int. Rev. Exp. Pathol. 5, 253.

Gore, I., and Goodman, M.L. (1967). Intimal thickening and dietary atherosclerosis. Arch. Pathol. 84, 49.

Hardin, N.J., Minick, C.R., and Murphy, G.E. (1973). Experimental induction of athero-arteriosclerosis by the synergy of allergic injury to arteries and lipid rich diet. III. The role of earlier acquired fibromuscular intimal thickening in the pathogenesis of later developing athero-sclerosis. Amer. J. Pathol. 73, 301.

Hass, G.M. (1955). Observations on vascular structure in relation to human and experimental arteriosclerosis. In "Symposium on Atherosclerosis." p. 24. National Academy of Sciences - National Research Council, Washington, D.C.

Hass, G.M., Trueheart, R.E., and Hemmens, A. (1961). Experimental atherosclerosis due to calcific medial degeneration and hypercholesterolemia. Amer. J. Pathol. 38, 289.

Haust, M.D. (1971). Arteriosclerosis. In "A Textbook of Pathology." (J.G. Brunson, ed.), p. 451. Macmillan, New York.

Kniker, W.T., and Cochrane, C.G. (1965). Pathogenic factors in vascular lesions of experimental serum sickness. J. Exp. Med. 122, 83.

McMillan, G.C. (This publication). Mesenchymal involvement in arteriosclerosis.

Minick, C.R., and Murphy, G.E. (1973). Experimental induction of athero-arteriosclerosis by the synergy of allergic injury to arteries and lipid-rich diet. II. Effect of repeatedly injected foreigh protein in rabbits fed a lipid-rich, cholesterol-poor diet. Amer. J. Pathol. 73, 265.

Minick, C.R., Murphy, G.E., and Campbell, W.G., Jr. (1966). Experimental induction of athero-arteriosclerosis by the synergy of allergic injury to arteries and lipid-rich diet. I. Effect of repeated injections of horse serum in rabbits fed a dietary cholesterol supplement. J. Exp. Med. 124, 635.

Moss, N.S., and Benditt, E.P. (1970). The ultrastructure of spontaneous and experimentally induced arterial lesions. II. The spontaneous plaque in the chicken. Lab. Invest. 23, 231.

Movat, H.Z., More, R.H., and Haust, M.D. (1958). The diffuse intimal thickening of the human aorta with aging. Amer. J. Pathol. 34, 1023.

Murphy, G.E. (Unpublished observations, 1973). Observations indicating that rheumatic injury to coronary arteries leads in some cases to precocious or later developing athero-arteriosclerosis in these arteries: A microscopic study of coronary arteries of infants, children, adolescents, and adults with rheumatic heart disease.

Murphy, G.E. (1960). Nature of rheumatic heart disease, with special fererence to myocardial disease and heart failure. Medicine 39, 289.

Murphy, G.E., Minick, C.R., and Alonso, D.R. (Unpublished observations, 1973). Comparative histologic study of the coronary arteries in human cardiac allografts and hearts of rabbits repeatedly injected with foreign protein and fed a lipid-rich diet.

Rössle, R. (1944). Über die Serosen Entzundungen der Organe. Virchows Arch. Pathol. Anat. 311, 252.

Ssolowjew, A. (1930). Experimentelle Untersuchungen über die Bedeutung von Localer Schädigung für die Lipoidablagerung in der Arterienwand. Z. Gesamte Exp. Med. 69, 94.

Taylor, C.G. (1955). The reaction of arteries to injury by
    physical agents, with a discussion of arterial repair and
    its relationship to atherosclerosis. In "Symposium on
    Atherosclerosis." p. 74. National Academy of Sciences -
    National Research Council, Washington, D.C.

Taylor, C.B., Trueheart, R.E., and Cox, G.E. (1963). Atheroscler-
    osis in rhesus monkeys. III. The role of increased
    thickness of arterial walls in atherogenesis. Arch. Pathol.
    76, 14.

Thompson, J.G. (1969). Production of severe atheroma in a
    transplanted human heart. Lancet 2, 1088.

Waters, L.L. (1955). The reaction of the artery wall to injury by
    chemicals or infection. In "Symposium on Atherosclerosis."
    p. 91. National Academy of Sciences - National Research
    Council, Washington, D.C.

Wilens, S.L. (1951). The nature of diffuse intimal thickening
    of arteries. Amer. J. Pathol. 27, 825.

Zeek, P. (1932a). Studies in atherosclerosis. I. Conditions
    in childhood which predispose to the early development of
    arteriosclerosis. Amer. J. Med. Sci. 184, 350.

Zeek, P. (1932b). Studies in atherosclerosis. II. Atheroma
    and its sequelae in rheumatic heart disease. Amer. J. Med.
    Sci. 184, 356.

DISCUSSION FOLLOWING THE PRESENTATION BY C. RICHARD MINICK

Dr. Stemerman: Dr. Gaynor has demonstrated in our
laboratory that the generalized Schwartzman reaction can, at
least in part, be explained by the immunologic injury of the
endothelium. Now I am wondering if this may be a possible
explanation for the lesions that you found, and that they might
result from the damage to be endothelium. Dr. Gaynor has been
able to find circulating endothelial cells in heparinized rabbits
following one dose of endotoxin. This might be a fruitful avenue
to explore.

Dr. Minick: We have not seen arteries denuded of endothelium in these relatively long-term experiments.

Dr. Ross: How soon after injecting?

Dr. Minick: The primary objective of our experiments to date has been to induce chronic atherosclerosis in rabbits that is like chronic atherosclerosis in man by means of the synergistic action of immunological injury and hypercholesterolemia. We are now utilizing transmission and scanning electron microscopy to examine acute arterial lesions. In this manner we may be able to learn more about the pathogenesis of this experimental atherosclerosis and, specifically, we may be able to answer Dr. Stemerman's and Dr. Ross's important question about the endothelium.

Dr. Ross: Just by way of responding, your studies are most interesting because your lesions strikingly resemble human atherosclerosis, and I think it would be worth going back and looking at some of your rabbits to see if after 24 hours, or after a week, or within the first week's time, you have marked de-endothelialization of those coronary vessels.

Dr. Wissler: Dr. Minick knows that I am very enthusiastic about his results which have given me new hope for the rabbit model. I had not been a great admirer of the rabbit model of atherosclerosis until I learned about these lesions, which certainly are remarkable and do resemble those in man. Having studied serum sickness arteritis for many years before I started studying atherosclerosis,[1] I would doubt if there is de-endothelialization in the period that Dr. Ross was talking about, but I think there is certainly injury to almost the entire vessel wall. I would like to ask Dr. Minick how he really interprets his results. How much of the disease in man has an immunological basis? How much of this mechanism is active in human atherogenesis?

Dr. Minick: This question cannot be answered at this time. To the best of our knowledge there have been no epidemiological studies reported that have examined this problem. The observations of Dr. Murphy and Dr. Zeek, which are cited in this paper, indicate that immunological injury in rheumatic fever attacks may in some instances lead to premature atherosclerosis. Furthermore, the experience with cardiac homotransplants certainly indicates that in some instances immunological injury to arteries may lead to rapidly developing atherosclerosis in man.

Dr. McGill: What is known about the effect of the experimental regimen on veins?

---

[1]Ebert, R. H., and Wissler, R. W. (1951). In vivo observations of the vascular reactions to large doses of horse serum using the rabbit ear chamber technique. J. Lab. Clin. Med. 38, 511.

Dr. Minick: We have not systematically looked at veins.
We do occasionally inspect the veins when we are looking at the
arteries. I certainly haven't seen gross atherosclerosis in the
veins and I haven't seen any microscopic changes in any of the
many sections I have.

Unidentified Speaker: You mentioned that antibiotics might
bring an allergic reaction. I wondered if you were going to do
anything along this line and possibly also include compounds such
as aspirin to determine if they produce allergic reactions. I
think you are really bringing up another subject, and that is,
the importance of cholesterol as compared with other atherogenic
stimuli.

Dr. Minick: I would like to respond to the last question
first. Results of our experiments certainly support the concept
that arterial injury, in this instance immunological injury, is
probably a primary causative factor in atherosclerosis. However,
I would like to emphasize that we are not suggesting that immunological injury leads to atherosclerosis in the absence of hypercholesterolemia. In general, our results indicate that immunological injury alone leads to fibromuscular intimal thickening,
but that the synergy of immunological injury and hypercholesterolemia, albeit more modest than that often used, is required to
induce atherosclerosis. In response to your question about drug
allergy, it should be pointed out that in the experiments we have
reported here, immune injury to arteries resulted from serum
sickness, presumably mediated by immune complexes or from graft
rejection. Dr. Carl Becker and I are now testing the hypothesis
that atopic allergy may result in increased endothelial permeability
and thereby lead to atherosclerosis. Although we have not tried
to induce lesions with drugs such as penicillin, both serum sickness and atopic allergy are important in drug allergy.

ENZYMIC VS NON-ENZYMIC FACTORS IN THE DETERIORATION OF CONNECTIVE TISSUE

Frank S. LaBella

University of Manitoba, Faculty of Medicine

Winnipeg, Manitoba, Canada

ELASTOLYTIC ENZYMES

Elastase, Elastinase

The term "elastase" has been used to designate enzyme activity that promotes dissolution, "elastolysis", of native elastic fibers or elastic lamellae and of the constituent elastic protein itself, irrespective of the state of purity of the substrate. Elastic structures consist of a reversibly extensible protein, elastin, embedded in a complex matrix of proteins, glycoproteins and glycosaminoglycans. The associations of elastin with these other substances range from weak electrostatic interactions to stable covalent bonds.

"Elastin" has been generally defined, in large part, on the basis of its relatively insolubility. It represents the tissue residue following the extraction, hopefully, of all other proteins and non-proteins. A reasonably reproducible protein component with rubber-like properties can be prepared from many tissues by this general procedure. However, it is clear that highly atypical "elastin" with respect, for example, to amino acid composition is yielded from elastic tissues of the very young (Keeley and LaBella, 1972; Cleary et al., 1965), the very old (LaBella et al., 1966; Hall, 1955; Lansing et al., 1951) and from uterine tissue (Downie et al., 1972). Even with elastin prepared from the same tissue and from animals of the same species, sex, and age, and often by the same procedure, controversy exists among laboratories concerning the chemical composition of the product.

Thus, assessment of claims for the identification of an "elastase" from one source or another is often difficult, because there may be little or no indication of the purity of the substrate. Sensitive methods for the detection of radioisotopically labelled, dyed, or fluorescent protein or of carbohydrate and lipid components may indicate that enzyme-induced solubilization is occurring, but it is usually not at all clear that the elastic protein is being attacked. The most reproducible procedure for preparing elastin of typical amino acid composition is extraction of de-fatted tissue with 0.1N NaOH at 100° (Lowry et al., 1941; Lansing et al., 1951). This drastic method may be validly criticized for its potential degradation of the primary structure of native elastin, but, in order to study this protein relatively free of other substances, some compromise must be achieved. There are sufficient data on the purification of elastin, that assays for enzymic hydrolysis of this protein with the use of substrate prepared by means other than with alkali may be considered as of doubtful validity.

On the other hand, solubilization of the carbohydrate, lipid, or glycoprotein components of native elastic fibers may be potentially as biologically significant as is dissolution of the elastic protein itself. However, the problem is confounded by the fact that the architecture of elastic fibers is such that a complex non-elastin matrix appears to have been incorporated throughout the period of fiber formation. Thus, the designation of elastomucase and elastolipoproteinase (Banga and Balo, 1956; Loeven, 1963; Hall, 1964) to individual fractions prepared from crude elastase preparations may not be appropriate, unless it can be shown that carbohydrate and lipid are covalently bound to elastin.

If "elastase", then, refers to enzymic activity which promotes elastolysis, i.e., dissolution of native elastic fibers or lamellae, "elastinase" might be a more appropriate designation for enzymes which attack and promote dissolution of the purified homogeneous elastic protein by cleavage of peptide bonds within the primary structure of the protein. For the purposes of the present review, these designations will be employed.

Enzymes which attack superficial and matrical elements of elastic microstructures, as well as those which hydrolyze the peptide bonds in purified elastin, have been clearly demonstrated in pancreas, certain plants, and some microorganisms. A major issue would appear to be whether or not endogenous elastase and/or elastinase of animals and man has a systemic physiological function in the metabolism of elastic tissues. Clarification of this point is crucial to our knowledge of the development and potential therapy of arterial and other connective tissue changes associated with aging and disease.

Mechanism of Elastolysis

Details of the mechanism of solubilization of elastin have
been elucidated with the use of pancreatic elastase and with
purified aortic or ligamental elastin as substrate. The enzyme
attaches to the insoluble substrate and through hydrolysis of peptide bonds promotes solubilization of the protein. The enzyme
degrades both soluble and insoluble moieties concomitantly.
LaBella (1961) and LaBella and Lindsay (1963) showed that bovine
or human aortic elastin is completely solubilized by elastase, but
30 to 40 percent was resistant to degradation by the enzyme and
remained non-dialyzable, i.e., mol wt > 10,000. The resistant
protein fraction was presumably highly cross-linked, a conjecture
supported by the observation that inherent fluorescence in elastin
was almost entirely associated with the non-degraded moiety. The
evidence for a cross-linking role of the fluorescent material in
connective tissue proteins has been reviewed (LaBella and Lindsay,
1963; LaBella and Paul, 1965; LaBella et al., 1968; LaBella, 1971).

The kinetics and soluble products of elastin solubilization
by elastase and organic acids are similar, suggesting the existence
of specific labile peptide bonds. Partridge et al. (1955) extracted
elastin serially with hot 0.25 M oxalic acid and obtained varying
proportions of two soluble fractions, an α-protein with mol wt
60,000-84,000 and a β-protein, mol wt 5500. The smaller component
is released in the early extracts, the larger one being solubilized
to a progressively greater proportion as the fiber structure is
weakened. The large soluble components may be further degraded
to the smaller by acids or enzymes. It is of interest that curves
of similar shape were found by LaBella (1961) who studied the action
of serial treatments with pancreatic elastase on a similar elastin
substrate as that used by Partridge et al. (1955). LaBella made no
estimates of mol wt but reported the rate of solubilization of
trichloroacetic acid soluble (β-protein?) and insoluble (α-protein?)
fractions.

Elastin can be considered as a unique protein insofar as it is
resistant to most proteolytic enzymes. The basis of this resistance
probably resides in the high density of peptide bonds formed between
non-polar amino acids. Because more than eighty percent of the
amino acids in elastin are non-polar, there may be an abundance of
peptide sequences which are absent or rare in most other proteins.
Elastases (elastinases), whether of animal, bacterial, or plant
origin, would appear to be highly specific enzymes because they
attack a unique substrate. They are, on the contrary, relatively
non-specific and hydrolyze many proteins.

Crude pancreatic extracts can be shown to contain a complex of
enzymes which attack the various components, e.g., glycoproteins

and lipoproteins, of native elastic structures and which act
synergistically in solubilizing the structures (Loeven, 1963; Hall,
1964).

Reported Sources of Elastolytic Activity in Animal Tissues

Aortic Wall (Loeven, 1969). Extracts of aortas were assayed
for elastase activity by incubation with beef aorta powder purified
by extraction with boiling 0.1N NaOH or by autoclaving in 2% acetic
acid. The formation of soluble protein was estimated by the biuret
reaction. There were "small but consistently present amounts of
the proteolytic elastase component."

Blood Platelets (Robert et al., 1970; Legrand et al., 1969).
Alkali purified elastin from aorta was labelled with radioiodine
or with various dyes. Solubilized protein was estimated from
measurements of the release of radioiodine or dye. The authors
reported the strongest activity occurred with 3.2 mg of a particular
preparation of platelet protein that caused solubilization of 15%
of the 10 mg of substrate in 2 hours.

Cultured Mammalian Cells (Gilfillan, 1968). The ingestion and
intracellular degradation of alkali-purified elastin from bovine
ligamentum nuchae by cultured cells was estimated by a microscopic
grading system (+1 to +4). All cell types examined consumed
elastin particles by phagocytosis.

Leucocytes (Janoff and Scherer, 1968; Janoff and Bosch, 1971).
Synthetic peptides known to be hydrolyzed by purified pancreatic
elastase were used as substrates. The authors assumed that
hydrolysis of the synthetic peptide substrates indicated the presence of elastase in the tissues and cells examined.

Blood Plasma (Hall, 1966). The action of plasma on dyed
elastin which had been purified from bovine ligamentum nuchae by
autoclaving in water and in 2% acetic acid was estimated by measuring release of dye.

Elastase Inhibitor in Blood. Proteinases elaborated by
exocrine glands of the gastrointestinal tract are inhibited by
substances present in blood. These proteinase directed inhibitors
also seem to be proteins. The presence of inhibitors in blood may
be an evolved mechanism for protecting the organism against the
systemic actions of proteinases which leak from tissues into the
circulation. The hypothesis that deficiencies in this protective
mechanism with age or disease could account for the deterioration
of, for example, arterial elastin has appealed to several investigators. Results of studies concerned with the levels of elastase

inhibitor as a function of age or arteriosclerosis have been
inconclusive. (See Hall, 1964 for a review of this subject).
A correlation has been reported between decreased elastase and
trypsin inhibitors in blood and the presence of severe pulmonary
emphysema (Turino et al., 1969). This same laboratory (Turino
et al., 1964) has reported that parenteral elastase alters the
mechanical characteristics of the lung.

Comment

Methodological deficiencies exist in each of the studies pur-
porting to show the presence of elastase or elastinase activity in
tissues, cells and blood. Some very sensitive methods are used to
detect the process of solubilization, such as the use of dye and
radioactive substrate. Even trace amounts of contaminating protein
conceivably could be hydrolyzed by proteolytic activity in the
extracts, thus giving a false positive for elastinase activity.
Furthermore, Banga and Ardelt (1967) showed that various proteins
caused non-specific displacement of Congo Red from insoluble
elastin. They also showed that no significant dissolution of
elastin, as determined gravimetrically, resulted from incubation
of the Congo Red-elastin with serum or plasma. Extremely sensitive
methods are available for determining the amino acid composition of
minute amounts of protein. Even the minimal amount of elastinase
activity should be capable of yielding a soluble elastin fraction
whose identity could be confirmed by its amino acid composition.
Probably the most significant deficiency in the various studies is
that in no case has complete dissolution of the insoluble elastin
substrate occurred, even after prolonged incubation. Pancreatic
elastase is known to cause rapid and complete solubilization even
of relatively impure preparations of elastin. The data of Robert
and his colleagues on elastase in blood platelets are, perhaps,
potentially the most important. Alkali-purified elastin was used
as substrate and 15% of the protein was reported solubilized.
Assays of elastase activity using synthetic peptides as substrates
are invalid, because it has been incorrectly assumed that small peptides which are hydrolyzed by pancreatic elastase are specific
substrates for other elastases. Pancreatic elastase is, in fact,
a relatively non-specific protease; it will attack many protein
and peptide substrates.

NON-ENZYMIC MODIFICATION OF CONNECTIVE TISSUE WITH AGE

Elastin

There is no convincing evidence of any type that a systemical-
ly active elastinase plays a physiological role in the turnover of

elastin. Even assuming undetectable levels of the enzyme in the
blood and connective tissues, the impact of the enzyme on elastin
turnover appears to be minimal. Radioisotopic studies show very
little or no turnover of elastin (Slack, 1954; Walford et al.,
1964). Furthermore, numerous histological observations indicate
no loss of elastin, but rather continuous alteration of existing
elastic structures.

If one prepares elastin from human aortas by conventional
extraction with alkali, gross inspection of the powdered product
shows a brilliant fluorescence under ultraviolet light and increased
yellow pigmentation with age (LaBella and Lindsay, 1963). Solubilized aliquots of the purified elastin show increasing fluorescence
(A/F 340-405 nm) with age (Figure 1). Others (Banga, 1969;

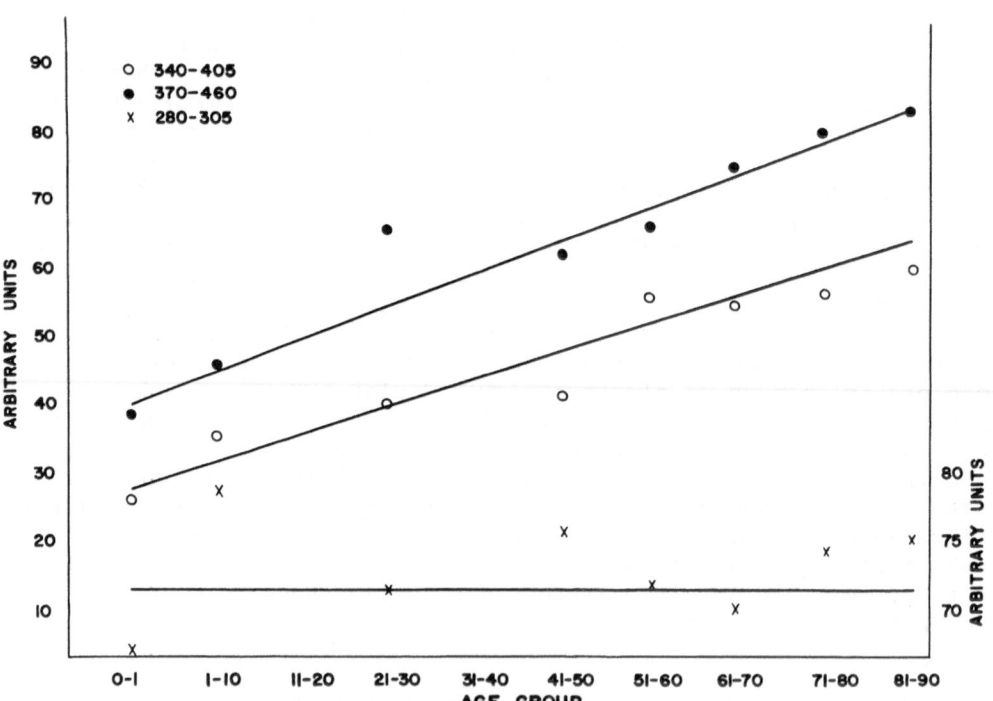

Fig. 1. Fluorescence of acid-hydrolyzed elastin purified from
pooled human aortas by alkali extraction. Fluorescence maxima at
405 and 460 nm probably represent the same unidentified substances.
The substance emitting maximally at 305 nm is tyrosine. The ordinate represents the fluorescence intensity (meter reading) per mg
protein. (from LaBella and Lindsay, 1963).

Blomfield and Farrar, 1969) have confirmed our findings on human
elastin; Banga (1969) has reported, in addition, that accumulation
of fluorescent material is greater in plaque areas of the aorta.
Several groups have reported that elastin becomes more susceptible
to the action of pancreatic elastase, as determined histologically
(Balo and Banga, 1955; Tunbridge, 1957) or _in vitro_ with elastin
purified by extraction with formic acid (Mull and Ram, 1965); our
own conclusion (LaBella and Lindsay, 1963) of a decreased susceptibility of elastin to the enzyme was probably erroneous because of
the presence of large amounts of mineral salts in the older preparations. In more recent unpublished work we extracted alkali-
purified elastin with formic acid to remove inorganic material;
there was little difference among the elastins from various age
groups with respect to susceptibility to elastase. Assuming that
elastin is, in fact, more readily solubilized by elastase, perhaps
due to its partial degradation _in vivo_, it is of interest that
exposure of purified elastin to ultraviolet irradiation results in
changes in the protein very similar to those reported above to occur in humans with age. The protein becomes more susceptible to
elastase digestion as u.v. irradiation is prolonged (Figure 2).

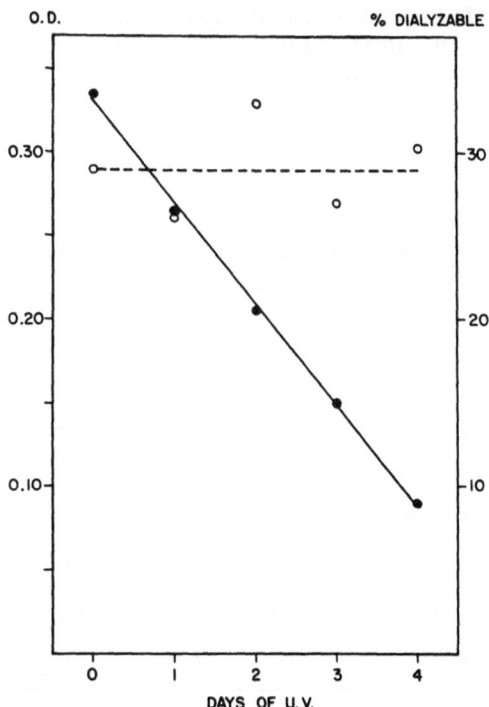

Fig. 2. Effect of 15 minute incubation with elastase on the solubilization (optical density at 500 nm) and degradation (dialyzable
nitrogen) of a suspension of elastin previously exposed to u.v. for
varying periods. closed circles: O.D.: open circles: % dialyzable
nitrogen.

Furthermore, u.v. causes changes in purified elastin very similar
to what is seen with both elastin and collagen during the aging
process in man (Table I, Figure 3; see below). The data in
Figure 3 support the hypothesis that the characteristic fluorescence of elastin (as well as of collagen and other connective tissue proteins) which increases with age is derived from tyrosine
residues. Whereas the amino acid composition of alkali-purified
elastin from younger individuals is "typical", that of older per-
sons show much higher contents of polar amino acids (Figure 4),
confirming the report of Lansing et al. (1951). On the other hand,
purification procedures which resulted in the dissolution of most
of the aortic powder from middle-aged individuals were required to
provide an elastin with composition similar to the youngest preparations. The oldest preparations, even after exhaustive extraction,
were contaminated with polar protein (Figure 5). It is significant
that, excluding the oldest preparation which is not pure elastin,
the only changes in amino acid composition with age occur with the
aromatic residues, tyrosine and phenylalanine (Figure 5). It was
concluded that an acidic contaminating protein becomes more firmly
bound with age and resists conventional extractive procedures for
isolating elastin. This contaminant could not be completely removed
from aortas of very old individuals. The amino acid compositions
of elastin in comparison with an alkali-soluble structural protein

TABLE I.   EFFECTS OF ULTRAVIOLET IRRADIATION ON ELASTIN*

	Days of u.v.			
	0	1	2	3
Rel. Fluor. (305 nm)	44	37	31	27
Rel. Fluor. (405 nm)	57	69	88	94
Yellowing	+1	+2	+3	+4
Schiff Reaction†	+1	+2	+3	+4
Rel. Absorbance (275 nm)	0.76	0.83	0.86	0.88

*Similar results were obtained with collagen except that
 Schiff positivity was not determined.
†Solubilization of elastin with acid or with elastase
 causes disappearance of the colour and prevents quantitation.
        (From LaBella and Thornhill, 1966)

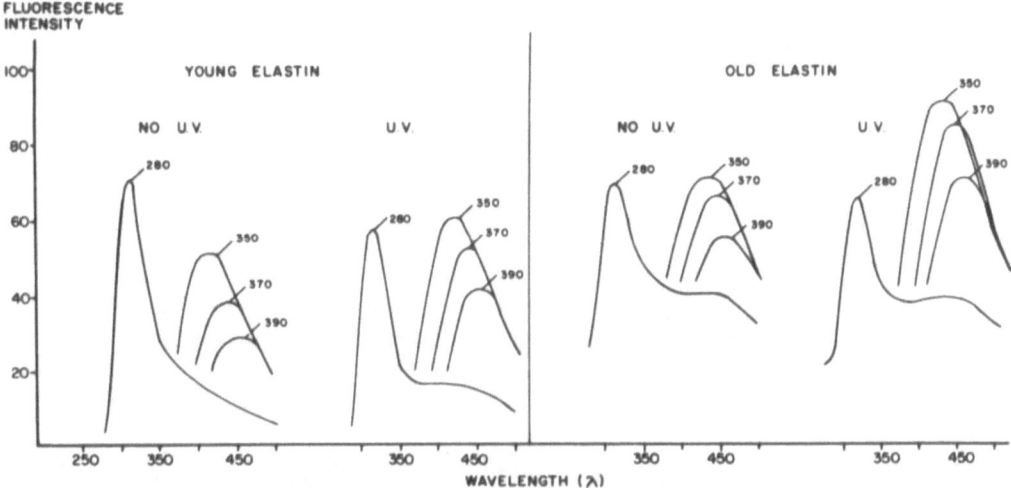

Fig. 3. Fluorescence spectra of human aortic elastin before and after 48 hr. exposure to u.v. Alkali-purified elastin powder was suspended in phosphate buffer, pH 7.4, at 37° and irradiated with a germicidal lamp. The elastin was washed and hydrolyzed with HCl and fluorescence determined on the hydrolysate. Young: pooled specimens from males aged 11-20 yr. Old: pooled specimens from males aged 81-90 yr. (from LaBella and Thornhill, 1966).

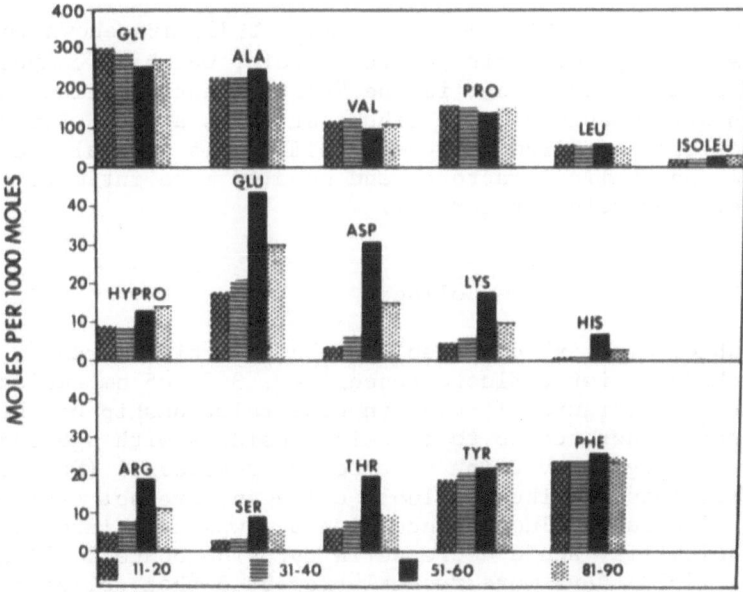

Fig. 4. Amino acid composition of alkali-purified elastin from human aortas of males of four age groups. (from LaBella et al., 1966).

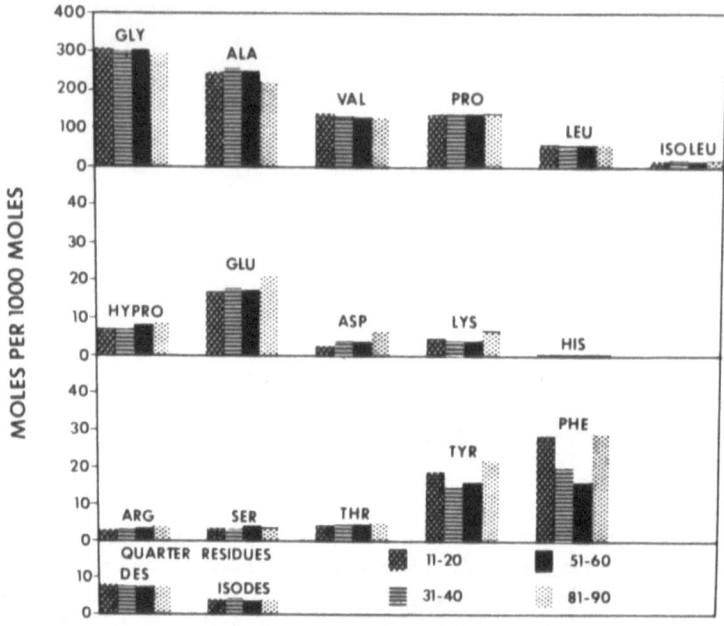

Fig. 5. Amino acid composition of the residue after exhaustive treatment of alkali-purified elastin with formic acid and 0.1N NaOH. (from LaBella et al., 1966).

(Keeley and LaBella, 1972a; Downie et al., 1972) are shown in Table 2. It seems likely that this acidic protein, which is composed largely of polar amino acids, is the "contaminant" in elastin. Thus, the non-renewable elastic fiber serves as a locus for continual deposition of circulating metabolites, is partially degraded by physical and chemical factors, and becomes more intimately bound to surrounding proteins (Figure 6).

Collagen

Insoluble, "matrix" collagen from human Achilles tendon also shows the characteristic fluorescence, i.e., 340/405 nm, which increases with age (Figure 7). The inverse relationship of the characteristic fluorescence to tyrosine residues with age suggests further the in vivo conversion of tyrosine residues. (Soluble collagen fractions, unlike insoluble collagen, are not visibly fluorescent). Increased fluorescence with age was associated with a decreased solubility and a decrease in tyrosine content (Figure 8). Deyl et al. (1970) have more recently reported that collagen from various tissues of the dog, cat, human, and beef is more fluorescent in older individuals. They reported that insoluble collagen was more fluorescent than were the soluble fractions. We find that soluble collagen is not visibly fluorescent.

TABLE 2.   AMINO ACID COMPOSITION OF MATURE ELASTIN AND ALKALI-
SOLUBLE PROTEIN

	ALSP	Elastin
	(Residues/1000 Total Residues)	
HPRO	0	19
ASP	102	4
THR	44	7
SER	54	5
GLU	129	13
PRO	60	127
GLY	98	361
ALA	84	177
BAL	70	166
CYS*	–	–
MET†	18	0
ILEU	45	19
LEU	87	50
TYR	26	11
PHE	37	20
LYS	61	3
HIS	19	1
ARG	43	5

*Not determined in these acid hydrolysates.
†Estimated as methionine plus methionine sulphone.
(From Keeley and LaBella, 1972a)

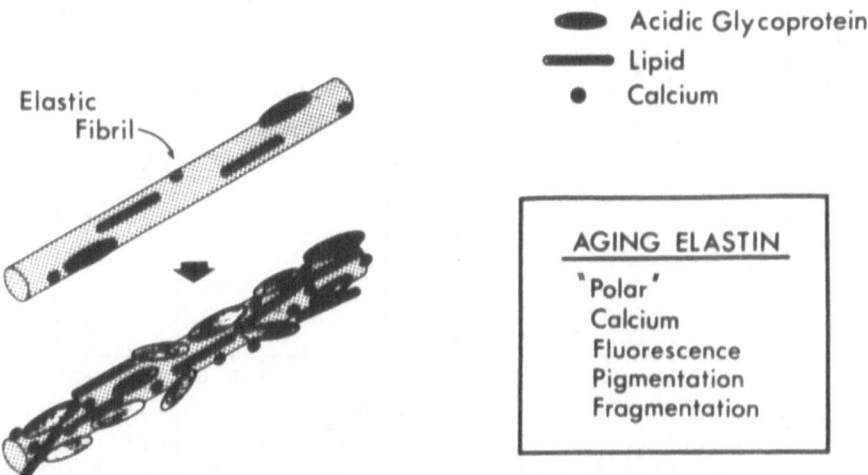

Fig. 6.   Diagramatic representation of processes of accretion in
elastic fibers which lead to observed changes with age.

Alkali-Soluble, Acidic Protein

The acidic protein which becomes more firmly bound to elastin has been isolated in our laboratory from aorta of several species, ligamentum nuchae, and uterus (Keeley and LaBella, 1972a, 1972b; Downie et al., 1972) and is apparently identical to structural glycoproteins isolated from various tissues by others (Barnes and Partridge, 1968; Robert and Compte, 1968; Timpl et al., 1968). Amino acid compositions of the acidic protein and elastin are presented in Table 2. Microfibrils which seem to be concerned with the orientation of newly synthesized elastin have been shown by Ross and Bornstein (1969) to be composed of this acidic protein; however, the abundance of this protein in connective tissues suggests that it may derive from the amorphous ground substance, as well. The acidic protein _in vivo_ appears to undergo progressive polymerization and becomes insoluble even in the 0.1N NaOH with which it is usually extracted (Downie et al., 1972; Keely, 1970).

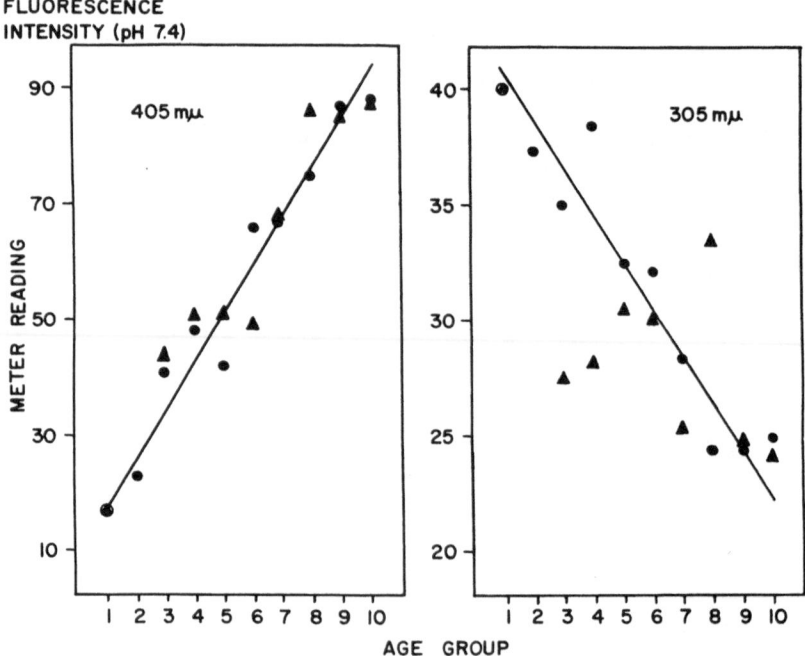

Fig. 7. Fluorescence intensity of acid-hydrolyzed, purified collagen power from human Achilles tendon. Meter readings of intensity of fluorescence at 305 nm (tyrosine) and 405 nm (unidentified substance) are plotted for males (circles) and females (triangles) of age groups 0-1, 2-10, 11-20, 21-30, 31-40, 41-50, 51-60, 61-70, 71-80, and 81-90 yrs. (from LaBella and Paul, 1965).

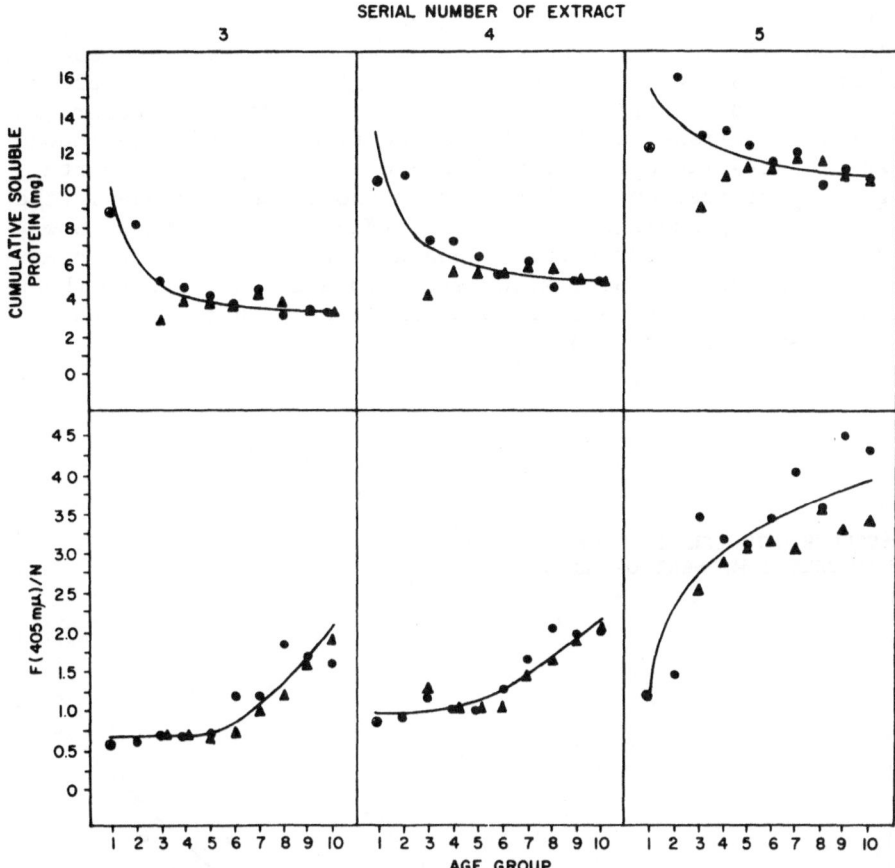

Fig. 8. Extraction of human tendon collagen by repeated autoclaving
(1 hr periods at 15 psi). Upper series of curves: cumulative soluble protein. Middle series of curves: fluorescence (405 nm) to
nitrogen ratios (F/N) calculated for protein solubilized in each
extract. Lower species of curves: tyrosine fluorescence (305 nm)
to nitrogen ratios (F/N) calculated for protein solubilized in each
extract. Symbols and age groups as in Figure 7. (from LaBella and
Paul, 1965).

        The alkali-soluble protein may be identical to the non-col-
lagenous beta protein characterized in several connective tissues
by means of X-ray diffraction (Little, 1973). This beta protein
species can be distinguished by its diffraction pattern from collagen and elastin and is present as a gel. Also, with age there is
a decrease in the water content and the amount of protein is seen
to increase in various tissues. Little (1973) interprets her observations to indicate that the matrix comprising the beta protein
becomes more crystalline, hence more stable, with age.

The acid protein is visibly fluorescent under u.v. light, and in solution, like elastin and collagen, emits maximum fluorescence at 450 nm when activated at 340 nm. Aging studies on this presumed intercellular matrix protein have not yet been done. However, in some earlier published work (LaBella and Lindsay, 1963) we showed that an alkali-soluble fraction obtained in collagen-free aorta during the purification of elastin also showed an increase in the fluorescence to protein ratio with age (Figure 9). We know now that this alkali extract probably contains the acidic protein as its major component. Thus, fluorescent moieties similar to those in elastin and collagen appear to accumulate in this other connective tissue protein with age.

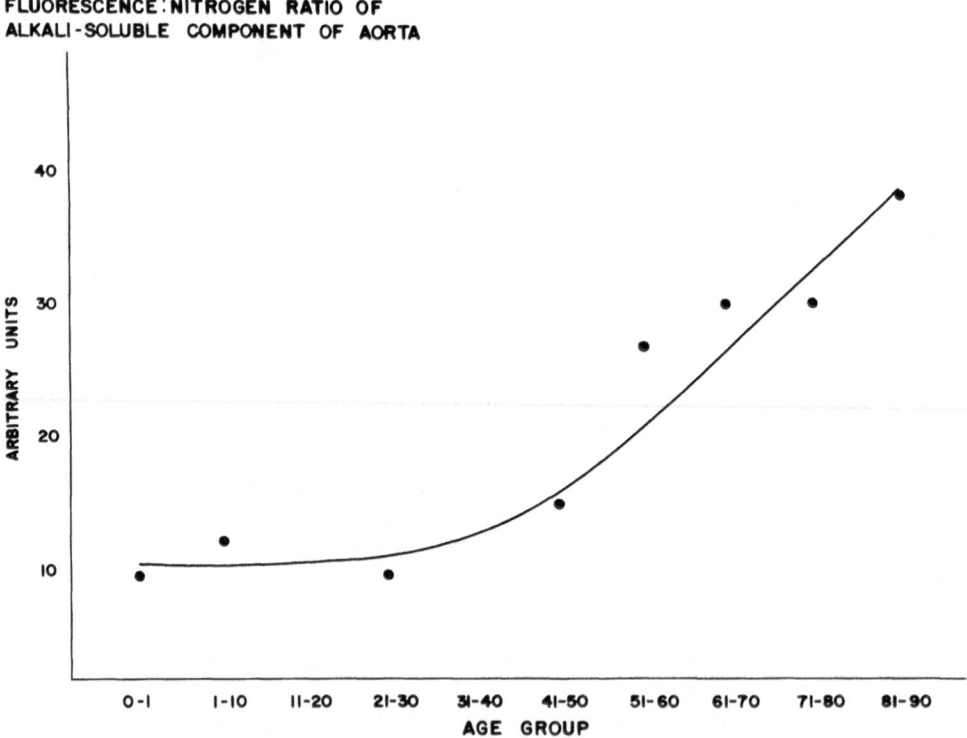

Fig. 9. Fluorescence (405 nm) in the alkali-soluble fraction of human aortas of various ages. The ordinate represents fluorescence intensity (meter reading) per mg nitrogen in the extracts. (from LaBella and Lindsay, 1963).

Nature and Significance of Fluorescent Moieties

<u>Fluorescence of Structural Proteins</u>. Most proteins do not
emit visible fluorescence when irradiated by ultraviolet light.
Visible bluish-white fluorescence is characteristic of structural,
relatively inert proteins of phylogenetically diverse organisms.
Purified fluorescent fractions from hydrolysates of all of these
structural proteins are apparently similar insofar as they emit
maximally at about 400 nm. In Figure 10, the appearances of several proteins under u.v. light are presented. Elastin from mature
(bovine ligament) and fetal (calf aorta) animals is brilliantly
fluorescent. The soluble form, and presumed precursor of elastin
obtained from copper deficient animals (provided by Dr. L. Sandberg)
is only very weakly fluorescent, although the characteristic 400 nm
fluorescence can be detected photofluorometrically. The other
three proteins shown do not visibly fluoresce; the apparent emission
is due to reflected light.

In Figure 11, additional protein preparations were photographed
under u.v. illumination. Gelatin derived from "insoluble," presumably mature, collagen fibrils is brilliantly fluorescent in
contrast to soluble collagen. This latter observation supports

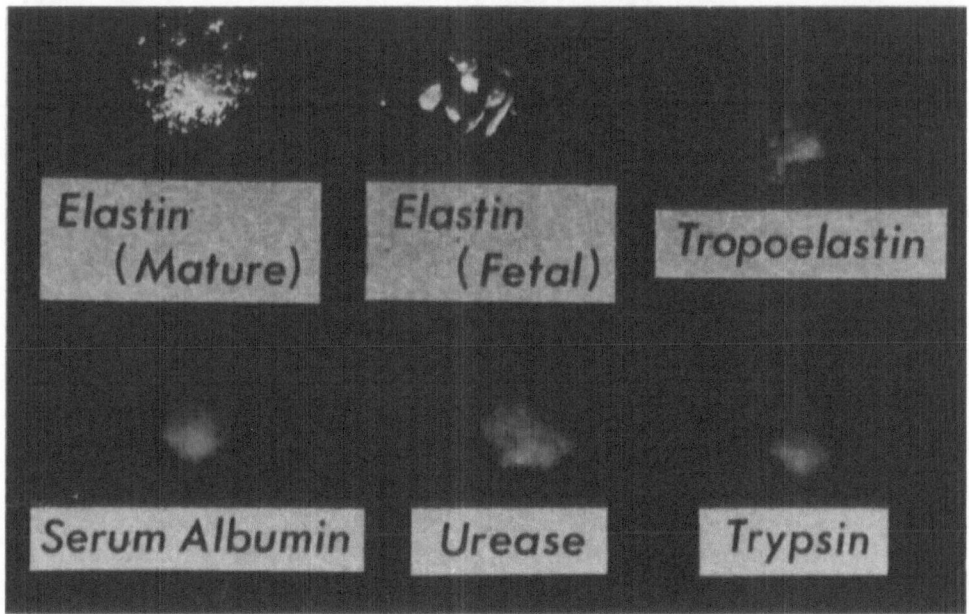

Fig. 10. Visible fluorescence of several purified proteins under
ultraviolet illumination.

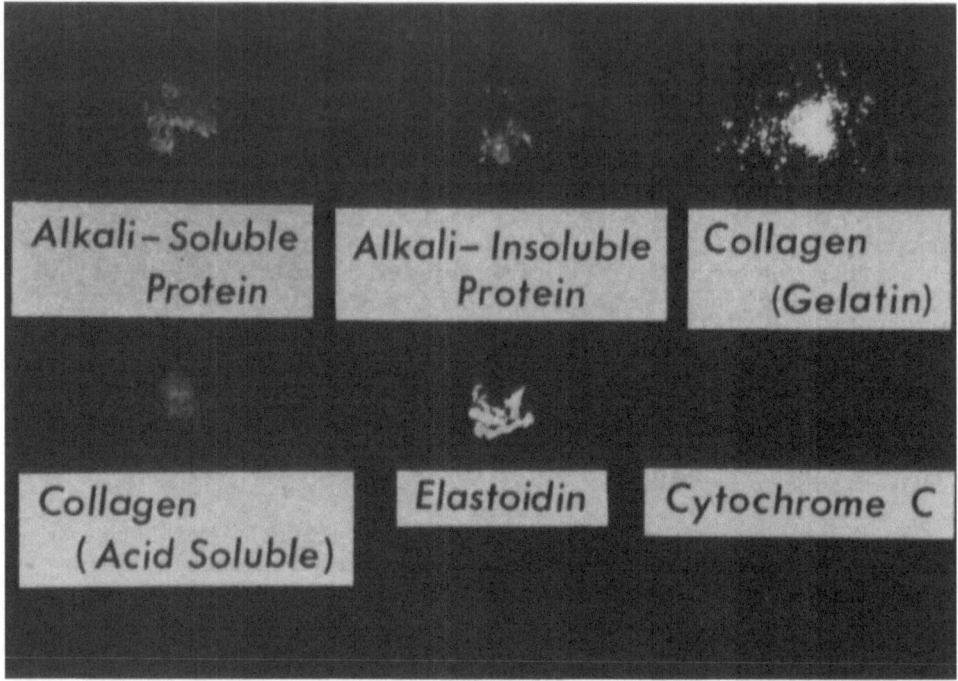

Fig. 11. Visible fluorescence of several purified proteins under ultraviolet illumination.

the notion that incorporation of fluorescent material contributes to the stability of the mature connective tissue proteins. The acidic protein, both alkali-soluble and alkali-insoluble forms, is definitely fluorescent, although not markedly so in the photograph; photofluorometric examination shows significant emission with a maximum near 400 nm. Another structural connective tissue protein, elastoidin from shark skin, exhibits visible fluorescence. Cytochrome C, on the other hand, like essentially all non-structural proteins, shows no visible fluorescence.

Other structural proteins exhibiting visible fluorescence include abductin, the hinge protein of the mollusc (Thornhill, 1971) eye lens albuminoid (LaBella, unpublished), dentin (Armstrong and Horsley, 1972) and resilin, a rubber-like insect protein (Andersen, 1966). Thus, it is significant that characteristic visible fluorescence is limited to stable structural proteins from diverse species. These proteins are, for the most part, permanent and non-renewable body constituents and their similar fluorescent properties suggest that they may be stabilized by common endogenous metabolites.

Evidence for the Aromatic Nature and Crosslinking Role of the Fluorescent Compounds. Several types of evidence, both from our laboratory and others, have led us to hypothesize that the fluorescent moieties in structural proteins are derived from tyrosine or some other aromatic compound and that these, as yet unidentified, substances serve as in vivo "tanning" agents. We have previously reviewed this aspect in some detail (LaBella, 1971) and only a summary of the evidence will be presented here.

The yellow fluorescent substances can be isolated from acid hydrolysates of the structural proteins with the use of charcoal or other adsorbents to which non-polar substances are strongly bound. Exposure of connective tissue proteins, such as elastin, collagen, and the alkali-soluble acidic protein, to agents which oxidize the tyrosine residues on the proteins results in a decrease in tyrosine content and an increase in the characteristic visible fluorescence. Thus, incubation with tyrosinase which is specific for phenolic residues, or with peroxidase plus hydrogen peroxide, causes an increased fluorescence and pigmentation of the proteins (Keely, 1970; LaBella et al., 1968). A similar phenomenon occurs upon exposure of suspensions of the proteins to ultraviolet radiation (LaBella and Thornhill, 1966). Also incubation of proteins with free tyrosine in the presence of these enzymes or ultraviolet radiation results in the covalent attachment of the amino acid to the proteins (Keeley, 1970). Treatment of soluble collagen with peroxidase plus hydrogen peroxide results in the rapid formation of rigid, insoluble gels and a concomitant increase in specific fluorescence and in the content of dityrosine a presumed crosslink (Figure 12) (LaBella et al., 1968). It is important to note,

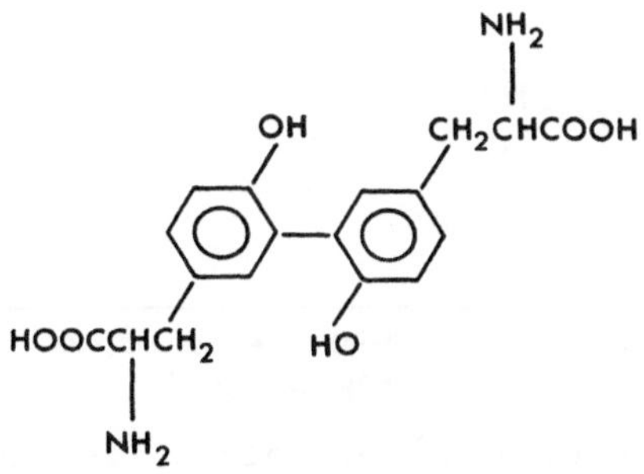

Dityrosine

Fig. 12. The structure of dityrosine isolated from alkali-soluble protein. Each of the constituent tyrosine residues was presumably in peptide linkage in the native protein and contributed to the formation of the dityrosine crosslink.

however, that in elastin and other structural proteins fluorescence
is associated with the enzyme-resistant, non-degradable protein
moiety (Figure 13) (LaBella and Lindsay, 1963; Thornhill, 1972;
Thornhill, 1971). This last observation is compatible with the
known resistance to enzymic digestion of artificially crosslinked,
i.e., tanned, proteins. As indicated in a previous section of
this paper, the increased fluorescence with age occurring naturally in human collagen and elastin is associated with a progressive
decrease in tyrosine residues. These latter observations suggest
that modification of the aromatic amino acid residues on the proteins, as well as incorporation of exogenous aromatic substances,
could result in the formation of links between peptide chains.
In elastin and collagen several distinct crosslinks have been
identified (see review; LaBella, 1971). These particular cross-
links are formed by the union of modified side chains of lysine

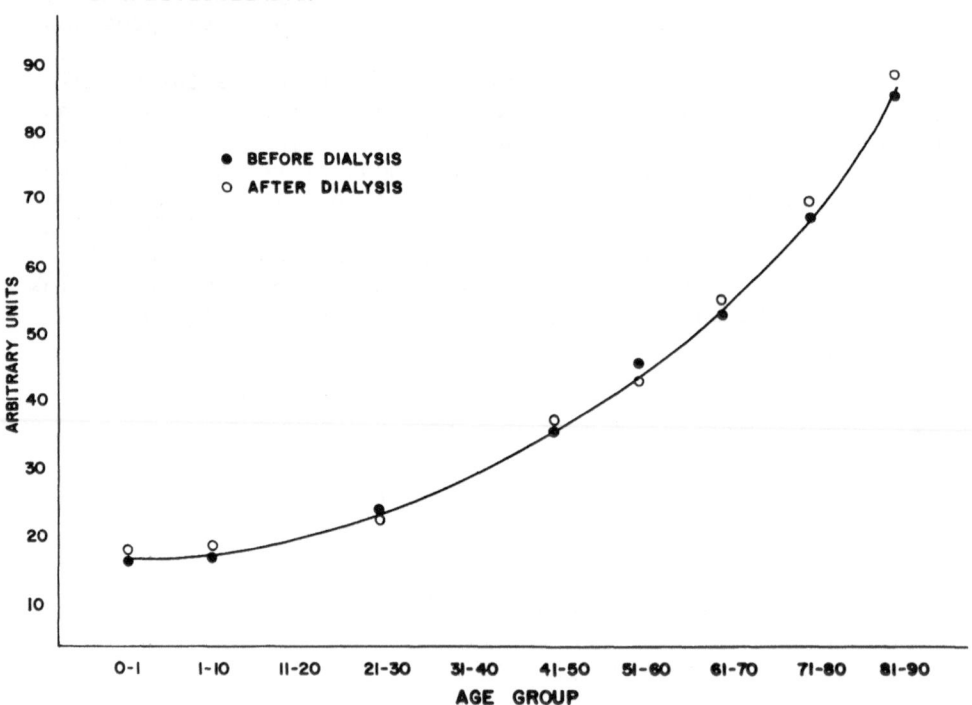

Fig. 13. Fluorescence (405 nm) of solubilized human aortic elastin
before and after dialysis. Enzymic digestion of the soluble protein has reached completion. Fluorescence was totally non-
dialyzable in all age groups, although varying proportions of the
solubilized elastin have been degraded to dialyzable fragments.
The ordinate represents the fluorescence intensity (meter reading)
per mg protein. (from LaBella and Lindsay, 1963).

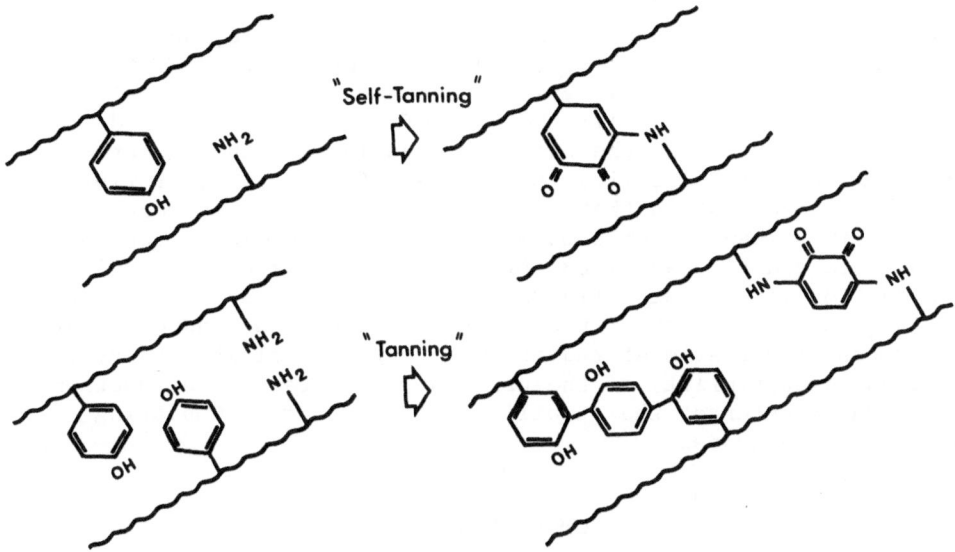

Fig. 14. Hypothetical tyrosine-derived crosslinks between peptide chains of connective tissue proteins. In "self-tanning" tyrosine residues within the protein participate in interchain bond formation. In the "tanning" process, exogenous aromatic molecules may combine with reactive groups on the protein and unite functional groups on two different chains.

residues in the proteins and they are produced during the early maturation phase of fiber development. In Figure 14 is presented a suggested sequence for crosslink formation via tyrosine residues.

Finally, there are well established examples in lower species of animals in which crosslinking of structural proteins occurs by means of aromatic compounds. For example, the presence of dityrosine and trityrosine have been shown to account for the fluorescence and stability of a rubber-like protein, resilin, in the locust (Andersen, 1966). Another aromatic substance derived from tyrosine, N-acetyldopamine, is a protein tanning agent in certain insect cuticles (Karlson and Sekeris, 1962). In this regard, it is of significance that dityrosine, a biphenolic compound, (Figure 12) has been isolated in our laboratory from several mammalian connective tissues (Keeley and LaBella, 1972b). Although dityrosine itself is a minor component and cannot account for all of the fluorescence in the mammalian proteins, its presence provides additional support for the participation of tyrosine and perhaps other aromatic compounds in connective tissue stabilization.

Although it appears highly likely that aromatic compounds play a crosslinking role in mammalian connective tissue proteins, other chemical species may also be involved and may contribute to overall

fluorescence of the structural proteins. For example, some aldehydes and lipid oxidation products, both of which are effective
protein crosslinking agents, are fluorescent (Chio and Tappel,
1969; see LaBella, 1971). In the case of collagen, increased
fluorescence with age in the human is associated with an increased
toughness and/or insolubility (LaBella and Paul, 1965); similarly,
there is some suggestion that an amorphous protein component, also,
in connective tissue becomes more stable and more fluorescent with
age (LaBella and Lindsay, 1963; Little, 1973; Peereboom, 1970).
The situation with elastic fibers may be complicated by the fact
that in vivo degradation of the elastin molecule, as indicated by
the effects of ultraviolet radiation on purified elastin or by the
increased susceptibility of the protein to elastase as a function
of age, may counteract the stabilizing effects of accumulating
fluorescent substances.

CONCLUSION

There is no convincing evidence that systemic elastase plays
a significant role in the degradation or turnover of elastin in
the mature or aged adult. This conclusion is based, on one hand,
on the extremely slow turnover of elastin as demonstrated by radio-
isotope studies and on the observation that, histologically, elastin
seems to be a permanent fixture in tissues and gradually deterio-
rates over the lifetime of the individual. Furthermore, assays for
elastase activity in blood and in tissues other than the exocrine
pancreas have relied on extremely sensitive procedures in attempting
to demonstrate substrate degradation. Solubilization of traces of
radioactivity or of dye from insoluble elastin substrate may represent non-specific action of tissue proteases on minor contaminants
of the fiber. Also, the proteolytic activity of tissue extracts
on synthetic peptide substrates cannot be taken as indicative of
the presence of an elastinase.

There is abundant evidence to indicate that physical and
chemical influences are major determinants of the progressive
modification of elastic tissues in the body. The incorporation
of fluorescent materials over the entire life span represents one
of these processes affecting connective tissue proteins. The
structural proteins from very diverse sources are for the most
part irreplaceable or only slowly replaceable and, as such, are
subject to continuous attack by a variety of chemical and physical
agents. The natural incorporation of endogenous crosslinking substances, which can be detected by their characteristic fluorescence,
during the formation and development of connective tissue appears to
be designed for producing strong, inert supporting tissues. These
stable proteins, however, are subject to the same influences
throughout the life span of the individual. Excessive crosslinking

may account for deleterious changes taking place in connective tissue with age.

The ultimate aim of research designed to elucidate pathological processes is to provide a basis for therapy or prophylaxis. The non-enzymic processes which appear to be more significant in the deterioration of elastin and other connective tissue proteins, may be, theoretically counteracted. For example, caloric restriction, which has been shown to dramatically increase the life span of experimental animals, may exert its demonstrated ability to maintain connective tissue in a "young" condition by minimizing the concentration of endogenous, potentially crosslinking metabolites. The reported beneficial effects of antioxidants on animal survival may, by their known property of free radical scavenging, prevent in vivo tanning reactions. Alternatively, enzymes or chemical agents may be discovered which can specifically cleave interchain protein linkages in highly crosslinked connective tissue. Finally, although endogenous elastase or related enzymes may be of little significance in determining connective tissue status in the mature individual, pharmacological preparations of the enzymes might be exploited for possible salutary effects in disease states.

ACKNOWLEDGMENTS

The study was supported by the Medical Research Council of Canada, the Manitoba Heart Foundation, and the Canadian Arthritis and Rheumatism Society. The author is a Medical Research Associate, MRC of Canada.

REFERENCES

Andersen, S.O. (1966). Acta Physiol. Scand. 66, Suppl. 263.

Armstrong, W.G., and Horsley, H.G. (1972). Calc. Tiss. Res. 8, 197.

Balo, J., and Banga, I. (1955). 3rd Internat. Congr. Biochem.,
    p. 120.

Banga, I., and Balo, J. (1956). Nature 178, 310.

Banga, I., and Ardelt, W. (1967). Biochim. Biophys. Acta 146, 284.

Banga, I. (1969). Intern. Symp. on the Biochemistry of the
    Vascular Wall, Fribourg, p. 18.

Barnes, M.J., and Partridge, S.M. (1968). Biochem. J. 109, 883.

Blomfield, J., and Farrar, J.F. (1969). Cardiovasc. Res. 3, 161.

Chio, K.S., and Tappel, A.L. (1969). Biochemistry 8, 2821.

Cleary, E.G., Jackson, D.S., and Sandberg, L.B. (1965). In "Biochemistry and Physiology of Connective Tissue." (P. Comte, ed.), p. 167, Societe Ormeco et Imprimerie du Sud-Est, Lyons, France.

Deyl, A., Sulcova, H., and Praus, R. (1970). Exp. Gerontol. 5, 57.

Downie, J.W., LaBella, F.S., and West, M. (1972). Biochim. Biophys. Acta 263, 604.

Gilfillan, R.F. (1968). Cancer Res. 28, 137.

Hall, D.A. (1955). Biochem. J. 59, 459.

Hall, D.A. (1964). "Elastolysis and Aging." Charles C. Thomas, Springfield, Ill.

Hall, D.A. (1966). Biochem. J. 101, 29.

Janoff, A., and Scherer, J. (1968). J. Exp. Med. 128, 1137.

Janoff, A., and Bosch, R.S. (1971). Proc. Soc. Exp. Biol. Med. 136, 1045.

Karlson, P., and Sekeris, C.E. (1962). Nature 195, 183.

Keeley, F.W. (1970). Ph.D. Thesis, Univ. of Manitoba.

Keeley, F.S., and LaBella, F.S. (1972a). Connective Tissue Res. 1, 113.

Keeley, F.W., and LaBella, F.S. (1972b). Biochim. Biophys. Acta 263, 52.

LaBella, F.S., Vivian, S., and Thornhill, D.P. (1966). J. Gerontol. 21, 550.

LaBella, F.S., and Thornhill, D.P. (1966). Studies on Rheumatoid Disease: Proc. Third Canad. Conf. Res. Rheum. Dis., Univ. of Toronto Press, 246.

LaBella, F.S. (1961). Arch. Biochem. Biophys. 93, 72.

LaBella, F.S., and Lindsay, W.G. (1963). J. Gerontol. 18, 111.

LaBella, F.S., and Paul, G. (1965). J. Gerontol. 20, 54.

LaBella, F.S., Waykole, P., and Queen, G. (1968). Biochem. Biophys. Res. Commun. 30, 333.

LaBella, F.S. (1971). In "Biophysical Properties of the Skin," (H.R. Elden, ed.), p. 243, John Wiley & Sons, New York.

Lansing, A.I., Roberts, E., Ramasarma, G.B., Rosenthal, T.B., and Alex, M. (1951). Proc. Soc. Exp. Biol. Med. 76, 714.

Lansing, A.E., Rosenthal, T.B., Alex, M., and Dempsey, E.W. (1951). Anat. Rec. 114, 555.

Legrand, Y., Pignaud, G., Robert, B., Robert, L., and Caen, J. (1969). Compte rend. Seances Soc. Biol. 163, 1104.

Little, K. (1973). J. Pathol. 110, 1.

Loeven, W.A. (1963). In "Internat. Rev. Connective Tissue Res." (D.A. Hall, ed.), p. 184, Academic Press, New York.

Loeven, W.A. (1969). J. Atheroscler. Res. 9, 35.

Lowry, O.H., Gilligan, D.R., and Katerspy, E.M. (1941). J. Biol. Chem. 139, 795.

Mull, J.D., and Ram, J.S. (1965). J. Gerontol. 20, 201.

Partridge, S.M., Davis, H.F., and Adair, G.S. (1955). Biochem. J. 61, 11.

Peereboom, J.W.C. (1970). Gerontologia 16, 352.

Robert, L., and Comte, P. (1968). Life Sci. (Oxford) 7, Part II, 493.

Robert, B., Szigeti, M., Robert, L., Legrand, Y., Pignaud, G., and Caen, J. (1970). Nature 227, 1248.

Ross, R., and Bornstein, P. (1969). J. Cell Biol. 40, 366.

Slack, H.G.B. (1954). Nature 174, 512.

Thornhill, D.P. (1971). Biochemistry 10, 2644.

Thornhill, D.P. (1972). Connective Tissue Res. 1, 21.

Timpl, R., Wolff, I., and Weiser, M. (1968). Biochim. Biophys. Acta 168, 168.

Tunbridge, R.E. (1957). In "Ciba Found. Colloq. Aging,"
     p. 92, Little, Brown, & Co., Boston.

Turino, G.M., Lourenco, R.V., and McCracken, G.H. (1964). J.
     Clin. Invest. 43, 1297.

Turino, G.M., Senior, R.M., Garg, B.D., Keller, S., Levi, M.M.,
     and Mandl, I. (1969). Science 165, 709.

Walford, R.L., Carter, P.K., and Schneider, R.B. (1964). Arch.
     Pathol. 78, 43.

DISCUSSION FOLLOWING THE PRESENTATION BY FRANK S. LABELLA

Dr. Kramsch: Dr. LaBella, in your study on changes in aortic
elastin due to aging, did you analyze the intima-media of whole
aorta in the different age groups?

Dr. LaBella: To prepare "elastin" from human aortas, the
intima and adventitia were stripped off and the media was defatted
and extracted with hot alkali.

Dr. Kramsch: Then you studied only the media of the aorta?

Dr. LaBella: Yes.

Dr. Kramsch: With regard to that, I cannot understand why in
our own analysis of plaques from aortas in young individuals (the
youngest was 26) we found increases of polar amino acids and lipids
in the elastin preparation. If they are age-related they should
not be there. The increased polar amino acids were clearly related
to atherosclerosis. The rabbits in our animal studies also were
actually quite young. We fed them an atherogenic diet, and again
only the elastin preparation from plaques showed a change in amino
acid composition and also in lipid content. This cannot be due to
aging. On the other hand, when we analyzed adjacent areas to
plaques in old human individuals, we could not find any such
dramatic increases in polar amino acids of the elastin preparations.
In fact, with some 80 year old and one 90 year old individual there
was no increase in the polar amino acid of elastin if we went far
enough away from severe plaques. I wonder if you feel that some
of the changes which you observed might be due to atherosclerosis.

Dr. LaBella: Dr. Banga in Budapest has confirmed our finding
of an increase in fluorescence in human elastin with age and in
addition that the increase is more pronounced in elastin prepared
from plaque regions. Our amino acid data suggest that with age
elastin becomes more and more associated with the surrounding

acidic protein, presumably derived from the intercellular matrix. This process is more prevalent in plaques, and in very old individuals there may be little "normal" elastin.

Dr. Partridge: Concerning the fluorescence, have you isolated the fluorescent compound?   Is it possible that there is a relationship here, one dityrosine per molecule of tropoelastin?

Dr. LaBella: Tropoelastin (provided by Dr. L. Sandberg) is very weakly fluorescent and gives a small emission peak at about 400 nm.   Dityrosine is not present in tropoelastin nor in mature elastin.   Its presence in fetal or embryonic elastin, as we have reported, is probably due to the presence of the acidic protein which cannot be dissociated from elastin in these developing tissues (Keeley, F.W., and LaBella, F. (1972).   Connective Tissue Res. 1, 113).   Fluorescence is associated with insoluble elastin and is implicated in cross-linking of this protein.   We have purified what appears to be a family of aromatic compounds, most of which are ninhydrin-negative.   This is all we can say definitively about these fluorescent substances.

Dr. Martin: You discounted the possibility that enzymes digest elastin in aging or in various diseases.   During development of the aorta in chicks, marked changes occur in the diameter of the aorta.   I would agree that the evidence for animal elastase is weak, but there must be a turnover of elastin.

Dr. LaBella: I too feel that there probably are enzymes concerned with the turnover of the structural proteins, including elastin.   In fact, Dr. Keeley and I have proposed an enzymic process concerned with elastin fibrogenesis (Keeley, F.W., and LaBella, F. (1972).   Connective Tissue Res. 1, 113).   This type of enzyme might serve as the necessary machinery for remodeling of growing blood vessels, as you suggest, and other maturing tissues.   In my talk the negative conclusion I drew, was based on the available data which purport to demonstrate elastase activity in serum, the aortic wall, and other tissues.

Dr. Robert: I would like to take issue with you as far as the statements you made concerning tissue elastases.   I believe that only tissue-elastases can act on aorta elastin, and I don't think that pancreatic elastase could be of any importance in this respect. I feel that pancreatic elastase is a sort of remnant of the prehistoric times when much elastin could have been eaten by man.   As far as human blood platelet elastase is concerned, its isolation, properties, and action on elastin were described (Biochim. Biophys. Acta 309: 406, 1973).

Dr. LaBella: I have tried to distinguish in my talk between "elastases" which act on native elastic fibers and may be solubilizing a variety of proteins other than elastin and "elastinase" which solubilizes the elastic protein. The issue I take with you is that only very sensitive methods, such as release of radioactivity or of dye, are capable of demonstrating solubilization of elastic tissue. To demonstrate the existence of a true elastase, i.e., elastinase, one must show that the highly purified protein with typical amino acid composition serves as substrate for the enzyme and that solubilization of this substrate does in fact occur.

Dr. Robert: Platelet elastase also acts on synthetic substrates such as trialanine methyl ester and others.

Dr. LaBella: Hydrolysis of synthetic substrates by proteases cannot be taken as evidence for the presence of an elastinase.

Dr. Robert: I cannot agree with this statement because synthetic substrates are very useful to establish the specificity of proteases, and none of the conventional digestive proteases (trypsin, chymotrypsin) did attack trialanine-methyl ester at a measurable rate (C.R. Acad. Sci., Paris 274, 1749-1752, 1972). These enzymes which did attack this and other synthetic substrates also attacked elastin.

Pathological elastolysis is a slow process. Elastin is slowly fragmented along the years and not diffusely lysed as by pancreatic elastase, not even in the atherosclerotic plaque. We do not need potent elastases giving fast and "complete" solubilization of fibrillar elastin to explain pathological in vivo elastolysis. The mechanism of action of platelet elastase is just about what we need for that.

CALCIFICATION PROCESSES IN ATHEROSCLEROSIS

Shiu Yeh Yu

Veterans Administration Hospital and Department of
Internal Medicine, Washington University School of
Medicine, St. Louis, Missouri

In atherosclerotic aortas, there are marked changes in the
structure of smooth muscle cells and elastic tissue in addition to
other intimal changes such as the focal accumulation of lipids,
mucopolysaccharides, blood, and blood products. These changes are
observed predominantly in the subendothelial space, around the
internal elastic lamina, as well as in the media.

The internal elastic lamina frequently is destroyed and the
elastic tissue of the media fragmented; then calcification of
aortic tissue takes place in these areas. Also, some of the early
fatty streaks may develop into fibrous plaques and eventually a
deposit of calcium develops, resulting in a complicated lesion.

NATURE OF INORGANIC COMPOUNDS IN AORTAS

With a systematic chemical analysis of the inorganic compounds
in whole human aortas (Table I), there is essentially a progressive
rise in percentage of ash, as well as of calcium and phosphate,
except the first and the last decade (Yu and Blumenthal, 1963a,b).
This increase is highly significant after the sixth decade. The
major constituents of the ash of highly mineralized aortas of the
fourth decade appear to be calcium and phosphate. If one calculates
the Ca/P mole ratio, there is a progressive rise that finally
approaches a maximum which is similar to the value of 1.67 of carbonate apatite. These data strongly suggest that a unique compound
is accumulating as calcium phosphate in aortas.

During the process of cellular fractionation of the aortic
homogenate, the major calcium phosphate compound was recovered in
the fraction of elastin. Subsequently, elastins were prepared by

403

TABLE I.   ASH, CALCIUM AND PHOSPHATE IN WHOLE HUMAN AORTA*

Age Group (Years)	No.	Ash†	Ca	PO$_4$	Ca/P Mole Ratio‡	Ca + PO$_4$ / Ash
0-9	5	2.67	0.13	0.92	0.36	0.39
10-19	13	1.86	0.10	0.65	0.36	0.40
20-29	10	2.86	0.29	0.93	0.78	0.43
40-49	15	4.30	1.10	2.07	1.21	0.74
50-59	27	4.98	1.51	2.52	1.46	0.81
60-69	20	8.63	2.49	4.44	1.36	0.80
70-79	25	15.83	5.45	8.10	1.58	0.86
80-89	26	12.66	4.21	6.50	1.56	0.84

* Defatted and dehydrated aortas from Caucasian patients.
† Calculated as gms per 100 gm of defatted dry tissue.
‡ The Ca/P mole ratio of carbonate apatite is 1.67.

TABLE II.   CALCIUM AND PHOSPHATE IN ELASTIN

Age (Years)	Race	No.	Ca(%)	PO$_4$(%)	Ca/P Mole Ratio*
10-20	Negro	10	0.27	0.37	1.66
40-49	Negro	12	6.70	10.27	1.56
50-59	Caucasian	14	6.25	9.04	1.64
60-69	Negro	13	9.22	12.93	1.70
60-69	Caucasian	18	11.95	17.53	1.64
80-90	Caucasian	10	17.10	24.51	1.65

* The Ca/P mole ratio of carbonate apatite is 1.67.

a hot-alkaline method from aortas from different age groups
(Yu and Blumenthal, 1963a). The calcium and phosphate contents
show a similar increase with progressive aging as in the entire
aortas (Table II). An interesting difference between the analysis
of elastin and entire aorta is that the Ca/P mole ratio of elastin
is almost identical in all age groups.

For the indentification of the crystalline structure of
calcium phosphate, X-ray diffraction analysis was used on aortic
elastin prepared by repeated autoclaving of calcified plaque of
aortas which had a high content of calcium phosphate. The
results of the analysis and comparison with the standard data from
carbonate apatite (Table III) show that the spectrum of the powder
specimen of the calcified plaque appeared to be nearly the same as

TABLE III. X-RAY DIFFRACTION DATA ON ELASTIN FROM CALCIFIED PLAQUE

Autoclaved Calcified Plaque		Carbonate Apatite*	
$\overset{o}{A}$	$1/1_1$	$\overset{o}{A}$	$1/1_1$
-	-	4.08	20
-	-	3.90	20
3.45	53	3.44	80
3.10	30	3.18	10
-	-	3.08	20
2.80	100	2.82	100
2.72	59	2.71	90
2.64	38	2.62	50
-	-	2.52	10
2.62	28	2.25	60
-	-	2.14	10
-	-	2.06	10
-	-	2.00	10
1.945	32	1.92	70
1.84	33	1.89	30
-	-	1.83	70
-	-	1.80	40
-	-	1.77	40
1.72	24	1.75	40
-	-	1.64	20

* From American Society for Testing Materials x-ray powder data file.

TABLE IV. CALCIUM, PHOSPHORUS AND CO_2 IN CALCIFIED PLAQUE OF HUMAN AORTAS* AND IN HUMAN BONE

Constituent	Autoclaved Plaque	Autoclaved Bone	Carbonate Apatite†
Ash	57.40%	65.40%	-
HCl Soluble Ca	27.95%	21.40%	-
HCl Soluble P	13.95%	10.50%	-
Ca/P Mole Ratio (HCl Soluble)	1.56	1.34	1.67
Total Ca	27.90%	21.40%	-
Total P	14.30%	10.44%	-
Ca/P Mole Ratio (Total)	1.52	1.34	1.67
CO_2	4.81%	3.42%	-
CO_2/P Molar Ratio	0.237	0.236	-

* Calcified plaques were collected from eight aortas from Caucasian individuals and pooled.
† Calculated from the file of the American Society for Testing Materials.

for the standard apatite crystal. The analysis of highly calcified plaques (Table IV) shows that both acid-soluble and total calcium and phosphorus were essentially the same. Acid solubility is indicative of inorganic calcium and phosphate, and the insolubility indicates the existence of these elements in organic binding. The data indicate that all of the calcium and phosphate in the plaque were in the form of inorganic compounds. Also, the plaque contained carbonate, which indicated the presence of carbonate apatite.

Although the unique characteristic of the crystalline structure of the apatite is expressed in the X-ray diffraction data, unfortunately the X-ray diffraction data do not distinguish between the difference of hydroxyapatite, $Ca_{10}(PO_4)_6(OH)_2$; carbonate apatite, $Ca_{10}(PO_4)_6CO_3$; calcium-deficient apatite, $Ca_{10-x}H_{2x}(PO_4)_6(OH)_2$; fluoroapatite, $Ca_{10}(PO_4)_6(F)_2$; chloroapatite, $Ca_{10}(PO_4)_6(Cl)_2$; and so forth. Also, it is impossible to detect minor inorganic minerals which might be present in the specimen in concentrations of less than 5%. Carbonate-apatite and probably a considerable amount of hydroxyapatite are present in these tissues.

TRACE ELEMENTS AND CALCIFICATION OF AORTAS

In addition to these apatite forms, there is the possibility of the presence of other apatites such as barium, strontium or lead apatite (Neuman and Neuman, 1958), since after analysis by emission spectroscopy the ash of aortas contains these elements (Table V).

In general, calcified lesions appear first in the iliac artery, then the abdominal aorta, and finally the thoracic aorta. Consequently, mineralization is greater in the iliac, abdominal, and thoracic aortas in descending order. When the trace elements in these aortic segments are compared during life, only calcium and phosphate accumulate in quantities. Since other trace elements such as magnesium, aluminum, copper, silicon, and others show no significant correlation with the degree of mineralization of the aortas, the possibility that some other inorganic compound(s) might play a role in seeding of apatite formation should be ruled out. In the presence of such a mechanism, it would probably be the predeposited apatite itself that serves as an epitaxy for the further introduction and deposition of calcium phosphate.

In addition, from the data of trace element analysis, the content of copper decreases significantly in the highly mineralized aortic tissues (Table V). Recently the copper ion was found to be essential for the normal synthesis of elastic fiber in aortas (Sandberg et al., 1971; Shields et al., 1962). A decrease of copper ion in aortic tissue may result directly in the formation of a lower cross-linked elastin, which may lead to the development of

TABLE V. MINERAL CONTENT IN DIFFERENT AREAS OF HUMAN AORTAS

Age	27 yr.	78 yr.	78 yr.
Area	Abdominal*	Abdominal[†]	Iliac[†]
Ash[‡]	1.44%	29.89%	42. 98%

Mineral Contents in Crude Ash (%)			
Mg	1.0	0.8	0.5
Al	0.005	0.001	0.005
Cu	0.005	0.001	0.010
Si	0.08	0.03	0.06
Sr	0.8	0.9	0.4
Fe	0.3	0.01	0.10
Sn	0.0036	trace	trace
Ni	0.01	trace	trace
Ag	0.00012	trace	trace
Zn	0.0576	0.028	0.012
Pb	0.0240	0.0032	0.0016
Ca	33.55	34.59	36.77
PO4	46.76	47.90	48.54
Na	11.16	1.43	1.19
K	5.91	0.14	0.08

* The aorta was obtained from a young female subject without
  arteriosclerotic lesions; the aorta grade was No. 1 - No. 2.
[†] The specimens were obtained from a similar subject with
  severe athero-arteriosclerosis; the degree of arteriosclerosis was grade No. 6.
[‡] Adventitial portion of aortic tissue was removed and the
  remaining intimal and medial portions were dried at 110°C
  and ash was calculated as gms per 100 gm of dry tissue.

arterial lesions and then calcification; or, highly mineralized
tissues may prevent transportation of copper ion into the areas,
which could contribute to the abnormal synthesis of elastic fibers
at the site.

ULTRASTRUCTURE OF CALCIUM CRYSTALS AND THEIR ORGANIC MATRICES

Because of the affinity of calcium crystals for a specific
ultrastructural site of collagen fibers, the structure of apatite
in aortic elastin was studied (Yu and Blumenthal, 1963a,c; Yu, 1967).
In calcified areas of human aorta (Figure 1), spherical masses are
located between elastic lamella and occasionally inside the elastic
fiber; others lie either on the surface of the fiber, where its
edges are frayed, or in degenerated material between the fibers.
Cellular elements are not seen in this specimen, probably because

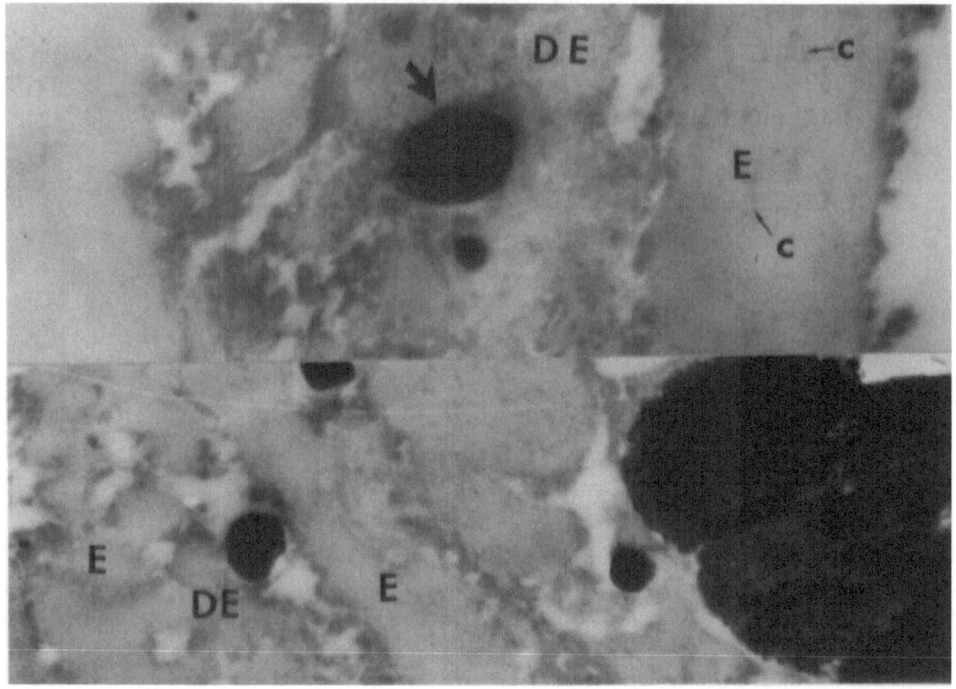

Fig. 1. Electron micrographs of section of human aorta. DE, areas of degenerating elastin; E, inact elastic fiber; C, collagen. Large arrow indicates spherical masses appear on the degenerated elastin or the surface areas of elastic fibers. (x 40,000).

of postmortem autolysis. It is important to notice that the entire elastin was not calcified, and only a certain area of elastic fiber carried different sizes and shapes of mineral.

Numerous large, needle-like crystals appeared in the preparation of a calcified plaque which had been treated with boiling 0.1 N NaOH. In some areas, crystals were seen on the surface of the elastic fibers (Figure 2). In other areas, microcrystals appeared in a random arrangement in fragmented elastin (Figure 3). This specimen was obtained from heavily calcified areas of human aorta. Some small crystals are polyhedral in form instead of large needle crystals, while others are microspherulites.

The calcified mass in isolated elastin-collagen preparations, which were obtained from human arteriosclerotic aortas, is observed more frequently on the surface of the fibers (Figure 4). Treatment of the elastin-collagen preparation with elastase revealed a pincushion-like structure of calcium apatite (Figure 5). The crystalline structure appeared initially as a microgranule, and in some sites eventually develops into the form of a spherically symmetrical mass in the degenerated or regenerated elastic fiber. In other sites microgranules and micropolyhedral crystals aggregate in fraying elastin.

Analytical data of the organic constituents of calcified human aortic plaques (Table VI) show that there are mucopolysaccharides, lipids, microfibrils, and elastin present. One should take into consideration that these materials, besides elastic fibers, may also play a role in the initiation of calcification, either by providing epitaxy or removing the inhibitor for calcification at a certain site (Sobel et al., 1960).

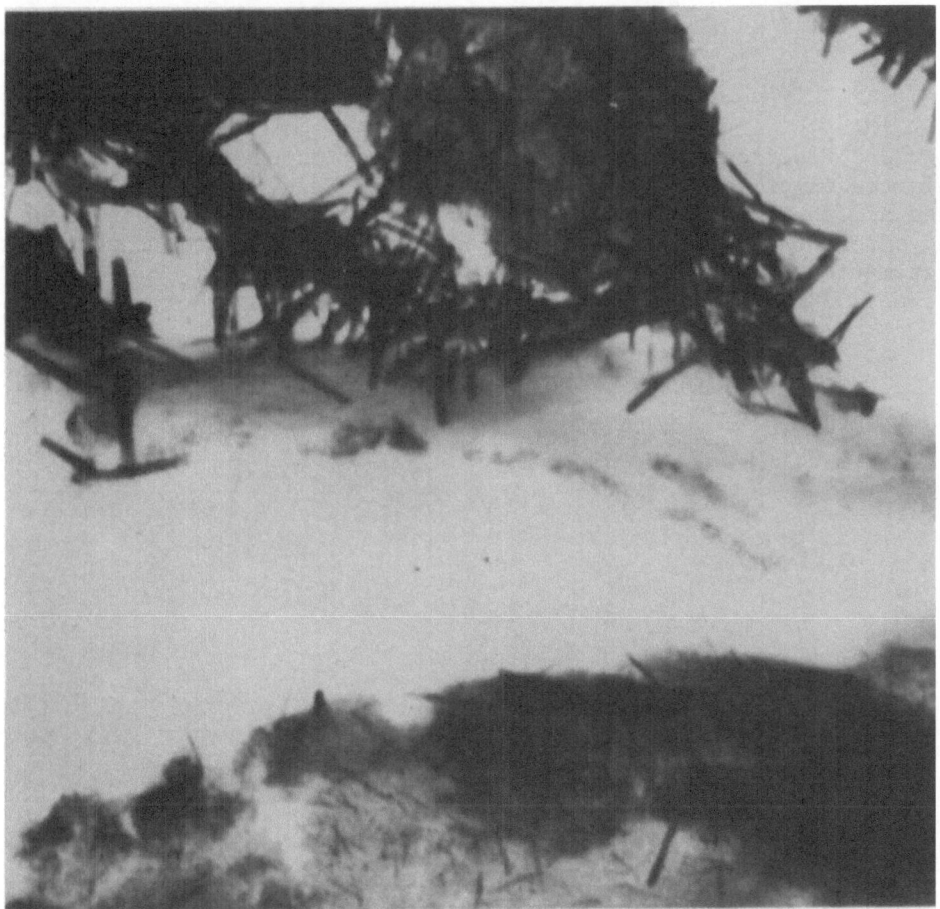

Fig. 2. Electron micrograph of a thin section of autoclaved, defatted, calcified plaque of human aorta. Numerous needle-like crystals are seen in the highly dense elastic fiber. The crystals arrange randomly with various sizes. (x 40,000).

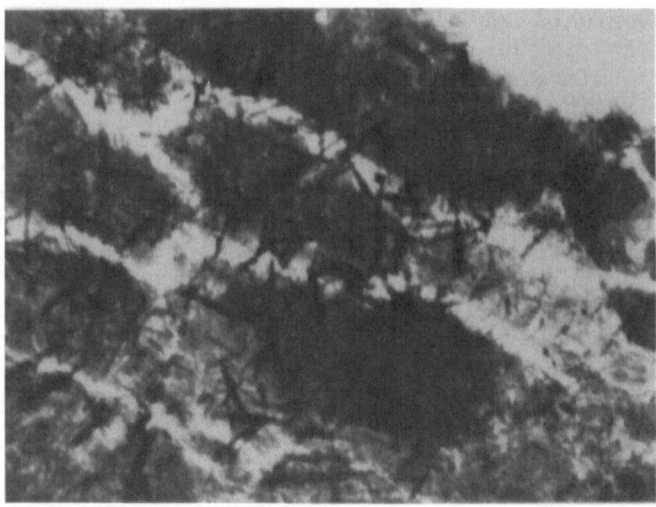

Fig. 3. Electron micrograph of a thin section of autoclaved,
defatted calcified plaque of human aorta. Heavy calcification is
seen and the organic matrices are not detectable. Numerous shapes
and sizes of calcium crystals are seen, which indicates that nonsystematic calcification takes place at the site. (x 40,000).
(Reduced 30% for reproduction).

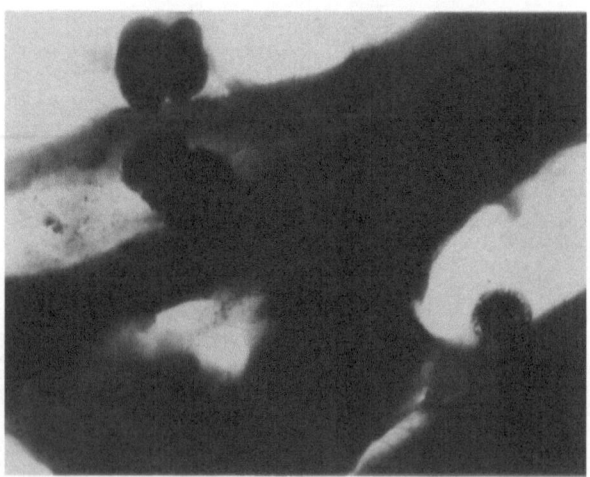

Fig. 4. Electron micrograph of elastin-collagen preparation from
homogenate of atherosclerotic aorta. Spherical nodules are seen
on the surface membrane of elastic fibers. (x 40,000). (Reduced
50% for reproduction).

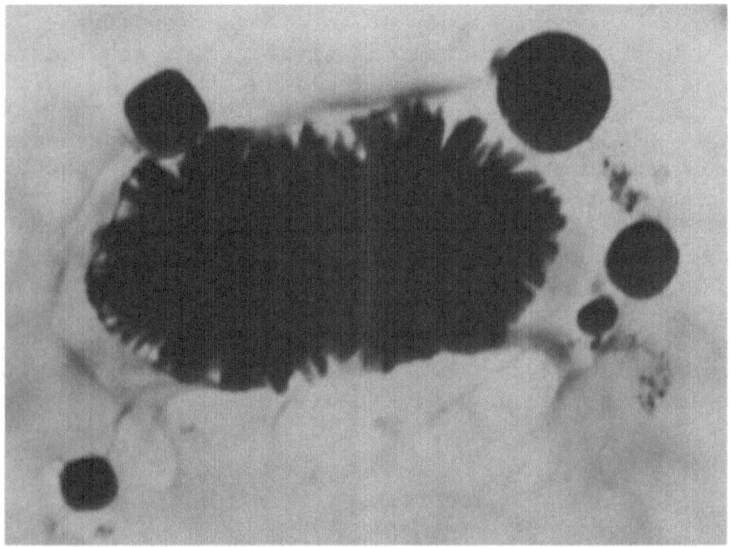

Fig. 5. Electron micrograph of spherical nodules which were
prepared by treating the elastin-collagen preparation with
elastase in glycine buffer pH 8.0 at 37 C. After the elastase
digestion, a pincushion-like structure of calcium apatite is seen.
(x 40,000). (Reduced 25% for reproduction).

TABLE VI. ORGANIC CONSTITUENTS OF CALCIFIED PLAQUE OF HUMAN AORTAS

Constituent	Percent
Ash	57.4
Protein	30.4
Mucopolysaccharides	
(as Chondroitin Sulfate)	3.6
Lipids	1.5
Total Cholesterol	1.2
Sulfur	0.09
Glucosamine	0.07
TOTAL	94.16

The mechanism of initiating arterial calcification is complex,
and one may conclude that the acidic mucopolysaccharides may play
a role in this process (Sobel et al., 1960). Normally in aortas,
the elastic lamina directly associates with glycoprotein (Robert
et al., 1972) and acidic mucopolysaccharides (Yu and Blumenthal,

1958). An autoradiographic study of aortic sections from $^{35}SO_4$-treated rats shows that concentrated silver grains are localized at the elastic laminae (Yu et al., 1968). Furthermore, acidic mucopolysaccharides have been demonstrated histochemically at the site (Moore and Schoenberg, 1959). Using a modified procedure of colloidal iron staining and electron microscopic technique (Yu et al., 1967), mucopolysaccharides appear localized at the surface of the isolated elastic laminae (Figures 6 and 7). Although it has been suggested that glycoprotein, which is believed to be firmly bound with the elastic fiber, may play a role in the process of calcification of aortas (Grant et al., 1971; Robert et al., 1972), there is no direct evidence to support this hypothesis. The precise mechanism of the action by mucopolysaccharides on calcification remains for further studies.

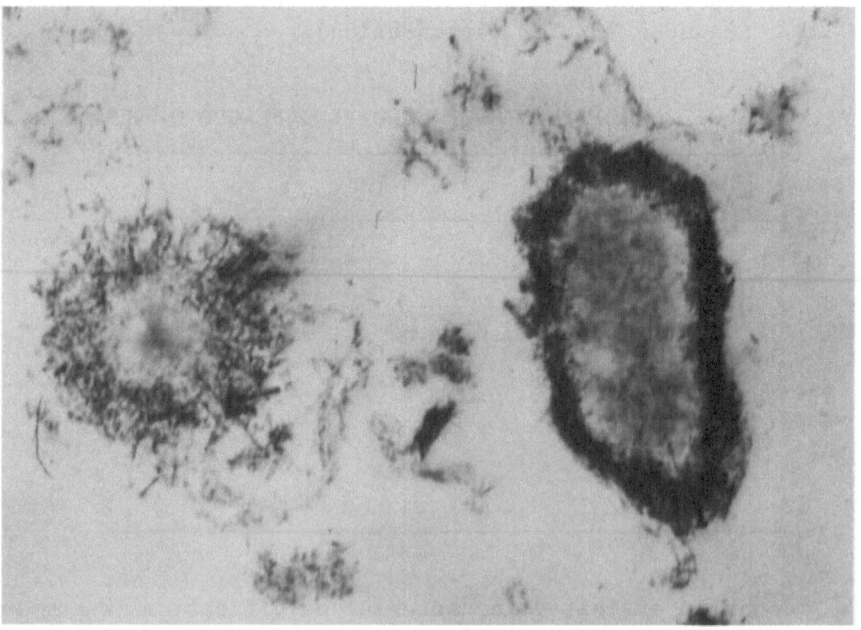

Fig. 6. Electron micrograph of section of elastic fiber preparation stained with colloidal iron. Iron crystals are seen on the surface of elastic fiber in which mucopolysaccharides occur in higher concentration. (x 40,000).

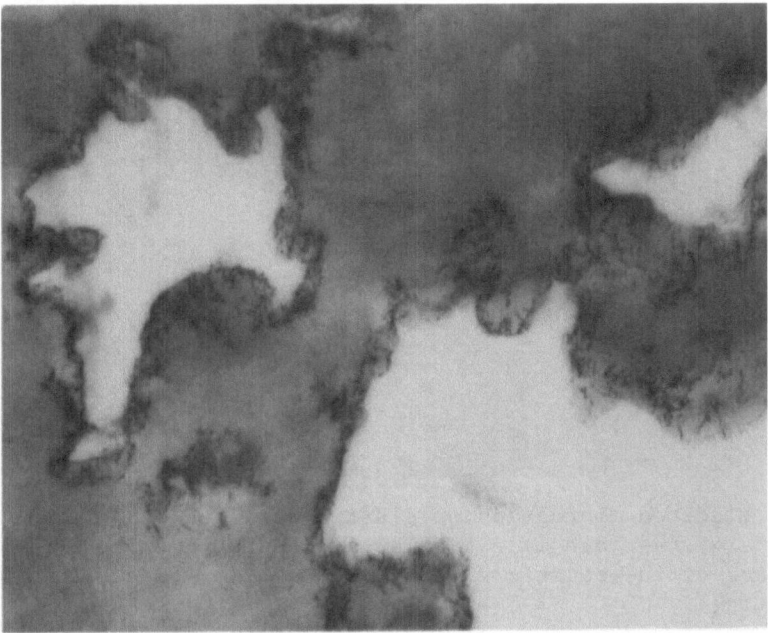

Fig. 7. Electron micrograph of section of elastic fiber preparation stained with colloidal iron. Denser areas are the matrix of
elastic fiber. High accumulations of iron are seen in the peripheral area of the fiber. (x 40,000). (Reduced 20% for reproduction).

ULTRASTRUCTURE OF DEGENERATED ELASTIC FIBERS

From the observation of electron micrographs of various
preparations of calcified elastin, it appears that the calcium
compounds are much more firmly bound with the elastic fiber
(Figure 8). Numerous knob-like densities are extended along the
surface of the elastic fibers. This specimen was prepared from
an arteriosclerotic aorta after treating an aortic homogenate
with cold Triton X-100 solution and cold saline, extensively. A
water suspension of the fibrous material was placed directly on a
coated-grid without cutting a thin section.

Further decalcification with EDTA solution of the above
specimen revealed that the elastic fiber had irregularities on its
surface (Figure 9). These surface or laminated areas of elastic
fiber significantly alter its structure. Aortic elastic fibers
characteristically have two morphologically distinguishable fibers,
one is a fibrous rod-like structure, and the other is a membrane
or lamella-like structure (Figure 10). The membrane-like elastin
frequently coats the surface of the rod-like fibrous elastin.

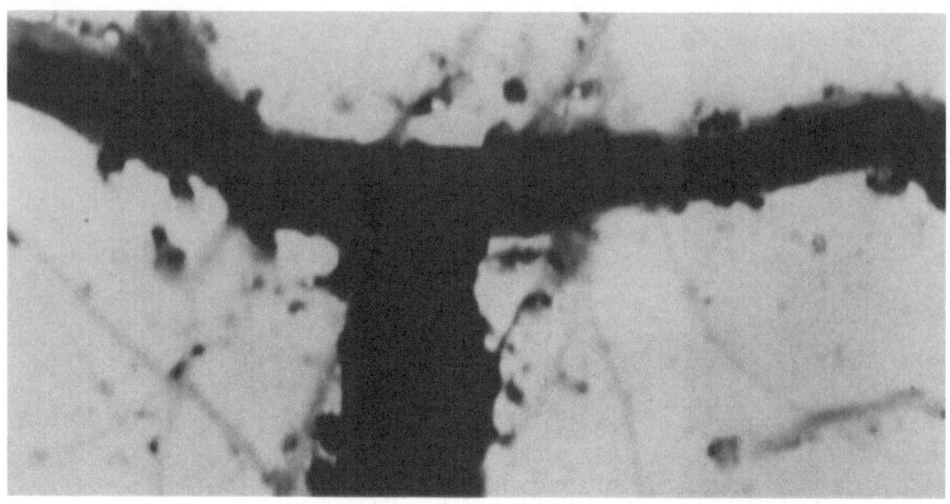

Fig. 8. Electron micrograph of elastin-collagen preparation of
aorta of a 45 year old male. Numerous nodules are seen only on
the surface of the elastic fiber. (x 60,000). (Reduced 40% for
reproduction).

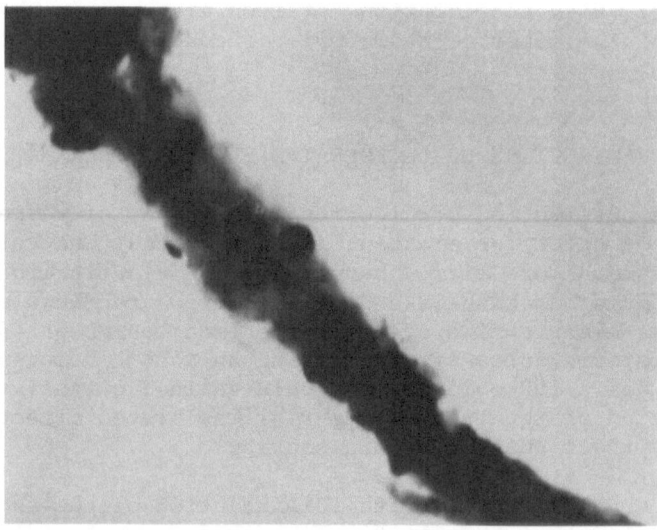

Fig. 9. Electron micrograph of isolated elastic fiber. The
specimen was prepared from an aorta of severe atherosclerosis,
autoclaved to remove collagen and decalcified with EDTA solution.
Highly degenerated elastic membrane is seen on the surface of the
elastic fiber. Some calcified nodules remain. (x 60,000).
(Reduced 30% for reproduction).

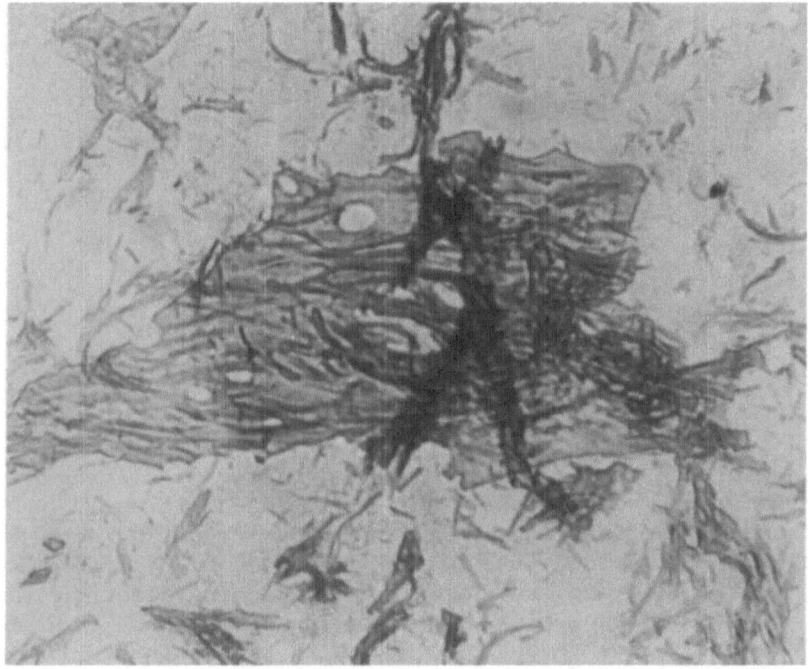

Fig. 10. Isolated aortic elastic fibers from a segment of human aorta. Both laminated and fibrous elastic fibers organize to form elastic lamella (Weigert stain; approximately x 500).

Scanning microscopic pictures show human aortic elastic lamellae and fibers which were prepared by treatment of aortic segments of arteriosclerotic aorta with formic acid for eight days at 45°C (Ayer et al., 1958) (Figure 11). The specimen contained no collagen and had been decalcified (Yu and Kuhn, 1972). It shows layers of elastic lamellae as they would be in aorta. It is not known whether multiple fenestrations of the laminated elastin or anchorage sites between smooth muscle cells and elastic fibers are the sites of calcified nodules. However, we propose that the membrane-like area of the elastic fiber is prone to calcification. Finally, in some areas, especially in heavily calcified femoral artery, collagen is also calcified (Figure 12). Unlike the bone system, calcification of collagen in aorta is nonsystematic. Collagen fiber can be seen with cross-striation, and microcrystals appear to be present on the collagen banding with corresponding striation. In some areas larger nodules similar to those seen on the surface of elastic fibers are attached to collagen fiber.

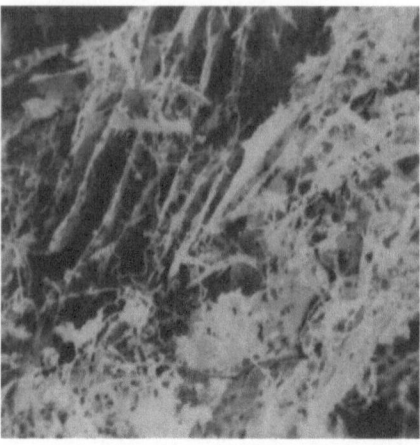

Fig. 11. Isolated aortic lamellae from atherosclerotic human
aorta. The structure of elastic fiber remains as it would be in
aortic tissue. The specimen was prepared by incubating segments
of aorta in formic acid by the method described by Ayer et al.
(1958), lyophilizing and examining with a scanning electron microscope. Note two morphologically distinguishable fibers -- laminated
and fibrous. Multiple fenestra are seen in the laminated fibers.
(x 500). (Reduced 35% for reproduction).

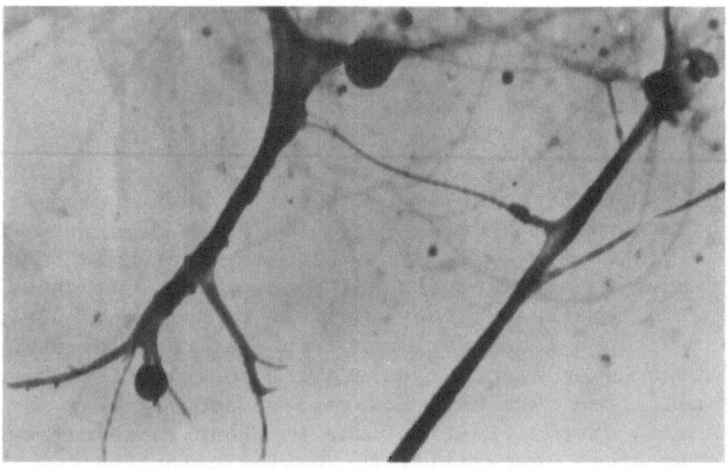

Fig. 12. Electron micrograph of collagen preparation from femoral
artery of an 85 year old male subject. The collagen preparation
in this area shows calcification takes place in denser areas of
the fibrous cross banding. Several large spheres are seen.
(x 51,000). (Reduced 40% for reproduction).

The rate of formation of the calcium compound, and the pattern of crystal deposition, as well as the structure of the apatite crystals, probably depend upon such factors as substrate concentration, its ratio to preformed apatite, and the presence of steric hindrance and various inhibitors of calcification. The latter two factors may affect the initiation of mineralization. The smallest and probably earliest deposits occur as spherules measuring 110 ± 20A in diameter. The spherical granules are conglomerated at specific sites, mainly the approximation to the surface of the elastic fiber, seen in Figure 13. The specimen

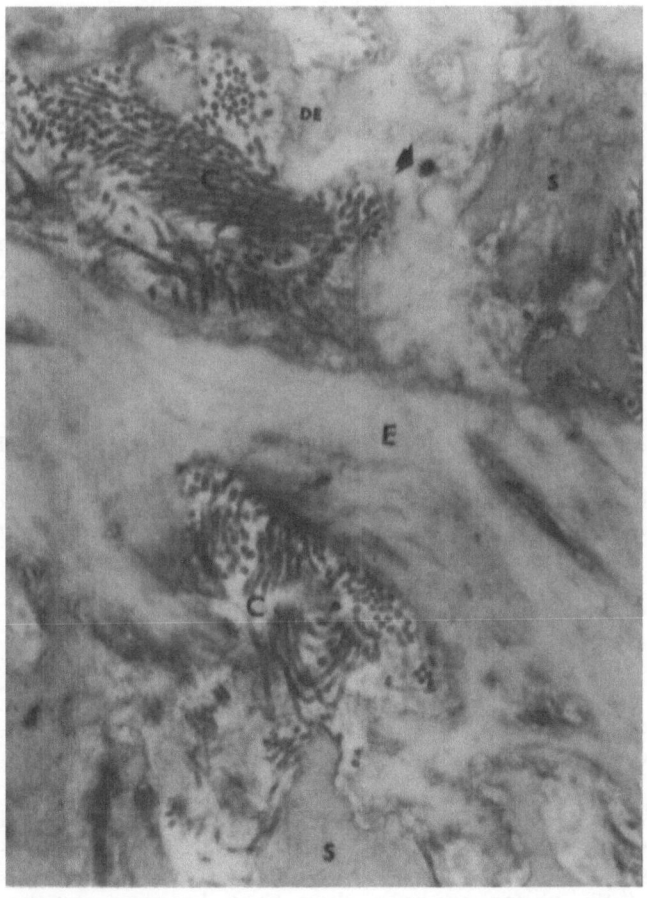

Fig. 13. Electron micrograph of an aortic section of an epinephrine treated rabbit. C, collagen; E, elastic fiber; S, smooth muscle. Arrow indicates a microgranule deposit in the area of degenerated elastin (DE). (x 44,000). (Reduced 30% for reproduction.)

was obtained from a subendothelial area of a section of aorta from
an epinephrine-treated rabbit. It is interesting that in this area
there is no evidence of accumulation of lipid materials in the
tissue. A definite site of earlier calcification in the degenerated
elastic fiber is indicated by arrow. These have no distinctive
pattern but more or less aggregate random fashion. There is also
the possibility that some colloidal calcium phosphate might accumulate at the site prior to the formation of small spherical bodies.
On the other hand, when apatite formation occurs relatively slowly
in the absence of steric hindrance and in low substrate concentration, the typical form is that of a large sphere in which the
crystals are coated with elastin protein. These crystals can only
be revealed by digestion with elastase.

Although calcification occurs predominantly in association
with elastic fiber and preformed microcrystals or small spherical
bodies, when massive mineralization is encountered, nucleation may
not be apatite, nor may seeding be limited to elastin. Minerals
can be found on other solid materials and be in other forms of
calcium, such as calcite, calcium oxalate, or complexes of iron
such as occurs in the calcification of lung tissue. Such forma-
tions are similar to those which occur in development of renal
stone. In the femoral arteries, crystal deposition also occurs in
collagen fiber, although the shape of the crystals is not uniformly
arranged, as those in bone collagen.

BIOCHEMICAL CHARACTERISTICS OF DEGENERATED ELASTIC FIBERS

The morphological observation on the affinity of calcium
apatite toward aortic elastin led us to believe that there may be
a qualitative difference in elastin from arteriosclerotic aorta.
In the following experiments some evidences are provided.

Calcification Process Studied by ^{45}Ca Uptake
(Yu and Wertalecki, 1965; Yu and Blumenthal, 1967)

The aortas of rabbits which have been treated with epinephrine develop severe calcification without accumulations of
lipids and cholesterol (Yu and Blumenthal, 1965). Also, after
injections of ^{45}Ca these animals show that isotope uptake in vivo
by aortic elastin is greater in epinephrine injected animals than
in normal controls (Table VII). This suggests that biochemical
differences in aortic elastin may contribute to alterations in its
affinity for calcification.

TABLE VII. ^{45}Ca UPTAKE IN ELASTIN

	Degree of Calcification	Ca in Aortic Elastin %	^{45}Ca in Aortic Elastin μmol /100 gm
Normal	0	0.091	1.43
Epinephrine (I)	+ + +	1.920	13.45
Epinephrine (II)	+	0.263	2.47
Epinephrine.(III)	+ +	0.366	3.86
Epinephrine (IV)	+	0.187	2.34

Calcification of Aorta and Amino Acid Composition of Elastins from Different Areas of Aorta of a Human Subject (Yu, 1971; 1972).

It is well known that various segments of the arterial tree differ in their susceptibility to atherosclerosis. Aortic tissue was obtained from a 70 year old male subject; the degree of arteriosclerosis corresponded to grade No. 6 of the American Heart Association grading system. The aorta showed high calcification in both abdominal and iliac segments and a lesser degree of calcification in the thoracic aorta. The elastins from each segment of the aorta were prepared by a series of exhaustive extractions, with at least six repeated extractions at each step with different solutions including saline, Triton X-100, decalcification with EDTA solution, guanidine-HCl solution, autoclaving, and a final treatment with 0.1 N NaOH solution for 1 hour at 98°C. It would be difficult to assume the possibility of contamination with other proteins or glycoprotein. Some of the amino acids of elastin from the thoracic aorta, such as glycine, valine, alanine, and proline were present in higher concentrations (Table VIII). In contrast, higher contents of aspartic, glutamic acids, and other polar amino acids were found in elastins of abdominal and iliac aorta than the corresponding amino acids of the elastin from the thoracic segment. It is not known whether this difference is due to contaminating protein in the elastin from arteriosclerotic aorta or a true difference in amino acid composition. Also, a significant difference was observed in the content of cross-linking amino acids of elastin among these preparations (Table IX). This observation has subsequently been confirmed by John and Thomas (1972). In the atherosclerotic aorta, both isodesmosine and desmosine contents are lower, and the concentration of lysine is higher in the elastins of abdominal and iliac segments compared with the corresponding compounds from thoracic aorta. It is possible that these elastins, having a lower degree of cross-linkage and coming from highly

TABLE VIII.   AMINO ACID COMPOSITION OF ELASTINS FROM DIFFERENT
AREAS OF A HUMAN AORTA

(Moles per 70,000 g of protein)

Amino Acid	Thoracic (A)	Abdominal (B)	Iliac	Difference (B-A)
Hydroxyproline	11.1	15.3	11.3	+4.2
Aspartic Acid	7.4	17.9	11.3	+10.5
Threonine	6.6	9.1	8.5	+2.5
Serine	5.7	10.5	8.3	+4.7
Glutamic Acid	16.5	29.7	21.2	+13.2
Proline	75.6	71.2	71.0	-4.4
Glycine	184.0	161.7	180.7	-22.3
Alanine	145.0	121.0	138.1	-22.0
Cystine (half)	-	-	-	-
Valine	88.8	62.2	85.4	-26.6
Methionine	1.5	4.3	2.5	+2.8
Isoleucine	16.6	19.2	17.3	+2.6
Leucine	40.6	44.7	41.2	+4.1
Tyrosine	14.0	13.5	14.8	-0.5
Phenylalanine	13.4	13.2	14.4	-0.2
Lysine	4.0	7.9	5.8	+3.9
Histidine	trace	trace	trace	-
Ammonia	26.9	23.8	26.0	-3.1
Arginine	7.7	12.6	9.9	+4.9

TABLE IX.   CROSS-LINKS OF ELASTINS FROM DIFFERENT AREAS OF HUMAN
AORTAS (Moles per 70,000 g protein)

	Young (without Atherosclerosis)			Old (with Atherosclerosis)		
	Upper Abdominal	Lower Abdominal	Iliac	Thoracic	Abdominal	Iliac
Isodesmosine	0.65	0.68	0.70	0.61	0.37	0.48
Desmosine	1.15	1.08	1.04	0.91	0.72	0.77
Merodesmosine	0.25	0.20	0.16	0.21	0.31	0.20
Lysinonorleucine	0.42	0.44	0.44	0.40	0.48	0.41
Total Cross-Links	(2.47)	(2.40)	(2.13)	(2.13)	(1.88)	(1.86)
Lysine	4.05	3.67	4.0	4.0	7.92	5.82

calcified areas, are either newly synthesized, chronologically
young elastin or an abnormal protein (Yu, 1970). A similar
technique was used to examine and compare the elastins from different areas of an aorta which was obtained from a 39 year old
human subject without atherosclerosis. The results show no significant difference in the degree of cross-linkage in elastin and
no significant differences in its amino acid composition. Although
we do not know whether glutamic, aspartic, and other amino acids

TABLE X. TRITIUM-HYDROGEN EXCHANGE OF ELASTINS FROM DIFFERENT AREAS OF HUMAN AORTAS*

Tissue	H(G-atoms) Exchanged per 70,000 g Elastin	Ash in Elastin (%)
Young, Normal, Upper Abdominal	1,596	0.0
Young, Normal, Lower Abdominal	1,561	0.0
Young, Normal, Iliac	1,652	0.0
Arteriosclerotic, Thoracic	1,456	0.5
Arteriosclerotic, Abdominal	4,011	62.0
Arteriosclerotic, Iliac	2,128	53.7

* The reaction was carried at $37^{\circ}C$ for 48 hrs in 0.025 M potassium phosphate buffer at pH 7.4.

contain a free carboxyl group or an amide group in the side chain of the elastin peptide, if the former is the case, it tends to support Urist's theory (Urist, 1966) of a triphasic mechanism of localization of calcium deposit. According to this theory, a calcium ion may be bound to two free carboxyl groups to initiate the first phase of calcification, followed by entrance of phosphate as the second phase, and finally released calcium phosphate as the crystal of apatite by influx of water and soluble protein as the third phase. A recent theory of calcification of elastin by Urry is most interesting. Calcium ion is apt to bind at neutral or hydrophobic sites of elastin, making the selection of calcium ion by elastin highly specific (Urry, 1971).

Structure of Elastic Fiber and Tritium-Hydrogen Exchange Reaction (Yu, 1972).

Hydrogen isotope exchange has been used as a tool to study the properties of protein structure (Bensusan and Nielsen, 1964; Grant et al., 1971; Leach et al., 1964; McBride and Harrington, 1967). This exchange reaction takes place more rapidly when hydrogen is bound to oxygen, nitrogen, or sulfur. The hydrogen of the amide in the protein will also exchange slowly with tritiated water. The degree of the exchange depends upon the location; some hydrogens are in full contact with the solvent. The difference in the magnitude of hydrogen exchange in the aqueous solvent in the protein may provide some information with regard to the protein structure. A tritiated water exchange reaction was carried out for 48 hours at $37^{\circ}C$ in 0.025M potassium phosphate buffer at pH 7.4 on the isolated elastins from different areas of human aortas. The exchanged tritium was measured and calculated as H-gram atoms per

the unit weight of elastin. The results show a markedly higher
exchange of hydrogen in the elastins from highly calcified areas
(Table X). Partridge (1962, 1966) postulated that an open space
of the macromolecular elastin may provide a nucleation center for
calcification of elastin. The degree of the cross-linkage of
elastin indicates the nature of the structure of the protein; on
the other hand, the hydrogen exchange reaction may indicate the
nature of the chemical reactivity. It may also inform us of the
hydrophilic and hydrophobic nature of elastin.

Numerous changes take place in elastic fibers in arteriosclerotic disease. These include accumulation of calcium deposits, a
decrease in degree of cross-linkage with degenerative change in
the protein matrix, an alteration of amino acid composition or
increase of the firmly bound glycoprotein in the prepared elastin,
a higher degree of hydrogen exchange, a change to a less resilient
and more rigid protein, and finally an increase of affinity for
cholesterol (Kramsch et al., 1970). However, we do not know how
these changes in elastin are related to the calcification process
in aortas, but this observation may be important in regard to
cellular activity which is expressed by mesenchymal cells of aortas
during the process of arteriosclerosis (Yu and Blumenthal, 1965).

SUMMARY

The process of calcification in aortas was reviewed. Mineralization in aortas is characterized by deposition of calcium
phosphate compound as a mixture of apatite. Other inorganic
elements, including trace elements, do not participate directly
in mineralization of aorta, and the apatite appears to form
initially on elastin. Although calcium apatite precipitates
primarily on elastin-containing structures, mineralization in vivo
is not uniform in all elastin. Apatite formation is prone to form
at the surface of the elastic fiber or more in the areas of the
laminated elastin. Calcification of collagen has been encountered
only when calcification of arteries is massive.

Degenerating and regenerating elastic fibers are favorable
sites for early crystallization of the calcium compound. The
preformed or predeposited calcium apatite provides seeds for
further accumulation of calcium phosphate, as well as for growth
of larger crystals of apatite. In the areas of mineralization,
accumulation and qualitative changes in acid mucopolysaccharides
may play a role in calcification. Change in amino acid composition
of elastin in arteriosclerotic aortas provides more polarized side-
chains on the peptide of elastin; this results in an increase of
more hydrophilic centers in the relatively insoluble elastin. A
progressively lower degree of cross-linkage in elastin is observed

in aortas with advancing arteriosclerosis. The elastins isolated from different areas of aorta obtained from the same human subject show different amino acid composition and different degrees of cross-linkage, which indicates new formation of elastin or abnormal protein is present with normal elastin in the areas of arteriosclerosis. The hydrogen exchange data show that the protein structure of elastin from the arteriosclerotic area is less shielded from the aqueous solvent. Therefore, it appears to indicate the possibility of entrance of calcium ion in the protein structure. These changes in elastin of arteriosclerosis are characteristic of degenerative-regenerative elastin.

ACKNOWLEDGEMENTS

Dr. H.T. Blumenthal directed my research and gave many helpful suggestions. The author wishes to thank Dr. Shiu Eng Lai, who assisted in certain phases of this work, and Miss Karen L. Dryoff who ably and patiently typed the manuscript. The author is indebted to Dr. M.S. Wang of the Monsanto Company, St. Louis, Missouri, for carrying out the emission spectroscopic analysis of the trace elements presented in Table V.

REFERENCES

Ayer, J.P., Hass, G.M., and Philpott, D.E. (1958). AMA Arch. Pathol. 65, 519.

Bensusan, H.B., and Nielsen, S.O. (1964). Biochemistry 3, 1367.

Grant, M.E., Steven, F.S., Jackson, D.S., and Sandberg, L.B. (1971). Biochem. J. 121, 197.

John, R., and Thomas, J. (1972). Biochem. J. 127, 261.

Kramsch, D., Franzblau, C., and Hollander, W. (1970). J. Clin. Invest. 50, 1666.

Leach, S.Y., Hill, J., and Holt, L.A. (1964). Biochemistry 3, 737.

McBride, O.W., and Harrington, W.F. (1967). Biochemistry 6, 1499.

Moore, R.D., and Schoenberg, M.D. (1959). J. Pathol. Bacteriol. 77, 163.

Neuman, W.F., and Neuman, M.W. (1958). "The Chemical Dynamics of Bone Mineral." Chicago University Press, Chicago, Illinois.

Partridge, S.M. (1962). Advan. Protein Chem. 17, 227.

Partridge, S.M. (1966). Fed. Proc. 25, 1023.

Robert, L., Robert, B., Moczar, E., and Moczar, M. (1972).
    Pathol. Biol. 20, 1001.

Sandberg, L.B., Weisman, N., and Gray, W.R. (1971). Biochemistry
    10, 52.

Shields, G.S., Coulson, W.F., Kimball, D.A., Carnes, W.H.,
    Cartwright, G.E., and Wintrobe, M.D. (1962). Amer. J.
    Pathol. 41, 603.

Sobel, A.E., Penni, L.A., and Burger, M. (1960). Trans. N.Y.
    Acad. Sci. 22, 233.

Urist, M. (1966). Clin. Orthop. 44, 13.

Urry, D.W. (1971). Proc. Nat. Acad. Sci. USA 68, 810.

Yu, S.Y. (1967). In "Cowdry's Arteriosclerosis" (H.T. Blumenthal,
    ed.), pp. 170-192. C.C. Thomas, Springfield, Illinois.

Yu, S.Y. (1970). Anal. Biochem. 37, 212.

Yu, S.Y. (1971). Lab. Invest. 25, 121.

Yu, S.Y. (1972). Fed. Proc. 31, 2436.

Yu, S.Y., and Kuhn, C. (1972). (Unpublished experiments).

Yu, S.Y., and Blumenthal, H.T. (1967). In "The Connective Tissue"
    (B.M. Wagner and D.E. Smith, eds.), pp. 17-49. Williams
    and Wilkins, Baltimore, Maryland.

Yu, S.Y., and Blumenthal, H.T. (1958). J. Gerontol. 13, 366.

Yu, S.Y., and Blumenthal, H.T. (1963a). J. Gerontol. 18, 119.

Yu, S.Y., and Blumenthal, H.T. (1963b). J. Gerontol. 18, 127.

Yu, S.Y., and Blumenthal, H.T. (1963c). Lab. Invest. 12, 1154.

Yu, S.Y., and Blumenthal, H.T. (1965). J. Atheroscler. Res. 5,
    159

Yu, S.Y., Lai, S.E., and Watson, E.D. (1967). Fed. Proc. 26, 1247.

Yu, S.Y., Watson, E.D., and Lai, S.E. (1968). Fed. Proc. 27, 143.

Yu, S.Y., and Wertalecki, C. (1965). Fed. Proc. 24, 311.

Yu, S.Y. (1972). Unpublished Experiments.

DISCUSSION FOLLOWING THE PRESENTATION BY SHIU YEH YU

Dr. Robert: I think I would like to state my agreement with Dr. Yu's very important finding that lipid deposition and calcification can go on independently of each other. I think we will learn more about this process this afternoon in Madame Renais' presentation concerning immunoarteriosclerosis. We found that one way of obtaining only calcified lesions is to immunize rabbits with elastin or structural glycoproteins (Arteriosclerosis 13, 427, 1971). Just a brief statement about this. Before we jump to the conclusions that there are different elastins, "normal" and "sclerotic" or "plaque-elastin," I think we should draw attention to the fact that 0.1 N sodium hydroxide even at 100°C is not enough to take out glycoproteins-microfibrils from elastin. Therefore, purified elastin samples always contain, besides polymeric elastin, variable amounts of structural glycoproteins-microfibrils. If the ratio of glycoproteins to elastin increases, and this happens in the atherosclerotic plaque, there will be a higher polar amino acid content as compared to "normal elastin." Careful extraction of purified elastin with urea-mercaptoethanol could diminish this error (Eur. J. Biochem. 21, 507-516, 1971). The importance of structural glycoproteins-microfibrils (Kadar, Robert, Robert. Pathol. Biol. 1973, in print) can hardly be over estimated in normal and pathological elastin biochemistry. Since the early 1960's when we first described these tissue or "structural" glycoproteins (Fed. Proc. 21, 172, 1962; Biochem. Biophys. Res. Com. 10, 209-214, 1963; C. R. Ac. Sci. 256, 323-325, 1963), we could demonstrate them in all connective tissues and establish their identity as the "microfibrils" seen by several investigators (Pathol. Biol. 20, 1001-1012, 1972). Throughout this meeting we saw projections of amino acid compositions of aorta extracts similar or identical to those we described for "structural glycoproteins" (Life Sci. 7, 493-497, 1968), but the denominations used to designate these extracts or substances were different. This makes me think of an old statement of Montaigne, I think, which is very à propos for the structural glycoprotein story: "When a new observation comes up, said Montaigne, the scientific community first reacts by telling that it is not true. Then when you produce more evidence in favor of your discovery, colleagues would say, it is true but it is not important. Then you produce even more evidence which is now reproduced by more and more people and now they say, it is true, it is important, but it is not new."

SUBJECT INDEX